# PARENTS' CULTURAL BELIEF SYSTEMS

CULTURE AND HUMAN DEVELOPMENT
*A Guilford Series*

**Sara Harkness**
**Charles M. Super**
*Editors*


PARENTS' CULTURAL BELIEF SYSTEMS:
THEIR ORIGINS, EXPRESSIONS, AND CONSEQUENCES
*Sara Harkness and Charles M. Super,* Editors

CULTURE AND ATTACHMENT:
PERCEPTIONS OF THE CHILD IN CONTEXT
*Robin L. Harwood, Joan G. Miller, and Nydia Lucca Irizarry*

SIBLINGS IN SOUTH ASIA:
BROTHERS AND SISTERS IN CULTURAL CONTEXT
*Charles W. Nuckolls,* Editor


*Forthcoming*

JAPANESE CHILDREARING:
TWO GENERATIONS OF SCHOLARSHIP
*David W. Shwalb and Barbara J. Shwalb,* Editors

HAVIN' A BABY FOR MAMA:
CULTURE, PSYCHE, AND TEENAGE PREGNANCY
*Anne L. Dean with Sarah J. Ducey and Mary M. Malik*

# Parents' Cultural Belief Systems

*Their Origins, Expressions, and Consequences*

Sara Harkness
Charles M. Super
*Editors*

THE GUILFORD PRESS
New York    London

©1996 The Guilford Press
A Division of Guilford Publications, Inc.
72 Spring Street, New York, NY 10012

Printed in the United States of America

This book is printed on acid-free paper.

Last digit is print number:  9  8  7  6  5  4  3  2  1

**Library of Congress Cataloging-in-Publication Data**

Parents' cultural belief systems : their origins, expressions, and
   consequences / Sara Harkness and Charles M. Super, editors.
      p.  cm. — (Culture and human development)
   Includes bibliographical references and index.
   ISBN 1-57230-031-0
   1. Child rearing—Cross-cultural studies.  2. Child development—
Cross-cultural studies.  3. Socialization—Cross-cultural studies.
I. Harkness, Sara.  II. Super, Charles M.  III. Series.
HQ769.P2728    1996
649′.1—dc20                                     95-36802
                                                      CIP

# Contributors

**Mary Field Belenky,** Ed.D., is Associate Research Professor at the University of Vermont, Burlington, Vermont.

**Lucinda Bernheimer,** Ph.D., is Key Investigator with Project CHILD, a longitudinal study of families who have children with developmental delays, at the University of California, Los Angeles.

**Lynne A. Bond,** Ph.D., is Professor of Psychology at the University of Vermont, and President of the Vermont Conferences on the Primary Prevention of Psychopathology, Inc.

**Toni V. Cook,** Ph.D., is Director of Community Programs at Rhino Foods, Inc., Burlington, Vermont.

**Jarissa Dijkstia** is a student in Education and Developmental Psychology at the University of Leiden, The Netherlands.

**Carolyn Pope Edwards,** Ed.D., is Professor of Family Studies at the University of Kentucky in Lexington.

**Patrice Engle,** Ph.D., is Professor and Chair of the Psychology and Human Development Department, Cal Poly State University, San Luis Obispo, California.

**Marinka Fintelman** is a student in Education at the University of Leiden, The Netherlands.

**Lella Gandini,** Ed.D., is liaison to the United States for the Reggio Emilia Children Foundation (Italy) and Adjunct Professor of Education, University of Massachusetts at Amherst.

**Lino Garcia M.** is a nutritionist who has worked for the Nicaraguan government.

**Suzanne Gaskins,** Ph.D., teaches in the Departments of Psychology and Anthropology at the University of Pennsylvania in Philadelphia.

**Donatella Giovannini** is Pedagogical Coordinator for the Municipal Infant-Toddler Centers of the city of Pistoia, Italy.

**Jacqueline J. Goodnow,** Ph.D., is a Professorial Research Fellow at Macquarie University, Sydney, Australia.

**Charles F. Halverson,** Ph.D., is Professor of Child and Family Development and Lifespan Psychology at the University of Georgia in Athens.

**Sara Harkness,** Ph.D., M.P.H., is Associate Professor of Human Development and Anthropology at the Pennsylvania State University in University Park.

**Valerie Havill** is a doctoral student in the Department of Psychology at the University of Georgia in Athens.

**Constance H. Keefer,** M.D., is Instructor in Pediatrics at Harvard Medical School and Director of Clinical Services in the Child Development Unit, Children's Hospital, Boston, Massachusetts.

**Myung-In Kim** is a doctoral student in Clinical Psychology at Fordham University in New York City.

**Elizabeth Kipp Campbell,** Ph.D., is Postdoctoral Fellow on the Bio-Behavioral Training Grant in Disability Studies at the Institute of Child Development at the University of Minnesota in Minneapolis.

**Geldolph A. Kohnstamm,** Ph.D., is Professor of Developmental Psychology at the University of Leiden, The Netherlands.

**Sara Latz,** M.D., is a psychiatrist and member of the faculty at the University of California, Los Angeles.

**Robert A. LeVine,** Ph.D., is Roy E. Larson Professor of Education and Human Development and Professor of Anthropology at Harvard University, Cambridge, Massachusetts.

**Sarah LeVine** is Research Associate in the Laboratory of Human Development at the Harvard Graduate School of Education, Cambridge, Massachusetts.

**Robert Levy,** M.D., Emeritus Professor of Anthropology, University of California at San Diego, and Research Professor at Duke University, Durham, North Carolina.

**Gorjana Litvinovic** is a doctoral student in the Developmental Psychology Program of the University of North Carolina at Chapel Hill.

**Betsy Lozoff,** M.D., is Director of the Center for Human Growth and

Development and Professor of Pediatrics and Communicable Diseases at the University of Michigan, Ann Arbor.

**Catherine Matheson,** Ph.D., is Research Associate with the Sociobehavioral Group in the Neuropsychiatric Institute at the University of California, Los Angeles, and a member of the faculty at Santa Monica Community College, California.

**Ann V. McGillicuddy-De Lisi,** Ph.D., is Associate Professor in the Department of Psychology at Lafayette College, and Research Scientist at Educational Testing Service, in Princeton, New Jersey.

**Yadira Medrano,** a trained nurse, is Professor in the Faculty of Medicine at the Universidad Nacional Autonoma in Managua, Nicaragua.

**Ivan Mervielde,** Ph.D., is Professor of Psychology at the University of Ghent, Belgium.

**Patrice M. Miller,** Ed.D., is Assistant Professor of Psychology at Salem State College, Massachusetts.

**María Carmen Moreno,** Ph.D., is Associate Professor in the Department of Developmental and Educational Psychology and the Assistant Dean for Academic Affairs at the University of Seville, Spain.

**Rebecca S. New,** Ed.D., is Associate Professor of Education and Coordinator of the graduate program in Early Childhood Education at the University of New Hampshire in Durham.

**Jesús Palacios,** Ph.D., is Professor of Developmental Psychology at the University of Seville, Spain.

**Roberto Paludetto,** M.D., is Associate Professor of Pediatrics and Chief of the Division of Neonatology at the Federico II University in Naples, Italy.

**Chemba S. Raghavan,** Ph.D., is Research Associate in the Sociobehavioral Research Group at the University of California, Los Angeles.

**Amy Richman,** Ed.D., is Director of Quality Management at Work/Family Directions, a Boston, Massachusetts research and consulting firm specializing in corporate work life services.

**Junichi Shoji,** a developmental clinical psychologist, is Senior Researcher in the Department of Child/Family Welfare at the Japan Aiiko Research Institute in Tokyo.

**Barbara Shwalb,** Ph.D., is Associate Professor in the Department of Languages at Nagoya Skoka University in Aichi, Japan.

**David Shwalb,** Ph.D., is Associate Professor of International Studies at Koryo Women's College in Nagoya, Japan.

**Irving Sigel,** Ph.D., is Emeritus Distinguished Research Scientist at the Educational Testing Service in Princeton, New Jersey.

**Subha Subramanian,** M.A., is a teacher at the International School of Tanzania in Dar es Salaam.

**Charles M. Super,** Ph.D., is Professor of Human Development and Family Studies at the Pennsylvania State University, and Associate in Practice at the Child, Adult, and Family Psychological Center in University Park, Pennsylvania.

**Jaan Valsiner** is Professor of Psychology at the University of North Carolina at Chapel Hill.

**Ellen J. van der Vlugt** is a graduate of the Developmental Psychology Program at the University of Leiden, The Netherlands.

**Nathalie M. van Tijen** is a developmental psychologist researcher at the Children's Hospital of the University of Utrecht, The Netherlands.

**Jacqueline S. Weinstock,** Ph.D., is a NIA Post-Doctoral Fellow at the Center for Developmental and Health Research Methodology, Pennsyvania State University in University Park.

**Thomas Weisner,** Ph.D., is Professor in the Departments of Psychiatry and Anthropology at the University of California, Los Angeles.

**Barbara Welles-Nyström,** Ed.D., is Senior Lecturer in Anthropology at the Department of Nursing, Stockholm University College of Health Sciences in Stockholm, Sweden.

**Abraham W. Wolf** is Assistant Professor of Psychology at the Case-Western University School of Medicine and is a Director of Outpatient Services at MetroHealth Medical Center in Cleveland, Ohio.

**Marian Zeitlin,** Ph.D., is Professor of Nutrition at Tufts University in Medford, Massachusetts.

# Contents

PART THREE

INTRACULTURAL VARIATION:
THE ROLES OF EDUCATION AND "EXPERTS"

## PART FOUR

### THE INSTANTIATION OF PARENTS' CULTURAL BELIEF SYSTEMS IN PRACTICE

## PART FIVE

### THE CONSEQUENCES OF PARENTS' CULTURAL BELIEF SYSTEMS FOR CHILDREN'S HEALTH DEVELOPMENT

# PARENTS' CULTURAL BELIEF SYSTEMS

# CHAPTER 1

# *Introduction*

Sara Harkness
Charles M. Super

The tropical sun burned brightly overhead but the air was cool and fresh on a day in July 1974 when one of us, accompanied by our senior research assistant Lila Grace, arrived at the homestead of the Mitei family in Kokwet. We had lived long enough as researchers in this Kipsigis farming community, located in the western highlands of Kenya, to know each family comfortably—and it was a help having a local mother as our guide and cultural interpreter. Mrs. Mitei, who we were interviewing on this occasion, was busy chopping wood outside her hut, wielding a large ax with practiced dexterity as she split a log into pieces small enough for the cooking fire inside. As usual, several of her seven children could be seen nearby doing other chores, playing, or sitting together. Our attention was immediately drawn to one child, however. Two-year-old Kibet was sitting by himself on a tree stump, wailing lustily and kicking his feet against the stump; his face was screwed into a picture of anger and misery even though few tears were in evidence. The scene was striking in the contrast between the agitation of the little boy and the calm lack of concern of his mother.

"What's the matter with Kibet?" Lila asked after the customary greeting. Mrs. Mitei's answer was succinct but expressive: *Kasinyin* (literally, "his work"). The child was "doing his thing," as we might have put it—there was nothing really wrong with him so no further attention was required, and he would soon enough get over it on his own.

On a hot summer evening in July 1988, one of us sat with Mr. and Mrs. D'Ambra on the deck at the back of their suburban Boston home, sipping iced tea while interviewing them about their ideas and observations on the recent behavior of 2-year-old Lucia.

"She does everything on her own," said Mr. D'Ambra.

"She's very single-minded and strong-willed," added his wife.

"She's very independent. What she wants is what she wants. There's no two ways about it," continued Mr. D'Ambra.

"She doesn't always get what she wants, but she makes it quite clear," explained Mrs. D'Ambra. She added, "We're getting tan-trummed a little bit early. Our only hope is that if she starts early with the tantrums, that maybe she'll end them early too."

Two-year-old tantrums are one of the great universals of human behavior, appearing expectably in simple as well as complex cultures. In Holland, there is a saying, *Ik ben twee, dus ik zeg nej* ("I am 2, so I say no"); in the United States, the "terrible 2's" are so widely recognized that a pediatrician can ask parents, without elaboration, "And is he beginning to get into the 2-year-old syndrome?" But whereas tantrums may be universally recognized by parents and other child care experts as part of normal 2-year-old behavior, the cultural meanings of this behavior vary considerably. Mrs. Mitei explained her son's tantrum by relating it implicitly to the innate characteristics of her child at this age. Individual differences in this context were not considered significant. Mr. and Mrs. D'Ambra also recognized the developmental basis of their daughter's tantrums, but related it further to an American cultural understanding of "independence" as manifested in this as well as other behaviors; in addition, they singled out their daughter's individual qualities of being "strong-willed." In Holland, meanwhile, parents we interviewed in the early 1990s often described their children as strong-willed, but tantrums were typically associated with a situational cause— the child's routine of sleep and regular daytime activities being disrupted.

Parents' understanding about the nature of children, the structure of development, and the meaning of behavior are to a large extent shared by members of a cultural group or subgroup. These under-standings are developed in the context of life in a particular cultural place and time, and they are related to understandings about other aspects of life as experienced by parents, including most immediately the nature and meaning of parenthood, the family, and the self in society. Because cultural understandings that parents hold are organized into larger categories of mutually supportive beliefs, we refer to them as *parents' cultural belief systems* or *parental ethnotheories*. These culturally organized understandings relate in systematic ways to action—including, for example, styles of talking to children, methods of discipline, or seeking advice from experts. Ultimately, parental ethnotheories exert a powerful influence on the health and development of children, and they are a key component in the development of parents themselves.

## Parental Ethnotheories

### *Intellectual Roots of Research on Parental Ethnotheories*

Parental belief systems have attracted increasing attention from researchers in human development in recent years, as attested to by the rapid growth of published work in this area. In 1985, Irving Sigel edited a volume, *Parental Belief Systems*, with the goal of identifying the field of parental beliefs, or parent cognition, as a major and legitimate area for empirical study. Five years later, interest had grown to such an extent that a review of the field, undertaken by Goodnow and Collins (1990), further defined its shape and potential for future development. Most recently, a second edition of *Parental Belief Systems* (Sigel, McGillicuddy-DeLisi, & Goodnow, 1992) has been published in response to rapid developments in theory and research, while the topic continues to receive increasing attention in scholarly journals and meetings.

The emergence of parents' cultural belief systems as a topic of study has been made possible by parallel trends in psychology, social anthropology, and related new interdisciplinary approaches to culture and human development. As a general area of concern, individual differences in parental belief systems have been a theme in psychological research since the field of child development emerged as an identifiable entity in the opening decades of this century. G. Stanley Hall, who is generally considered the first to move from philosophy to developmental psychology (White, 1992), began to apply his methods and talents to preparing "topical syllabi" for the education of parents, among other audiences, prior to the turn of the century (Sigel & White, 1982). The child study institutes that flourished in the subsequent decades, and Lawrence K. Frank's even more ambitious parent education movement, were explicit in their attempt to change at least some parents' thoughts and behavior regarding their children (Schlossman, 1983). The core model, however, was that parents lacked certain knowledge and needed expert help to gain it. In general, this orientation continued through the 1950s, when a large literature emerged on parental "attitudes," exemplified by Schaefer and Bell's (1958) Parent Attitude Research Instrument. Although this widely used instrument assessed beliefs about appropriate child behavior and developmental needs, the results were generally taken in contemporary theory as broad attitudinal dispositions such as parental control and affection.

There was an assumption that such attitudes were directly translated to parental behavior, but minimal empirical support for this assumption eventually contributed to a decline in interest in this approach.

Current psychological research on parents' beliefs as cognitive structures traces its roots especially to work on "naive psychology" in the 1960s (e.g., Baldwin, 1965). Although behaviorist and developmental (e.g., Piagetian) paradigms dominated the quest for a new developmental psychology at that time, the field eventually stepped back from these two conflicting views and a more dynamic, interactive model of parent and child interaction emerged (Bronfenbrenner, 1979; Kessen, 1979; Sameroff & Chandler, 1975). The subsequent growth of cognitive science in general then contributed to an appreciation of parental thinking as a process. Thus the current resurgence of psychological interest in parents' beliefs draws on two general recent trends: a reorientation toward cognitive aspects of human functioning and a recognition that understanding of the child's behavior and development requires knowledge of the dynamic context.

With the increase in psychological research on parents' beliefs has also come growing recognition that much of parental cognition is itself socially or culturally organized. Interest in the cultural dimensions of parents' beliefs was stimulated by studies of ethnic differences in developmental expectations (Ninio, 1979) and the identification of cultural themes in childrearing (Reid & Valsiner, 1986). Nevertheless, as Sigel et al. (1992, p. xviii) commented, "It is only recently that developmental psychologists have begun to pay systematic attention to how cultural belief systems are instantiated in parent cognition and actions."

Anthropological interest in how parents think dates back at least to classics such as Mead's studies of childrearing in Pacific societies (see Mead, 1972). Research by the Whitings and their colleagues also attended to parental beliefs and values, both as formed by the socioeconomic "maintenance systems" that parents themselves adapt to and as instrumental in the ways that parents organize settings of daily life for their children (Whiting & Edwards, 1988; Whiting & Whiting, 1975). More recently, LeVine and his coworkers (LeVine, 1974; LeVine, Miller, & West, 1988) have called attention to parental goals as organizers of behavior at the cultural level. Most significant for the development of new research on parental ethnotheories, however, is the recent rise of cognitive approaches in anthropology, especially the concept of "cultural models." As developed by Quinn and Holland (1987), cultural models are shared understandings that "frame experience, supplying interpretations of that experience and inferences about it, and goals for action" (p. 6). The power of cultural models as sources of motivation has been further recognized in recent work in this area (D'Andrade & Stauss, 1992).

Emerging interdisciplinary approaches also provide key resources for the study of parental ethnotheories. The rise of developmental paradigms based on the work of Vygotsky is especially important; it provides an intellectual framework for relating individual development to cultural meaning systems. The focus of this school on action or on practices as psychocultural mediators (see, e.g., Holland & Valsiner, 1988; Lave & Wenger, 1991; Miller, 1990; Rogoff, 1990) lays a foundation for research linking parenting behavior to symbolic systems. The "developmental niche" framework elaborated by Super and Harkness (1986; Harkness & Super, 1992, 1994a, 1994b) is also useful for conceptualizing relationships among parental belief systems, customs, and practices of childrearing and the organization of physical and social settings for children's daily lives. In recent writings using this framework, Harkness and Super (1992, 1994b; Harkness, Super, & Keefer, 1992) have assigned a leading role to parental ethnotheories as they influence the childrearing choices parents make within the constraints offered by the culture. Similar to this framework, the idea of the "ecocultural niche" developed by Weisner and his associates (Gallimore, Weisner, Kaufman, & Bernheimer, 1989; Weisner, Bausano, & Kornfein, 1983) relates parents' cultural belief systems to the ecology of the family in the community on the one hand and to parental behavior on the other. In "constructing and sustaining a daily routine of life that has meaning for culture members" (Weisner, Matheson, & Bernheimer, Chapter 21, p. 504, this volume), parents implicitly express cultural beliefs and values.

## Why Study Parental Ethnotheories?

Given the diverse intellectual sources of research on parents' cultural belief systems, it is not surprising that there are a good many reasons why they provide a rich and interesting research domain. Goodnow (Chapter 13, this volume) has summarized four reasons for considering parents' ideas: (1) parents' ideas are an interesting form of adult cognition and development, (2) parents' ideas provide a way to help understand parental action, (3) parents' ideas are one aspect of the idea of "context" in child development, and (4) the study of ideas held by two generations can provide some insight into processes of culture transmission and culture change.

All these points bear some elaboration from a cultural perspective. Parents' cultural belief systems, first, provide not only an interesting focus for studies of adult cognition but also a window into the culturally constituted self. This is particularly evident, of course, in societies in which virtually all socially mature persons become parents; but the field also has room for the study of people who advise parents or who interact with children in parent-like roles. Moreover, the study of parental ethnotheories as they evolve from *before* parenthood and through the course of parenting and grandparenting can provide a new dimension to understanding the development of the cultural self over the life course. Second, parents' ideas and action are particularly relevant to a cultural perspective as the most clearly observable link between beliefs and behavior at the cultural level. In contrast, individual situational and personal style factors sometimes make it harder to predict individual behavior from beliefs. Nevertheless, as Goodnow shows in her analysis of parents' ideas and practices related to household chores (Chapter 13, this volume), understanding the meaning of practices to their participants can take us a long way in improving our more general understanding of links between beliefs and behavior. The third point, parents' cultural beliefs as an aspect of "context," gains importance particularly in those cases in which the context of child life and development is problematic. For example, Zeitlin's analysis of Nigerian parents' ethnotheories (Chapter 17, this volume) helps to clarify the basis of feeding practices that in and of themselves would seem counterproductive. At the opposite extreme, Weisner, Matheson, and Bernheimer (Chapter 21, this volume) suggest that American parents' beliefs about the importance of "stimulation" for optimal child development may lead to an unnecessary concern about the earliest possible interventions for children with developmental delays. Finally, Goodnow's last point concerning the study of ideas of two generations as an entry into processes of culture transmission and change can apply not only across generations but across other categories of social role difference. As several chapters in this volume suggest, the formation of parental ethnotheories has a great deal to do with interactions among parents and others whose perspectives matter—for example, teachers and pediatricians. Furthermore, as LeVine, Miller, Richman, and LeVine (Chapter 10, this volume) and Palacios and Moreno (Chapter 9, this volume) illustrate, differences in educational experience during childhood and adolescence may sow the seeds of intracultural differences in parental ethnotheories.

Taken together, the various perspectives described here suggest that the study of parents' cultural belief systems can address important theoretical issues that cut across several disciplines. As belief systems that are socially shared yet constructed in the minds of individual parents, parental ethnotheories represent the basic paradox of mind and culture, and they offer an opportunity to address questions that have implications beyond the study of parenthood in itself. What are the nature and sources of parental ethnotheories? To what extent are parental ethnotheories similar or distinctive in different times and places, both within and across cultures? What are the roles of culturally appointed "experts" and individual experience in the development of parental ethnotheories? What is the relationship between parents' cultural belief systems and behavior? And finally, how do parental ethnotheories influence children's health and development?

This volume presents the collected observations and thinking of scholars from variety of disciplinary backgrounds—including developmental psychology, social anthropology, education, nutrition, and pediatrics—as they address these key questions. The chapters are concerned with the sources and consequences of parental ethnotheories in a worldwide sample of societies and employ a wide array of methods including interviews, questionnaires, behavioral observation techniques, ethnographic methods, and discourse analysis. Topics also vary widely, from general conceptualizations of parenting and childhood to specific developmental expectations or ideas and practices related to particular aspects of child development and family functioning. We now offer an overview of the issues as they are addressed in this volume and then describe how the book is organized.

## Issues, Perspectives, and Themes

### The Nature and Sources of Parental Ethnotheories

The most fundamental issue addressed in this volume is the nature of parents' cultural belief systems. The choice of terminology is in itself indicative. Goodnow and Collins (1990) reject the term "belief systems" or even "beliefs" in favor of "parents' ideas," because the term "beliefs" raises many other philosophical issues. Nevertheless, we have adopted the term "parents' cultural belief systems" for the title of this volume because it may be most easily interpretable by the general reader. We also favor the term "parental ethnotheory," since it acknowledges the intellectual roots of this construct in anthropological studies of indigenous belief systems or folk theories.

Regardless of what term we choose, what is the nature of parents' cultural beliefs?

Sigel and Kim offer a definition of beliefs that links them to knowledge on the one hand and to affect, intentionality, value and action on the other. In their view, beliefs are "knowledge in the sense that the individual knows that what he (or she) espouses is true or probably true, and evidence may or may not be deemed necessary; or if evidence is used, it forms a basis for the belief but is not the belief itself" (Sigel, 1985, p. 348, quoted in Sigel & Kim, Chapter 4). To relate this definition to cultural beliefs or knowledge, evidence is often not deemed necessary because such beliefs are taken for granted ideas about the nature of reality. Thus, cultural beliefs are arrived at without scientific sifting of the evidence and in fact are not perceived as beliefs at all. Weisner et al. (Chapter 21), like D'Andrade (1987), note the implicit nature of parents' cultural beliefs as a characteristic of cultural models that is particularly important in directing behavior. They comment "One reason cultural models . . . are so powerful is that they are implicit or procedural rather than explicit, formalized, and declarative" (p. 500). These beliefs are related to behavior without the mediating influence of conscious decision making.

How are parents' cultural beliefs related to other kinds of cultural knowledge or beliefs? Several authors suggest that parental ethnotheories are derived from more general belief systems. Bond, Belenky, Weinstock, and Cook hypothesize that women's beliefs about parenting are shaped by their "assumptions about how people learn and their conceptions of *themselves* as knowers" (Chapter 20, p. 467). Parental ethnotheories can also be related to more general cultural belief systems, as Welles-Nystrom suggests. In particular, she argues that in Sweden, equality as ideology is "a dynamic thread in society connecting family policy and legislation, health care programs, and the special status of the child to maternal theories of child development" (Chapter 8, p. 193). In this regard, parents' cultural beliefs seem to be organized in hierarchical relationships with other beliefs, as D'Andrade (1987) has suggested. Parents' cultural models about children are related to ideas about themselves or to more generally shared cultural ideas on the one hand, and on the other hand to ethnotheories for special purposes or circumstances, such as those related to children with developmental delay as discussed by Weisner and his co-authors. New and Richman cite LeVine et al.'s (1988) typology of cultural beliefs that also appears to represent a hierarchy: Parents hold long-term goals for their children's development, which are represented in the short term by a "pragmatic design" consisting of beliefs about the maternal role and typical infant development; these in turn are put into action through "conventional scripts" that dictate culturally appropriate behavior in various kinds of situations.

McGillicuddy-DeLisi and Subramanian (Chapter 6) provide an overview of conceptualizations of the relationship between culture and individual beliefs, suggesting that these can be grouped into three main typologies. In the first, specific beliefs (e.g., developmental expectations) are adopted wholesale from the culture and become internalized with the process of socialization. In the second conceptualization, different cultural settings provide qualitatively different kinds of experience, from which the individual derives generalizations leading to beliefs; the intracultural consistency of experience leads to the emergence of similar beliefs held by various members of the cultural group. In the third approach, culture is seen as knowledge and individuals co-construct beliefs interactively within the system of beliefs that constitutes the culture. According to this conceptualization, "Beliefs are constructed through the exchange of social meanings among peoples as individuals integrate personal experiences with their participation in the parenting role suggested by the culture at a particular point in history" (Chapter 6, p. 147). This third approach is elaborated by Valsiner and Litvinovic, who argue that culture is not an "independent variable" as implied by some psychological research paradigms but rather "serves as the main semiotic vehicle to organize both the conduct and reasoning of the actors in the role of parents" (Chapter 3, p. 57). In this view, parental reasoning is the product of both individual interpretations of specific situations and previously learned social directions. Insofar as parental interpretations and actions in particular situations feed back into the collective culture of ideas and expectations about children, they also contribute to the construction of that culture.

In summary, parental ethnotheories have some universal dimensions but are constructed within cultural belief systems, and they are often implicit. As such, they are powerful sources of affect and motivators of behavior. Parental ethnotheories are seen as relating to cultural beliefs and individual behavior in hierarchical fashion, with more general beliefs subsuming more specific ones that, in turn, entail scripts for action. The role of culture in the constitution of individual parental thinking and action can be conceptualized in several different ways, each of which allows for the possibility of variations within the culture; that is, differences in contact with a cultural knowledge base, in culturally facilitated experience, or in individual interactions can lead to the formation of different kinds of internal representations about children and parenting. All these ideas about the nature and sources of parental ethnotheories provide a basis for the other principal perspectives and themes developed in this volume: cross-cultural comparisons, cultural homogeneity versus variability, the instantiation of parental ethnotheories in practices, and finally their developmental consequences.

## Cross-Cultural Comparisons

The chapters in this volume are concerned with a wide variety of cultural groups in different parts of the globe, including the United

States, Western Europe, the Far East and Pacific, Africa, and Latin America. Not surprisingly, the United States is most strongly represented, both in single-sample analyses and in cross-cultural comparisons. A somewhat unusual feature of this volume is the relatively large number of cultural analyses of European groups, including three chapters that include Italian samples, two concerned with Dutch-American comparisons, and one each about Sweden and Spain. One of the Italian-American cross-cultural comparisons also includes a Japanese sample, while another chapter focuses primarily on Japan but includes comparisons with the United States. The Far East and Pacific are further represented in a comparative study of parental ethnotheories in Tahiti and Nepal, as well as studies undertaken in Australia. Reports of research in Africa include Tanzania and Nigeria. Latin-American studies are concerned with parents and children in Mayan and Ladino communities of Mexico, and Ladino mothers in Nicaragua. Several of the chapters—especially those by Welles-Nystrom (Chapter 8), Gaskins (Chapter 14), Shwalb, Shwalb, and Shoji (Chapter 7), and Zeitlin (Chapter 17)—focus primarily on an analysis of the culture in its own terms, providing rich ethnographic contextualization for a consideration of parental ethnotheories. It is worth noting that all these accounts are based on many years of experience in the cultures described.

Cross-cultural comparisons are undertaken, first, to delineate the role of cultural beliefs as modulators of practices and child outcomes. A basic benefit of this approach is to render the "invisible" culture of which the reader or researcher is a member more evident through comparison with a different culture. Thus, for example, Wolf, Lozoff, Latz, and Paludetto's cross-cultural comparison of beliefs and practices related to infant sleep in the United States, Italy, and Japan demonstrates the cultural specificity of culturally normative American white, middle-class approaches (Chapter 15). The cross-cultural approach is further enriched here by cultural comparisons *within* the United States, involving a group of African-American families as well as white families. In a related analysis, New and Richman (Chapter 16) demonstrate that differences between Italian and American practices related to infant motor activity, sleep, and eating can be traced to overarching differences in cultural belief systems regarding independence and interdependence in the family. Super, Harkness, van Tijen, van der Vlugt, Fintelman, and Dijkstra, in a study of the "three R's" of Dutch childrearing (Chapter 19), likewise, use an American comparative sample to demonstrate the effects of parental ethnotheories on practices and child outcomes related to infants' patterns of rest and state of arousal— aspects of infant development that might otherwise be assumed to be innately or developmentally determined.

An underlying issue in cross-cultural comparisons is that of universality versus cultural specificity. Several chapters directly address the question of universality as it relates to ways that parents think and act. Kohnstamm, Halverson, Havill, and Mervielde (Chapter 2) examine patterns of cross-cultural similarity and difference in how parents describe their own children, finding that although the "big five" dimensions of personality emerge in several cultures, their relative salience varies. This result is provocative in that it challenges the common present-day assumption that personality and culture are independent; although this may be the case, parental *perceptions* of children's personality or temperament seem to have both universal and culturally specific qualities. Levy (Chapter 5) suggests that "essential differences" in parental beliefs and practices may be traced to differences in level of societal complexity such as those exemplified in Tahiti and Nepal. If Levy is correct, it may be that parental ethnotheories (and accompanying practices) could be conceptualized in terms of typologies rather than as qualitatively unique. Edwards, Gandini, and Giovaninni (Chapter 11) raise the possibility of another kind of cultural universal in parental ethnotheories, based on the "universal culture" and similar experience of training and employment in early childhood education, in contrast to parents whose experience may be more culturally distinctive. Another issue related to universality is raised by Shwalb et al. (Chapter 7), who critique the constructs of temperament used for research with parents as being actually an expression of Western cultural ideas.

Studies of cultural organization and cross-cultural comparisons naturally tend to emphasize the internal consistency of each cultural group. Further, it may be that parents' cultural belief systems in some societies do exhibit a high degree of homogeneity. For example, Shwalb et al. suggest that in Japan, cultural beliefs about mothers' roles are based on historical continuity of several hundred years. Equally important to the study of parental ethnotheories, however, is the issue of intracultural variability.

## Intracultural Variability

Palacios and Moreno present the issue of intracultural diversity as a yet-unmet challenge in the study of culture and human development. They comment:

> According to Cole (1990), common to the different formulations existing within cultural psychology is a conception of culture as the unique *medium* of human existence. But cultures are not monolithic or homogeneous

entities, and any attempt to describe cultural processes and products should be accompanied by an attempt to describe and understand both what is common and what is diverse within a given cultural group. Otherwise, a part would be taken as if it were the whole and some of the most critical aspects of the culture would be ignored (namely, its heterogeneity and the maintenance of its diversity over the generations). Some of the formulations currently available in cultural psychology fail to recognize the existence of intracultural diversity, as if "culturalism" were the only alternative to individualism. (Chapter 9, p. 216)

Palacios and Moreno's declaration evokes Wallace's (1961) argument that culture should be conceptualized as the "organization of diversity" rather than the "replication of uniformity." The point is particularly relevant for research on parental ethnotheories insofar as studies are concerned with beliefs and practices of individual parents rather than general ethnographic characterizations. When faced with variation among actual individuals within a culture, the challenge is to characterize the nature and sources of individual differences without losing sight of their cultural basis.

The contributors to this volume take several different approaches to dealing with this issue. One, used by Engle, Zeitlin, Medrano, and Garcia (Chapter 18), is to identify "positive deviants" among mothers within a cultural community—women who, for whatever reason, differ from their peers in beliefs and practices that are related to desirable child outcomes. Another, used by Palacios and Moreno, is to identify different groups of parents based on their profile of beliefs about children. Three groups are found: traditional, modern, and "paradoxical." Among the first two groups, there is a high level of integration of specific beliefs into systems; the third group, true to its name, is distinguished by a characteristic profile of beliefs that do not appear to be internally consistent. Examination of the correlates of different parental belief groups shows that education and residence are strong predictors of difference, whereas experience as a parent is not. Although the constellation of modern ideas seems cognitively more complex (and is espoused by the more educated parents), Palacios and Moreno suggest that intracultural variation is like "a tree with different branches" (Chapter 9, p. 236) rather than a single developmental trajectory in the Piagetian sense. In contrast to this view, Bond et al. propose that the five different epistomologies they identify among low-income rural mothers in Vermont do constitute a developmental sequence, in which "each subsequent position seems more differentiated and more adequate for full participation in a society such as ours" (Chapter 20, p. 473).

LeVine, Miller, Richman, and LeVine also find intracultural differences in parental ethnotheories that are related to educational differences among Mexican mothers. They suggest that although these parents share a common background of traditional cultural models, they are "differentiated by personal histories of social participation" (Chapter 10, p. 254). Schooling, in particular, seems to foster the development of mothers' adoption of different beliefs about infants as communicative partners, with more educated mothers having earlier expectations. These beliefs are linked in turn to differential maternal communicative behavior and child outcomes. LeVine and his colleagues note that the apparent effect of schooling is found in many cultures, but it is not the only cultural source of these maternal beliefs.

The effects of education on parents' developmental expectations are approached from a somewhat different angle by Edwards et al., who studied parents and preschool teachers in two cultural communities: Amherst, Massachusetts, and Pistoia, Italy. In this case, culture rather than professional training and responsibilities emerges as the strongest predictor of developmental expectations, with the two groups of parents strongly differentiated (Amherst parents have earlier expectations) whereas the two groups of teachers occupy an intermediate position. Edwards et al. suggest that parents are more influenced by cultural models of child development in their own communities, whereas teachers participate in "a sort of professional culture shared internationally with other practitioners of parallel or equivalent education and training and experience with children" (Chapter 11, p. 285).

An important question raised by Edwards et al. is how cultural experts in child development, such as teachers, may influence the beliefs of parents with whom they interact. In the U.S. context, pediatricians also play a special role as providers of culturally based "expert" advice to parents, as Harkness, Super, Keefer, Raghavan, and Kipp (Chapter 12) note. They show that differences between parents and pediatricians in relative use of different underlying "root metaphors of development" in conversations during pediatric well-child visits create opportunities for the "negotiation" of cultural models. In these conversational interchanges, the formation of culturally based understandings about child behavior and development can actually be observed.

In summary, the issue of intracultural diversity in parental ethnotheories is a central one for the study of culture and human development. Among the chapters of this volume, schooling emerges as a particularly important factor in intracultural variation, although its effects are not always in the same direction: preschool teachers, who have more formal education related to child development than anyone else, have later (and probably more accurate) developmental expectations than do parents in some cultural settings. The importance of parental contact with "experts" in their communities is also addressed in the context of intracultural variation, with pediatricians playing an especially important role for American middle-class parents; in other cultures, as Wolf et al. suggest, grandparents and other elders may be more influential. Intracultural differences among parental ethnotheories may be conceptualized in terms of their quality, complexity, or "adequacy" for dealing successfully with childrearing issues or in society more generally, or they may be conceptualized as simply different. In either case, intracultural diversity seems to be a universal characteristic of societies and it is important for both the accommodation of individual differences at any given historical moment and as a resource for cultural change over time.

It is important to note that intracultural diversity does not replicate cross-cultural variability, as Bond et al. indicate in proposing their developmental sequence of epistomologies *within modern American society*. Even differences associated with "universal" variables such as schooling are related to qualitatively different belief systems in different societies—the less educated Mexican mother does not share the cultural belief system of the less educated Vermont mother, although there may be some common elements. The cultural specificity of parental ethnotheories is expressed in practices that instantiate or represent them in action, another major theme of the chapters in this volume.

## The Instantiation of Parental Ethnotheories in Cultural Practices

The choice of the term "instantiation" to describe the relationship of idea to action signals a departure from both traditional anthropological approaches (in which ideas and behavior were treated as inextricably interwoven aspects of culture) and psychological research paradigms (which have tended to ignore parental thinking altogether). Goodnow sets forth the view taken by many of the contributors to this volume, in relation to the domain of beliefs and practices surrounding household work:

> I propose that all cultures contain ideas about the contributions to the family that each member should make and about the connections, if any, that should exist between what people contribute and what they receive. All cultures also contain practices—in the form of words or deeds—that concretize these ideas, introduce newcomers to the ideas they should hold, provide rationales for why actions and beliefs take the form they do, and indicate where some flexibility or negotiation is possible or out of the

question. Where cultures differ, I suggest, is in the kinds of contribution expected, the connections promoted between what is given and received, the related practices, and the areas of flexibility or negotiation. (Chapter 13, p. 313)

Goodnow's statement includes several key points. First is the idea that some domains are represented in some form in all cultures, making possible sytematic cross-cultural comparisons. This idea is captured by Wolf et al.'s study of sleep practices. As they note:

How a child is allowed to fall asleep is one of the earliest forms of culturally determined interaction with the child. Sleep practices are embedded in a set of childrearing behaviors that reflect values about what it means to be a "good" parent and how the parents are to prepare the child for entry into the family and the community. (Chapter 15, p. 377)

Several chapters in this volume are concerned with such universal domains of childrearing, especially in relation to infants and young children: in addition to the management of sleep (also discussed by New & Richman and Super et al.), feeding practices (New & Richman; Engle et al.; and Zeitlin), motor activity (New & Richman), and play (Gaskins). Like "developmental timetables" that parents everywhere have in mind, practices related to the basic universal tasks of childrearing provide a natural basis for examining the cultural specificity of beliefs and behavior.

A second issue that Goodnow alludes to is how "practices" should be conceptualized: She suggests a broad definition that includes both language and behavior. The practices discussed in this book include aspects of mother–child interaction, routines for daily living, and even governmental policies as instantiations of cultural belief systems. Although they vary greatly in scale, however, all these kinds of human action are culturally regulated bearers of meaning for their participants. As such, they provide a point of entry to the understanding of cultural ideas not only for the researcher but also for the child or cultural novice.

Perhaps the most challenging issue that Goodnow's statement brings to mind is just how cultural beliefs and behavior relate to each other, and how one can explain the variations in these relationships both between and across cultural settings. Goodnow herself suggests that the appearance of individual consistency or inconsistency between beliefs and practices may be a function of the relative strength of opinion held on two or more principles that may come into conflict with each other, as well as of the characteristics of particular situations. The plurality of parents' cultural ideas also offers a way to understand intracultural diversity and its transmission across generations. As Goodnow states:

> Parents' ideas can accommodate several positions, just as the general culture often does, with the degree of attachment to one or the other shifting from time to time as circumstances change. The same point might also be made with regard to children. Rather than adopting the one position held by their parents, children may be more fruitfully regarded as hearing several messages and taking these over or drawing upon them to various degrees at various times. (Chapter 13, p. 336)

In summary, the analyses of practices as instantiations of cultural belief systems in this volume move the question of beliefs and behavior beyond the level of dialogue that has prevailed in both anthropology and psychology. The authors in this volume do not expect a perfect correspondence between cultural or even individual beliefs and behavior, but they offer a great deal of evidence that behavior can appropriately be seen as the expression of beliefs that are to a large extent culturally organized.

## Consequences for Children's Development

One of the most important reasons for studying parents' cultural belief systems is to understand how they may affect child health and development, both contemporaneous and subsequent. That such belief systems *do* influence child outcomes would seem self-evident, yet the relationship is not easy to demonstrate empirically. Monocultural studies of parental beliefs and child (or later adult) outcomes, such as those typical in the "culture and personality" movement in anthropology from the 1940s through the 1970s (see Harkness & Super, 1995), rely on the internal coherence of the information presented, and they run the risk of circularity in logic. As Levy comments in relation to the similar issue of relating childhood experience to later adult behavior in the community:

> If one is concerned about the relation of child experience to the shapes of community life, there is considerable circularity in our assertions. Working from both directions—childhood experience up and adult behaviors down—we should not be too surprised that they seem to fit. But our connections should be plausible, and the data we are observing rich and properly placed in context, and informed, ideally, by a strong "intuitive" sense of things. (Chapter 5, p. 124)

Within the framework of one culture, it is possible to construct a coherent explanation, but it may erroneously assign cause and effect; this danger is reduced in cross-cultural studies, but each culture increases the sample by only one, regardless of how many individuals are studied in each place. Furthermore, if we are interested in the effects of parental ethnotheories per se, cross-cultural studies can never provide a perfect natural laboratory as many other aspects of cultures also vary along with belief systems. Nevertheless, much of the power of parental belief systems to influence child outcomes derives from their cultural basis—both in terms of the individual motivational component of parental beliefs and in terms of the reinforcement of parental beliefs by other societal institutions such as schools, churches, political organization, or the media. Even with its limitations, thus, the analysis of child outcomes related to parental ethnotheories can provide valuable insights and, in some cases, a basis for culturally sensitive interventions.

The chapters in this volume take several different approaches to the issue of child outcomes. Zeitlin (Chapter 17) provides a detailed account of Yoruba beliefs about child development in order to explain patterns of underfeeding and consequent malnutrition and child deaths. Although her focus is primarily on one culture, her reasoning is enhanced by contrasting patterns of beliefs and child status from several other cultures. At a more interpretive level, Levy (Chapter 5) hypothesizes that differences in *adult* cognition, discourse, and the creative arts may be the result of different culturally organized childhood learning experiences in the two communities he describes. Although his analysis certainly does not "prove" the proposed relationships, it is important in pointing out the different kinds of cultural constellations in which differences in behavior, thought, and cultural expression arise.

Another way to measure child outcomes related to parents' cultural belief systems is to assess samples of parents and children in two or more culturally contrasting communities. Gaskins (Chapter 14) uses this approach in comparing infant exploratory play in a Yucatec Mayan community with data from same-age U.S. infants, and finds that although Mayan infants spend as much time as U.S. infants playing with objects, their play is less complex. She uses this finding to challenge the Western assumption that infant exploratory play is universally motivated by a desire to master the environment and to engage in social interactions. Super, et al. (Chapter 19) also compare findings from two cultures to study the developmental impact of different ethnotheories and practices—especially the Dutch "three R's" of childrearing—on the regulation of infant state. This research raises the intriguing question whether cultural beliefs, instantiated in such practices, may influence not only immediate behavior but even its biological foundations.

A third approach to the study of parents' cultural belief systems and child outcomes extends the study of intracultural variation in parental ethnotheories to variability in child outcomes. Engle et al. (Chapter 18) use this method in their study of maternal feeding beliefs and child nutritional status in Nicaragua. Interestingly, they are able to find a statistically significant relationship between maternal beliefs and child outcomes, although measures of maternal feeding behavior are not related to beliefs as expected. As Engle et al. comment, this result illustrates the difficulty of establishing valid measures for the behavioral instantiation of beliefs that evidently do have developmental consequences. The approach used by LeVine et al. (Chapter 10) to examine the developmental consequences of maternal beliefs in a Mexican sample is similar to Engle et al.'s, but they conceptualize individual differences in terms of relative involvement in culture change: More educated mothers, they propose, are further along the path of cultural change toward adaptation to modern life with its higher demands for literacy and changed personal interaction norms. The series of analyses they lay out, from maternal beliefs regarding the infant's communicative abilities, to maternal–infant responsiveness, and finally to developmental measures at $2\frac{1}{2}$ years, constitutes a coherent sequence of hypothesized causes and consequences.

In summary, demonstrating relationships between parents' cultural belief systems and child outcomes is a complex challenge, but one worth undertaking as the major variations in development are to be found at the level of cultural rather than individual differences. The chapters in this volume illustrate three approaches, each offering its own strengths and limitations: ethnographic analysis, systematic cross-cultural comparisons, and the study of intracultural variation. The results of all these studies offer not only evidence of the power of parental ideas to shape children's environments and development but also new avenues for the exploration of culture and human development.

## Organization of the Volume

The principal themes of this volume are represented, to varying degrees, in all the chapters. However, we have grouped them together based on which theme or issue seems most important or distinctive in each chapter in order to convey to the reader our sense of this emerging field as a set of questions in the process of being elaborated rather than as a descriptive grid to be filled in. Thus, the first section following this Introduction consists of three chapters that are concerned with the development of different theoretical perspectives on parental ethnotheories. Kohnstamm, Halverson, Havill, and Mervielde (Chapter 2) address the question of universality and cultural specificity in parents' concepts of the child, referring to constructs from personality psychology and the study of temperament. Valsiner and Litvinovic (Chapter 3) focus on conceptualizing the *process* of parental reasoning as both personally and culturally constructed. Sigel and Kim (Chapter 4) grapple with the issue of how the method of elicitation of parental beliefs affects the kinds of answers obtained, and how these interactions relate in turn to culture.

The second section of the book focuses on the cultural construction of parental ethnotheories. Levy (Chapter 5) describes "essential contrasts" between the beliefs of parents in two different societies—Tahiti and Nepal—as they relate to other dimensions of difference between the two settings. McGillicuddy-DeLisi and Subramanian (Chapter 6) propose three different models for the relationship of parental beliefs and culture, illustrating with a comparative study of Tanzanian and U.S. mothers. Shwalb, Shwalb, and Shoji (Chapter 7) relate Japanese concepts of infant temperament to cultural meaning systems and thereby highlight the cultural basis of the standard temperament constructs used in research. Welles-Nystrom (Chapter 8) describes the roots of Swedish parental ethnotheories in traditional beliefs as well as national government policy.

The third section of this volume highlights the issue of intracultural variation, especially the role of schooling and parents' interactions with "experts." Palacios and Moreno (Chapter 9) discuss the relative roles of schooling and parental experience in the formation of three different profiles of beliefs among Spanish parents. LeVine, Miller, Richman, and LeVine (Chapter 10) analyze the role of schooling in differences in maternal beliefs and behavior in Mexico. Edwards, Gandini, and Giovaninni (Chapter 11) are concerned with intracultural as well as cross-cultural variability in their comparative study of U.S. and Italian preschool teachers' and parents' developmental expectations. Harkness, Super, Keefer, Raghavan, and Kipp (Chapter 12) analyze differential usage of "root metaphors" of development in the explanatory systems that parents and pediatricians employ in jointly negotiating cultural understandings of child behavior in a U.S. health care setting.

The instantiation of parental ethnotheories in cultural practices is the focus of the fourth section of this book. Goodnow (Chapter 13) describes the historical development of her own thinking about parents' ideas through the study of household practices related to family tasks in Australia. Gaskins (Chapter 14) discusses the cultural origins of developmental differences in infants' exploratory play in Yucatec Mayan and U.S. samples. Wolf, Lozoff, Latz, and Paludetto (Chapter 15) discuss the complex relationships between general cultural themes such as "autonomy" or "interrelatedness" and the management of young children's sleep routines in Japan, Italy and the United States. New and Richman (Chapter 16) describe the role of cultural values in Italy and the United States as they relate to maternal practices in three domains: motor activity, sleep, and feeding.

The last section of the book explores the consequences of parental ethnotheories for child health and development. Super, Harkness, van Tijen, van der Vlugt, Fintelman, and Dijkstra (Chapter 19) analyze differences in Dutch and U.S. infant patterns of sleep and state of arousal while awake to cultural beliefs and practices. Zeitlin (Chapter 17) describes cultural belief system among the Yoruba of Nigeria as they affect child health and nutritional status. Engle, Zeitlin, Medrano, and Garcia (Chapter 18) analyze maternal beliefs about feeding in relation to nutritional status in Nicaragua. Bond, Belenky, Weinstock, and Cook (Chapter 20) discuss the role of mothers' epistemologies in interactions with children among socioeconomically deprived families in Vermont, and they propose that this perspective be used in developing more effective parent training programs. Finally, Weisner, Matheson, and Bernheimer (Chapter 21) discuss the role of U.S. cultural models of child development in parents' efforts to cope with the challenges of bringing up developmentally delayed children.

# Acknowledgments

This volume is a product of the efforts of many organizations and individuals, and we would like to offer here a word of thanks. The development of our own thinking about parental ethnotheories was originally supported by a grant from the National Science Foundation, and more recently by two grants from the Spencer Foundation. The Fulbright Commission of The Netherlands and the University of Leiden provided, respectively, a Senior Research Fellowship to one of us (C.M.S.) and generous hospitality to both of us during a wonderful period of cross-cultural research and teaching in spring 1992. The Pennsylvania State University has also provided essential support for data analysis through grants from the Cognitive Studies Program and the Center for the Study of Child and Adolescent Development. The continuity of support provided by all these sources is more than the sum of its parts.

Several colleagues in Europe have contributed to the development of this work through their interest and hospitality. We are grateful to Dolph and Rita Kohnstamm, Tom van der Voort, Marinus van IJzendoorn, Pieter and Ineke

The Culture and Human Development series of which this volume is a part owes its existence to the enterprise of Editor in Chief Seymour Weingarten. We greatly appreciate his faith in establishing an outlet for the new perspectives represented here and in other series publications.

A special word of thanks goes to the contributors to this volume, who have put great care into crafting works that will, we hope, speak to a wide audience of readers, in voices that are both scholarly and personal.

And finally, thanks to our children, Maggie, Kate, Betsy, and John, who have made it possible for us to develop and reflect upon our own parental belief systems in the varying cultural contexts of rural Kenya, Cambridge, Massachusetts, central Pennsylvania, and Holland. You are what this book is all about.

# References

Baldwin, A. (1965). A is happy—B is not. *Child Development, 36,* 583–600.

Bronfenbrenner, U. (1979). *The ecology of human development.* Cambridge, MA: Harvard University Press.

D'Andrade, R. G. (1987). A folk model of the mind. In D. Holland & N. Quinn (Eds.), *Cultural models in language and thought* (pp. 112–148). New York: Cambridge University Press.

D'Andrade, R. G., & Strauss, C. (Eds.). (1992). *Human motives and cultural models.* New York: Cambridge University Press.

Gallimore, R., Weisner, T. S., Kaufman, S. Z., & Bernheimer, L. P. (1989). The social construction of ecocultural niches: Family accommodation of developmentally delayed children. *American Journal on Mental Retardation, 94,* 216–230.

Goodnow, J. J., & Collins, W. A. (1990). *Development according to parents: The nature, sources, and consequences of parents' ideas.* Hillsdale, NJ: Erlbaum.

Harkness, S., & Super, C. M. (1992). Parental ethnotheories in action. In I. E. Sigel, A. V. McGillicuddy-DeLisi, & J. J. Goodnow (Eds.), *Parental belief systems: The psychological consequences for children* (2nd ed., pp. 373–392). Hillsdale, NJ: Erlbaum.

Harkness, S., & Super, C. M. (1994a). The developmental niche: A theoretical framework for analyzing the household production of health. *Social Science and Medicine, 38,* 217–226.

Harkness, S., & Super, C. M. (1994b). The developmental niche: Implications for children's literacy development. In L. Eldering & P. Leseman (Eds.), *Early intervention and culture: The interface between theory and practice.* Paris: UNESCO Publishing.

Harkness, S., & Super, C. M. (1995). Culture and parenting. In M. Bornstein (Ed.), *Handbook of parenting* (pp. 211–234). Hillsdale, NJ: Erlbaum.

Harkness, S., Super, C. M., & Keefer, C. H. (1992). Learning to be an American parent: How cultural models gain directive force. In R. G. D'Andrade &

C. Strauss (Eds.), *Human motives and cultural models* (pp. 163–178). New York: Cambridge University Press.

Holland, D. C., & Valsiner, J. (1988). Cognition, symbols, and Vygotsky's developmental psychology. *Ethos, 16,* 247–272.

Kessen, W. (1979). The child and other cultural inventions. *American Psychologist, 34,* 815–820.

Lave, J., & Wenger, E. (1991). *Situated learning: Legitimate peripheral participation.* New York: Cambridge University Press.

LeVine, R. A. (1974). Parental goals: A cross-cultural view. *Teachers College Record, 76,* 226–239.

LeVine, R. A., Miller, P. M., & West, M. M. (1988). *Parental behavior in diverse societies* (New Directions in Child Development, No. 40). San Francisco: Jossey-Bass.

Mead, M. (1972). *Blackberry winter: My earlier years.* New York: Simon & Schuster.

Miller, P. (1990). Narrative practices and the construction of self in childhood. *American Ethnologist, 17,* 292–311.

Ninio, A. (1979). The naive theory of the infant and other maternal attitudes in two subgroups in Israel. *Child Development, 50,* 976–980.

Quinn, N., & Holland, D. (1987). Culture and cognition. In D. Holland & N. Quinn (Eds.), *Cultural models in language and thought* (pp. 3–40). New York: Cambridge University Press.

Reid, B. V., & Valsiner, J. (1986). Consistency, praise, and love: Folk theories of American parents. *Ethos, 14,* 282–304.

Rogoff, B. (1990). *Apprenticeship in thinking.* New York: Oxford University Press.

Sameroff, A., & Chandler, M. J. (1975). Reproductive risk and the continuum of caretaking casualty. In F. D. Horowitz (Ed.), *Review of child development research* (Vol. 4, pp. 187–294). Chicago: University of Chicago Press.

Schaefer, E. S., & Bell, R. Q. (1958). Development of a parental attitude research instrument. *Child Development, 29,* 339–361.

Schlossman, S. L. (1983). The formative era in American parent education: Overview and interpretation. In R. Haskins & D. Adams (Eds.), *Parent education and public policy* (pp. 7–39). Norwood, NJ: Ablex.

Siegel, A. W., & White, S. H. (1982). The child study movement: Early growth and development of the symbolized child. *Advances in Child Development and Behavior, 17,* 233–285.

Sigel, I. E. (Ed.). (1985). *Parental belief systems: The psychological consequences for children.* Hillsdale, NJ: Erlbaum.

Sigel, I. E., McGillicuddy-DeLisi, A. V., & Goodnow, J. J. (Eds.). (1992). *Parental belief systems: The psychological consequences for children* (2nd ed.). Hillsdale, NJ: Erlbaum.

Super, C. M. & Harkness, S. (1986). The developmental niche: A conceptualization at the interface of child and culture. *International Journal of Behavioral Development, 9,* 545–569.

Wallace, A. F. C. (1961). *Culture and personality.* New York: Random House.

Weisner, T. S., Bausano, M., & Kornfein, M. (1983). Putting family ideas into practice: Pronaturalism in conventional and non-conventional California families. *Ethos, 11,* 278–304.

White, S. H. (1992). G. Stanley Hall: From philosophy to developmental psychology. *Developmental Psychology, 28*(1), 25–34.

Whiting, B. B., & Edwards, C. P. (1988). *Children of different worlds: The formation of social behavior.* Cambridge, MA: Harvard University Press.

Whiting, J. W. M., & Whiting, B. B. (1975). *Children of six cultures: A psychocultural analysis.* Cambridge, MA: Harvard University Press.

## PART ONE

# THEORETICAL PERSPECTIVES

# CHAPTER 2

# Parents' Free Descriptions of Child Characteristics

## A Cross-Cultural Search for the Developmental Antecedents of the Big Five

Geldolph A. Kohnstamm
Charles F. Halverson, Jr.
Valerie L. Havill
Ivan Mervielde

It is well known that there is little consensus on the main dimensions of temperament and personality in childhood. Several competing theories exist and each theory has generated instruments to measure dimensions of specific interest to that particular theory. Although the variety of theories and instruments is not as overwhelming as in adult personality psychology, progress in developmental psychology is impeded by the fact that individual differences in temperament and personality are conceived and assessed in so many different ways. More often than not, the outcomes of research in which temperament measures play a major role cannot be compared because measures used to operationalize individual differences are themselves incomparable. Progress in this field would be facilitated if consensus were reached on what the most important and "basic" dimensions of temperament are in infancy, in childhood, and in adolescence.

One way to pursue such a goal is to bring theorists together at conferences and attempt to reach consensus by discussing the merits of each individual theory. Although such conferences (e.g., the 10 successive "Occasional Temperament Conferences" held in the United States) have been very stimulating and rewarding, the goal of achieving consensus remains distant. While struggling to obtain uniformity in theory and assessment of temperament in childhood, we came across the new development in adult personality psychology known as the Big Five or the Five-Factor Model (see Goldberg, 1993, for a short history and overview).

The Five-Factor Model is generating consensus among researchers of adult personality and is stimulated by theory based on the study of language—more precisely on the study of adjectives that are used for denoting individual differences in personality. These adjectives have been selected from dictionaries but also, in recent years, from free descriptions of personality given by adults. The five main dimensions are usually labeled (I) *Extroversion*, (II) *Agreeableness*, (III) *Conscientiousness*, (IV) *Emotional Stability/Instability*, and (V) *Intellect, Culture, or Openness to Experience* (see also Digman, 1990; John, 1990a, 1990b).

Until recently, the studies by Digman and his associates (Digman, 1963, 1990; Digman & Inouye, 1986) were the only ones to explore the validity of the Five-Factor Model for assessing individual differences in personality among children. Now, the number of studies exploring this area further is rapidly growing (e.g., Halverson, Kohnstamm, & Martin, 1994).

When we began to think about the possibility of adapting this approach to the field of temperament and personality in childhood, we were hampered by the fact that no word lists of adjectives (or other words) used to express temperamental differences in childhood exist. A dictionary-based approach, as was used in adult personality psychology, seemed cumbersome and inadequate for the field of temperament in childhood. One of us had already experimented for some years with free parental descriptions of temperamental characteristics of children. These characteristics had been categorized in a temporary category system that was in continuous development. Encouraged by the fact that John (1990a, 1990b) and Church and Katigbak (1988; 1989) had used a similar free descriptions approach to validate some aspects of the Big Five theory (in particular its claim of sufficiently covering the major dimensions of personality), we decided to embark on a major expedition to collect parental free or natural language descriptions of children in several languages and cultures.

The first goal of this project is to create an alternative kind of dictionary (in each language) of expressions used by parents to describe the characteristics of their children. These dictionaries can then be used, in the second phase of the project, to select representative words, expressions, or phrases, for the construction of a series of experimental questionnaires. Factor-analyzing data from these questionnaires should then result in an *n*-factor model underlying the group variance in child descriptors. The resemblance between this *n*-factor model for temperamental differences in childhood and the Five-Factor Model for personality differences in adulthood can then be studied. These are, in a nutshell, the goals we are pursuing.

But why this emphasis on languages and different cultures? We propose that the traits parents come to see in their children depend partly on the saliency of those traits in their children, partly on what they expect to see based on their particular family history and partly on the prevailing belief systems about what traits are important for children in their particular culture. Just as different cultures make variable social distinctions, so may parents in specific cultures discern different personality traits in children. Constraints are made by the traditions of a culture, by the demands placed on children, and by the expectations a culture has for the future of its children.

Cultures may differ in their belief systems about the traits of well-adapted personalities. Cultures may also differ also in their views on ideal traits as a function of gender and age (see Williams & Best, 1990; Yang & Bond, 1990; Yik & Bond, 1993 for good examples of cross-cultural variability). Enthusiastic adherents of the Big Five expect to find the same major personality dimensions in most or all cultures and languages—thus, cultural universality. Others, however, expect that when samples are studied in other cultures where people speak different languages, this Five-Factor Model may not be replicated—thus, cultural specificity.

Dictionary-based studies in psychological research of adult personality are now under way in many different countries and languages. From such studies answers may be found to the question of cultural universality of the Big Five for adult individual differences psychology. Our work, however, is directed at the question of cultural universality of major dimensions of temperament and personality in childhood. From our developmental interest follows the next question: How do the major dimensions of infancy and childhood gradually evolve into the Big Five?

## Temperament and Personality in Childhood

Individual differences in traits ascribed to children have been studied at length since the beginning of this century. When young children are the subjects of such studies, most authors use the word "temperament." As children get older the word "personality" becomes more popular. These two concepts have fuzzy boundaries. The latter includes the former, but the reverse is not true. For example, personality also includes moral and intellectual traits (Strelau, 1983). (In this chapter we limit our discussion to the questionnaire approach to temperament. In the case of children, this means ratings by parents or teachers on tests with somewhere between 20 and 100 printed items. Other approaches, based on laboratory observations or experimental situations, are not be discussed here.)

Since Thomas and Chess (e.g., 1977) popularized the concept of temperament in childhood, a large number of studies devoted to temperamental differences among children have been published; the nine-dimensional structure devised by Thomas, Chess, and their collaborators has attained textbook status. Initially for babies, but later for older children as well, this approach categorizes temperamental differences into nine more or less independent traits: activity level, rhythmicity, approach–withdrawal, adaptability, threshold of responsiveness, intensity of reaction, quality of mood, distractibility, attention span, and persistence. Above this first-order level, a second order-level was constructed consisting of the three clusters *easy*, *difficult* and *slow to warm up*. The first-order categorization was based on clinical experience and commonsense knowledge. The second-order clustering was based on a preliminary factor analysis of the nine scales.[1]

Because of their clinical usefulness, the temperament scales developed by Thomas and Chess and by Carey (e.g., Carey & McDevitt, 1978) became well-known instruments for assessing temperamental differences in infancy and childhood. It is essential for the discussion in this chapter to realize that parents (and teachers) rated their children (and pupils) "subjectively" on questions posed orally or, mostly, in a printed form, allowing them no freedom to rate their children on traits other than the nine dimensions incorporated in these instruments.

This rating procedure is not unusual in the field of personality research. All questionnaires, Q-sorts, or other kinds of instruments begin with a priori ideas their authors have of how the hundreds or even thousands of different trait terms should be summarized into the most important and most relevant dimensions. These low-level theories guide them in searching for behavioral descriptions to phrase into items. The selection of items for their initial questionnaires is guided by researchers' implicit or explicit beliefs about which traits are important enough to include and which are not. Even if they let some form of factor analysis decide what dimensions can be shown to structure the data statistically—as opposed to clinically—the final result still depends on the selection of items made in the initial stages of work.

In the case of the scales by Thomas and Chess (1977) and Carey (e.g., McDevitt & Carey, 1978), other authors showed that only five to seven replicable factors result from factoring the scores on their individual items, before aggregation into the nine scales (e.g. Martin, Wisenbaker, & Huttunen, 1994). But certainly this does not mean that the original nine dimensions are necessarily useless either in clinical assessment procedures or in research programs.

Because most temperament and personality questionnaires are developed in the United States, translation into languages other than English implicitly assumes that North American notions about core individual differences of temperament in childhood are similar to the notions held by the culture for which the translation is made. Anthropologists and cross-cultural researchers have begun to demand justification for such cross-cultural applications of psychological instruments (e.g., Malpass & Poortinga, 1986; Shwalb, Shwalb, & Shoji, 1994). Such justifications are central to cross-cultural psychology.

Translated questionnaires can both facilitate and blind researchers in studying temperament in different cultures. Brislin (1983), referring to Berry (1980), described the distinction between concepts as facilitators and concepts as impositions, or blinders:

> Given the relatively rare opportunity of doing field research in other cultures, observations can be sharpened and time used most productively if the researcher starts with well-developed concepts. Of course, the concepts can also act as blinders. Especially for concepts with well-established operational definitions (e.g., a scale or experimental procedure), borrowing from general psychology can lead to the imposition of a framework and to an oversight in and for a given culture. . . . (p. 350)

The phrase "general psychology" in this context means the psychological theorizing and consequent methodology of the ruling scientific community that is presently located in North America and northwestern Europe, and that communicates in English at conferences, in journals, in edited volumes (such as this one), and in various monographs.

Although it may seem that cultural homogeneity is on the increase at the same time that cultural uniqueness is on the decrease, a world in which cultural differences have diminished into one big melting pot has not yet arrived. Thus, the appropriateness of translation and application of psychological instruments across cultures should be questioned more frequently than is presently done. Thus far, cross-cultural studies in the field of temperament have mostly consisted of comparisons of means and variances on scales originated in England (e.g., Eysenck Personality Questionnaire; Eysenck & Eysenck, 1975) or the United States and translated into other languages. Although this work has produced many interesting results (Super & Harkness, 1986; Kohnstamm, 1989), we decided to follow a different approach first to assess some major questions about cultural concordance and discordance.

## Free Descriptions of Adult Personality

As stated earlier, we were encouraged by John (1990a), who called for more studies using free descriptions to test for the possibility that the Big Five structure was "too parochial." He was concerned

> that the reliance on experimenter-imposed variable sets to define the universe of descriptors, may have unduly excluded important characteristics from consideration. To assess the importance of this limitation, studies are needed that select characteristics on the basis of new criteria. Findings that item sets assembled according to clinical expertise, such as the California Q-Sort (Block, 1961) or the Myers–Briggs Type Indicator yield dimensions similar to the Big Five are definitely encouraging. However, given that the Big Five were intended to represent the major dimensions of natural-language personality descriptions, another option is to investigate the characteristics people use in free descriptions of themselves and others. Would the Big Five be replicated if the set of descriptors factored was based on the content of subjects' free descriptions, rather than on those sets of terms selected by the taxonomers themselves? (p. 92)

John (John, 1990a, 1990b) asked more than 300 American college students to describe their own personalities and to generate terms for both their desirable and their undesirable characteristics. This first phase of collecting, categorizing, and counting descriptors was then followed by a second phase in which the most frequently used descriptors were put in a questionnaire and given to a new sample of subjects. John focused on 60 of the most frequently used descriptors and then factor-analyzed self-ratings on these descriptors made by a new sample of students. The fact that these analyses yielded five factors that closely resembled the conceptual definitions of the Five-Factor Model (FFM) lends support to the hypothesis that these five factors are indeed the most salient dimensions of personality for U.S. college students.

In these studies, spontaneously mentioned personality characteristics are valued as expressions of implicit beliefs on what characteristics are important enough to mention. The presupposition is that subjects will mention those characteristics they think are most relevant. A second presupposition is that they will give more exemplars from categories, or dimensions, that they think are important or basic. A third presupposition is that aggregating spontaneously mentioned descriptors over groups of individuals yields a collection specific for person perceptions in the culture to which the subjects belong.

The following is a general outline of the steps necessary to collect and categorize free descriptions of personality. First, when many people have been interviewed, the large collection of personality descriptors obtained must be ordered. This can be done by judges using a well-tested categorization system that has good interjudge reliability.

Once the system of categories has been "filled" with the descriptors produced by the participants, we can assess which categories contain many descriptors and which categories include only a few descriptors or none at all. Then, under the presupposition that frequency of use indicates the degree of salience of a personality category in a particular culture, exemplars are sampled from the best filled categories. This is done to prepare for the second phase of such studies in which a representative selection of descriptors is put into questionnaires which are then given to new samples of subjects from the particular culture involved. They may be asked to rate the personalities of themselves or others on the items selected. Finally, some form of factor analysis is then used to reveal the underlying dimensions in the set of characteristics.

## Free Descriptions of Child Personality

We know of one cross-cultural study using free descriptions of college students to test the applicability of the FFM in an Asiatic culture. Church, Katigbak, and Castaneda (see Church & Katigbak, 1988; 1989) conducted in-depth interviews with 41 Filipino bilingual college students (English and Tagalog). Students responded to open-ended questions to provide general descriptions of healthy and unhealthy Filipinos in several broad areas of functioning (e.g., attitudes and feelings toward others; actions with others; attitudes and feelings toward humans in general; attitudes, feelings, or thoughts about themselves; goals or values; and mood). Responses were recorded verbatim and transcribed as general verbs (e.g., "is concerned for others"), situation-specific verbs (e.g., "when told by her father not to go to the party, she obeys"), or adjectives (e.g., "obedient" and "understanding").

The 1,516 nonredundant descriptors obtained were reduced to 54 semantic categories. These categories were derived inductively. The authors could allocate almost all these 54 categories to one of the five dimensions of the FFM. There were, however, exceptions to the five dimensions. For example, a dimension relating to nationalism and societal awareness emerged. Although these descriptors could fit in category III (Conscientiousness) in the FFM, the authors suggested that their saliency in the personality descriptions was in response to the emphasis on social and political awareness in the Philippines during the time of the research.

In his own search for the major dimensions in the parental perceptions of temperament and personality of their children, the first author (G.A.K.) and his students since 1988 did some pilot studies using free parental descriptions. This series of pilot studies developed and refined the methodology of eliciting and coding parental free descriptions. In these pilot studies the sensitivity of the free-response format to detect both social class and informant differences (e.g., mother vs. father) within the Dutch language and culture was demonstrated. They also made us aware of the potential use of the FFM for categorizing descriptors given by parents in interviews. Until 1990, only one study had explored the structure of perceived personality in late childhood and adolescence from a FFM perspective. In Digman's work (Digman, 1963, 1990; Digman & Inouye, 1986) teachers rated their pupils on a set of scales derived from adult personality psychology. His results could not reveal developmental trends because his samples were composed of children in late childhood only; also, the number of subjects was too small to allow for separate analyses of different age groups.

By exchanging the usual theoretically based or lexicon-based collections of personality words for a collection of descriptors that appear with some frequency in free descriptions of temperament and personality by parents, confidence is increased in the "ecological" representativeness of the verbal material to use in our search for the antecedents or precursors of the Big Five.

Thus, inspired by the examples given by Church and Katigbak (1989) and Yang and Bond (1990), an international group of researchers was formed with the first goal to collect free descriptions of children's personality characteristics in different languages and cultures. Aside from us this group now consists of researchers from the Polish Academy of Sciences and from the universities of Louvain (Belgium), Athens (Greece), Wroclaw (Poland), Bielefeld (Germany), and Beijing (People's Republic of China). It is assumed that our method of collecting free descriptions will give somewhat different results over cultures and languages. To quote Church and Katigbak (1989): "By starting with a taxonomy of personality concepts generated independently in each culture, culture-relevant dimensions are allowed to emerge independently, providing a more convincing test of universality when comparable dimensions emerge" (p. 870).

## Method

In all participating countries, free personality descriptions are collected, given by parents of children ages 3, 6, 9, and 12. This will give us insight in eventual developmental trends, as it can very well be that the structure of the FFM develops only with growing age and cannot yet be discerned in the structure of free parental descriptions of young children. In some countries, parallel to the parental descriptions, teacher descriptions and young adolescent self-descriptions are collected. The interviews with the parents and teachers are held in the absence of their children and pupils.

The project has four phases. In the first phase the free descriptions are collected and the descriptors identified in these descriptions are categorized by trained coders into a system developed for this purpose. In more than 20 categories those descriptors that belong together in meaning are put together. Each category receives a share of all descriptors mentioned by the parents in a specific (national) sample. This share is expressed in a proportion. For example, for the 3-year-olds in a Dutch sample, 2% of the descriptors were coded in a category named Rhythmicity.

In the second phase, questionnaire items are written by the research teams, based on the descriptors coded in each category. These items are preferably phrased in the words used by the parents themselves, syntactically simple, and easy to read and understand, even for less educated subjects. The frequency of items written for each category is roughly in proportion to the percentages of descriptors coded in each category (in phase I).

The third phase begins with a long list of about 250 experimental items given to samples of parents who are asked to rate their child's temperament/personality on these items. A first factor analysis reduces these long lists to lists of about 100 items, which are then given to larger samples of parents of children of the ages indicated earlier.

Finally, in a last phase, the resulting factor structure is analyzed for its resemblance to the Five-Factor Model. Both exploratory and confirmatory techniques will be used in this phase, and the structure found in the collections of descriptors will be compared with both existing theories of temperament in childhood and structures empirically found in data sets with a totally different origin.

## The First Phase: Categorizing Free Descriptions

To categorize the expressions generated by these parents, we have developed a coding system that has now been tested on several samples of parental free descriptions. Although the system of categories was inspired by the FFM framework, with several subcategories in each of the five dimensions, an additional eight categories have been added to date. Thus, the fact that the category system partly follows the FFM model does not preclude the possibility that we will discover dimensions outside the FFM. Because the goal of a free description protocol is to select words or expressions from any category with a sufficient number of elements, no category has been precluded on an a priori basis.

Because homogeneous subcategories have been created within the five dimensions and eight other categories have been added, there is ample opportunity for factors other than FFM factors to emerge from the ratings done by groups of parents (in different languages and cultures) in the second phase of our project. One of our assumptions therefore is that our category system will be broad enough to be sensitive to sociocultural differences in parental views of individual differences.

The category system we are using consists of 14 main categories and up to 3 subcategories per category. Each major category is designated by a Roman numeral paralleling the FFM usage where appropriate. The subcategories or facets are inductively derived. Responses are coded as "positive," "neutral," or "negative" as well. For example, "enthusiastic" is coded as IA+; "tends to shut herself of" is coded IA−. Table 2.1 shows the total system. No examples are given for responses coded as neutral.

The oral interviews with the parents are first tape-recorded and then transcribed verbatim. Next, decisions are made on which utterances are to be used as units for coding and which utterances can be discarded. Detailed instructions have been developed for this step in applying the categorization scheme.[2] The unitizing procedure has proved to be more subjective than the subsequent procedure in which the units are coded into categories or subcategories.

## Rationale for Categories Included

The origin of the first five main categories has already been explained. The subcategories within those five are our own inventions, based on

**Table 2.1.** Categories for Coding Descriptors from "Free" Personality Descriptions and Examples of Descriptors

### I. Extroversion

1A: Sociability

| 1A + | 1A − |
|---|---|
| Enthusiastic | Tendency to shut self off |
| Totally thrilled to be alive | Inhibited and withdrawn |
| Likes to be with others | Shy, prefers to play alone |

1B: Dominance, Leadership, Assertiveness

| 1B + | 1B − |
|---|---|
| A leader | Passive |
| Strong character | Follows everyone |
| Assertive | Doesn't stand up for self |

1C: Activity, pace, tempo, energy, restlessness, vitality

| 1C + | 1C − |
|---|---|
| Active | Quiet |
| Energetic | Not physically active |
| Always on the move | Doesn't do much |

### II. Agreeableness

2A: Helpfulness, cooperation, amiability

| 2A + | 2A − |
|---|---|
| Loving, sweet child | Selfish |
| Good natured | Impatient |
| Caring | Not a good helper |

2B: Manageable for parents and teachers

| 2B + | 2B − |
|---|---|
| Well-behaved | Argumentative |
| Never belligerent | Stubborn |
| Cooperative | Rebellious |

2C: Honest, sincere

| 2C + | 2C − |
|---|---|
| Sincere | Lies |
| Honest | Can be deceiving |
| Trustworthy | Insincere |

### III. Conscientiousness

3A: Carefulness

| 3A + | 3A − |
|---|---|
| Long attention span | Forgetful |
| Good concentration | Daydreamer |
| Responsible | Careless |

*(cont.)*

**Table 2.1** *(cont.)*

### III. Conscientiousness *(cont.)*

3B: Dependability

| 3B + | 3B – |
|---|---|
| Very loyal to his/her friends | No examples |
| Stands up for his/her friends | |
| Reliable | |

3C: Diligence, industriousness, persevering

| 3C + | 3C – |
|---|---|
| Determined | Needs motivation |
| Hard worker | Lazy |
| Competitive | Unwilling to work |

### IV. Emotional Stability

4A: Emotional reactivity and stability

| 4B + | 4A – |
|---|---|
| Under control | Cries a lot |
| Very resilient | Sensitive to words from others |
| Rarely loses temper | Needs to control temper |

4B: Self-confidence

| 4B + | 4B – |
|---|---|
| Confident | Lacks self-confidence |
| Self-assured | Insecure |
| Certain | Tentative in own assessment of abilities |

4C: Anxious, fearful

| 4C + | 4C – |
|---|---|
| Doesn't exhibit a lot of fears or nervousness | Afraid of the dark, afraid of dogs, etc. |

### V. Openness to Experience, Intelligence

5A: Openness to experience, adventure seeking

| 5A + | 5A – |
|---|---|
| Curious | Afraid of failure |
| Inquisitive | Not too open (to new things or ideas) |
| Easily interested in new things | Hesitant to do things |

5B: Interested in things, good at . . .

| 5B + | 5B – |
|---|---|
| Interested in computers | Dislikes reading |
| Likes music, plays piano very well | Not interested in . . . |

*(cont.)*

**Table 2.1** *(cont.)*

5C: Intelligence, language proficiency, reasoning capacities

| 5C + | 5C– |
|---|---|
| Bright | Difficult in understanding |
| Quick to learn | Slow to learn |

### VI. Independence, Ability to Do Things Independently

| 6 + | 6 – |
|---|---|
| Independent | Doesn't do things on his/her own |
| Often involved in activities on | Too dependent on mom |
| Likes to do things on his own | |

### VII. Mature for Age

| 7 + | 7 – |
|---|---|
| Mature | Babyish behaviour |
| Precocious | Emotionally immature |
| Intelligent for age | Young for his peer group |

### VIII. Illness, Handicaps, and Health

| 8 + | 8 – |
|---|---|
| Healthy | Sickly |
| | Severe allergy problems, attention deficit disorder |

### IX. Rhythmicity of Eating, Sleeping, etc.

| 9 + | 9 – |
|---|---|
| Likes things to run on regular schedule | No examples |

### X. Gender-Appropriate/Physical Attractiveness

| 10 + | 10 – |
|---|---|
| He's all boy | He only likes to play with girls |
| Attractive, handsome | |

### XI. School Performance, Attitudes toward School

| 11 + | 11 – |
|---|---|
| Eager about school | Talks when he is not supposed to in school |
| Excellent student, self-motivated at school | Not challenged at school |

*(cont.)*

**Table 2.1** *(cont.)*

---

### XII. Contact Comfort, Desire to Be Cuddled, Clinging

12 +                                    12 −

Cuddly, huggable                        Clinging to mom

### XIII. Relations with Siblings and Parents

13A: Sibling relationships

| 13A + | 13A − |
|---|---|
| Helps with siblings | Ignores sister |
| Watches out for brother, problems with siblings | Will not play with brother |

13B: Interaction with parents and family

| 13B + | 13B − |
|---|---|
| Likes to do things with the family | Not too eager to do things with family |
| Oriented to her family |  |
| Good father–daughter relationship |  |

### XIV. Ambiguous, Phrases and Descriptions That Cannot Be Coded in Other Categories

Strong spiritual character
Persnickety
Too materialistic
He can charm people

---

clusters of high-loading items, or "facets" as published in several FFM studies (e.g., Goldberg, 1993). For the location of some of the subcategories (e.g., Manageable for parents and teachers—category II), we have no empirical basis because no adjectives for manageability were included in FFM adjective studies as they did not deal with children. It is very possible that in the second phase of this project, items dealing with manageability will not cluster with a higher-order factor recognizable as the FFM's Agreeableness.

We do not necessarily expect to find a neat FFM structure once large samples of parents have rated their children on the items we will select from the best filled categories. This will be particularly true for the ratings of young children below 6 years of age. At the end of this chapter, we will return to the question of what project outcomes we do expect.

Next, we describe some of the rationale for the coding that has been done in our pilot studies regarding the additional categories to the FFM (i.e., categories VI through XIV). We are coding the Independence (VI) category separately from the Big Five for two reasons. First, when parents describe their children as being independent (or as being too dependent) they seem to mean something we see as different from being high or low on Extroversion, Conscientiousness, Emotional Stability/Instability, or Openness to Experience. Second, in the adult FFM literature, repeatedly a factor labeled Autonomy or Independence has been discerned as having independent status. So, on rational grounds, John (1990a, 1990b) made a separate category "independence" when categorizing personality descriptors generated by his students. Also, Costa and McCrae (1988), on empirical grounds, saw sufficient indications for a separate factor Autonomy in the Personality Research Form (PRF). Whether being independent and autonomous *in childhood* will attain independent factorial status remains to be determined in the following phases of our project.

Mature for Age (VII) is a category that a student of adult personality characteristics would never think of as relevant to personality. Few adjectives of this kind have ever been included in FFM adjective studies using self or other ratings of adults; therefore, it is impossible to tell whether and where Mature for Age would fit in the factor analytically derived model. It is included for coding comprehensiveness and possible links to other categories.

It is questionable whether the fact that a person is often or never ill or is handicapped is a personality characteristic in the strict sense. The reason Illness, Handicaps, and Health (VIII) is included in our system is that parents of ill or handicapped children often mention this fact first and foremost in the beginning of the interview. They consider it fundamental background information for understanding their child's further characteristics.

Rhythmicity (IX) is included as a coding category because it is one of the nine dimensions of the Thomas–Chess model. In the Thomas–Chess derived Dimension of Temperament Survey–Revised (DOTS-R) questionnaire (Windle & Lerner, 1986), rhythmicity is even operationalized in three separate scales (for eating, sleeping, and daily habits). Angleitner and Ostendorf (1994) demonstrated that when students rate themselves on many different personality questionnaires, including the DOTS-R, Rhythmicity obtains independent status as a sixth factor outside the FFM domain. However, as we shall see in Table 2.3, only 1 or 2% of the descriptors generated by parents have to do with rhythmicity. Therefore, it will be difficult to justify including rhythmicity items in the second phase of our project because parents do not use rhythmicity descriptors often enough to consider the construct an important characteristic of children. For us, it makes little sense to develop standardized instruments to measure parent-rated traits that are not seen as important by parents. Others may be of the opinion that psychologists and psychiatrists know better about the importance of rhythmicity than lay parents do. They will not accept our layperson approach as decisive for what items to include in questionnaires and what not. Furthermore, it is also possible that parents from other cultures will generate more descriptors indicating aspects of rhythmicity than we have found so far.

Gender-appropriate Behavior and Physical Attractiveness (X) are not usually included in the concept of temperament and personality, though one can easily see them as important personal characteristics that may cluster with other important personality traits in childhood. Certainly there is a taboo, at least in Western cultures, against mentioning physical attractiveness or lack thereof of one's child in a conversation with a stranger. Nevertheless, we all know how important physical attractiveness may be, both in the life of children and in the life of adults. This personal characteristic is important for triggering positive or negative reactions from parents and peers; for being popular in class; for being hired in jobs; for careers in television, in the performing arts, and in politics; for finding a spouse; and for developing depressive disorders (e.g., Cavior & Dokecki, 1973; Hartup, 1983; Langlois & Downs, 1979; Ritter, Casey, & Langlois, 1991). Recently, Lanning (1994) found an independent attractiveness factor, the first one after the Big Five, when factoring a sample of 940 California Q-set (CAQ) ratings. As for the observations made by parents of their child as typically behaving according to their gender, there are indications in the adult FFM literature that femininity–masculinity is a trait sufficiently independent of the Big Five to obtain separate factorial status (Lanning, 1994).

We also included a category for descriptors indicating *How Well Children Are Doing in School*, for example, if their marks are good, average, or bad (XI). Typically, in the history of personality testing such qualities are measured by instruments other than personality questionnaires. However, by keeping school performance and attitudes apart in our category system, we have somewhat reduced the number of 'descriptors' coded in category III, Conscientiousness, notably those describing the child as being industrious or lazy at school.

Cuddliness and Clinging Behavior (XII) have something of a history in the temperament literature (e.g., Bates, Freeland, & Lounsbury, 1979). Thus far this category has attracted few descriptors. The low frequency of terms in this category may not warrant the inclusion of cuddliness and clinging behavior in the second phase of this project.

A separate category (XIII) was set up to code descriptions of *Relations Between the Target Child and His or Her Siblings*, and between the child and his or her parents. When such characteristics are referenced to a particular family member rather than as general characteristics of interactions with people outside the family, they are coded XIII and not, for example, II (Agreeableness) or IV (Emotional Stability/ Instability). Here, the same remark applies as made above in connection with category XI, School Performance. By setting this category apart we may have reduced the number of descriptors that otherwise would have gone to I, II, or IV.

The last category, XIV, needs no clarification. If coders hesitate about coding a descriptor in any of the 13 categories, they may decide to put it in this category. As it turns out, some coders make more use of this category than others do.

Our group has collected parental free descriptions of child characteristics in several countries and languages. The largest samples thus far have been collected in the United States, Holland, (Flemish) Belgium, Poland, Greece, and China. Smaller samples were obtained from Surinam, a former Dutch colony on the northern coast of the South American continent, and from Germany and French Belgium. Also, within the United States and Holland, smaller samples of a specific nature were obtained. Furthermore, free descriptions of pupils by their teachers have begun to be collected by Martin in Georgia (United States) and Mervielde in Belgium (Mervielde, 1994).

For this chapter, we limit the presentation and discussion of results to the samples of parental descriptions from the United States (Athens, Georgia), Holland, and (Flemish) Belgium. But we also present results of a smaller black sample, collected both in Surinam and in Holland.[3] A complete overview of results, obtained in all participating countries, will be published in a separate volume (Kohnstamm, Halverson, & Mervielde, in press).

## Participants

In some samples, if possible both mothers and fathers were interviewed, separately. Such was the case in the samples from the United States and Holland. In other samples, only mothers (Surinam) or either of both (Belgium) were interviewed. In addition, some parents described two of their children, so the total number of children described may be larger than the total number of parents interviewed. The children varied in age from 3 to 12. We tried to include as many children as possible around the target ages of 3, 6, 9, and 12, so that the larger samples could be split into clearly distinct age groups. The socioeconomic status of the parents was recorded so that the larger samples could also be split into separate groups based on socioeconomic status, in order to study the effects of socioeconomic status both within and between samples.

## Procedure

In the American sample, parents were asked simply "to tell us about your child." In the Dutch and Belgian samples, after an introduction in which the word "personality" was mentioned, the parents were asked, "Can you tell me what you think is characteristic of your child?" All the interviews were audiotaped or videotaped. Elaborate coding manuals were available for coders, which included instructions regarding units of analysis, division of phrases, repetitions, and synonymy.

For our purposes, a unit of analysis was defined as an adjective, verb, noun, or phrase referring to a description of behavior, personality characteristic, or ability. Phrases referring to situational causes of behavior or to physical attributes were not coded. Because a unit of analysis could be a phrase, it was sometimes helpful to split the phrases into simpler, easily codable parts. Adjacent words or phrases could be divided and coded separately as two individual units if the meaning of each part was understood when considered independently. If a coder judged that meaning or context is lost by splitting the phrase, the unit was coded as one single description. For example, the phrase "she likes to play outdoors with neighbor kids" can be separated into two distinct parts: (1) "she likes to play outdoors" and (2) "plays with neighbor kids." The first phrase would be coded as referring to physical activity level and the second phrase would be coded as indicating extroversion or sociability. The phrase "she's so quick, her head works very, very fast" would be coded as a single unit because breaking the description into two parts could conceivably lead the coder to misinterpret "she's so quick" as referring to physical activity instead of cognitive proficiency.

In free-language interviews, respondents often elaborate on a single characteristic by mentioning concrete, situation-specific behaviors to illustrate the personality characteristic. In such cases, the elaborative phrase or phrases were taken with the personality descriptive word or phrase and were coded as one unit of analysis. Respondents may also mention a descriptive characteristic in the past tense and contrast this with a similar descriptive characteristic in the present tense to illustrate how a child is now with respect to a younger age. In this case, the past tense phrase was not coded separately but was included in one unit with the present tense phrase. The part of the phrase in the present tense was the subject of analysis; the past tense word or phrase, however, may have helped the coder to assess the meaning or importance of the unit as a whole.

Words and phrases that were not coded as descriptive phrases included those referring to a person other than the target child or to children in general. These were considered nonrelevant phrases and were therefore not coded. Phrases offering peripheral information were also excluded. These were phrases including information connected to the main issue but so remote as to have no immediate relevance to the target child (e.g., "her parents are friends of mine," or "you have a lot of temper tantrums and things with all kids, you know, that is not specific to Susie, but that is something that would bother me about her"). If there was any reasonable doubt as to whether a respondent was referring to the target child directly, the word or phrase was not coded.

When words or phrases were repeated verbatim or if phrases expressing the exact same literal meaning were used more than once in a single interview, these units were recorded and coded as repetitions but were not included in frequency analyses more than once.

### Training of Coders and Coding Reliability

Intensive communication between the coding teams in the United States, Holland, and Belgium has helped to find solutions to most of the discrepancies and uncertainties encountered in coding the verbal protocols. The students from Leiden University who collected and coded the Surinam (black) sample were of Surinamese background. They were trained and supervised by the Dutch team. After training, coders' percentages of agreement over the 14 main categories were between 80 and 90. When agreement on the 15 subcategories in the first five (Big Five) main categories was also analyzed, reliabilities ranged between 70% and 80%. More detailed information regarding coding reliability has been presented elsewhere (Kohnstamm, Mervielde, Besevegis & Halverson, 1995).

## Results

In Table 2.2 the proportions of descriptors coded in the first five main categories are presented over four different samples. The total proportions for these five main categories range between 76 (Surinam) and 81 (United States). The distributions over the five categories are remarkably similar, though there are discrepancies of 5–7% in the first two categories.

The average number of codable descriptors generated in the interviews (line above bottom line of Table 2.2) differs considerably. This number reflects the average duration of the interviews, the verbal expressiveness of the parents, and the level of differentiation regarding

**Table 2.2.** Proportions of Child Descriptors Given by Parents, over the First Five Main Categories of the Coding Scheme

| Country | U.S. (Georgia) | Belgium | Holland | Surinam |
|---|---|---|---|---|
| Language | English | Flemish | Dutch | Surinam/ Dutch |
| Age of children | 3–13 | 3–12 | 3–12 | 6–10 |
| N of children described | 711 | 427 | 324 | 120 |
| Categories | | | | |
| I.   Extroversion | 32 | 27 | 28 | 25 |
| II.  Agreeableness | 21 | 19 | 19 | 24 |
| III. Conscientiousness | 6 | 8 | 7 | 7 |
| IV.  Emotional Stability | 6 | 9 | 11 | 6 |
| V.   Intellect, Culture, Openness to Experience | 17 | 13 | 13 | 14 |
| Total I–V | 82% | 77% | 78% | 76% |
| Total N of descriptors coded over all categories I–XIV, disregarding repetitions | 8,667 | 9,607 | 6,672 | 2,102 |
| Mean N of descriptors per interview, disregarding repetitions | 12.2 | 22.5 | 20.6 | 17.5 |
| Percentage of fathers interviewed | 35% | 18% | 41% | 0% |

their children's personalities that parents were capable of expressing. In the U.S. sample from Georgia, the parents were interviewed in all sorts of situations, some of these so informal (e.g., at the school door or in the playground) that the interviews could only be of short duration. This caused the relatively low average number of descriptors in the U.S. (Georgia) sample.

In Table 2.3 the proportions of descriptors over the remaining categories are given. Because of the small proportions, decimals are also presented. Table 2.3 can be read as a continuation of Table 2.2.

Next, in Table 2.4, the distribution of descriptors over the subcategories in the first five main categories is given, for the three larger samples only. Table 2.4 should thus be read as a specification of Table 2.2. Overall, the proportions over categories obtained from the descriptions by parents in these samples are remarkably similar.

Concerning the ages of the children described, some categories of

**Table 2.3.** Proportions of Child Descriptors Given by Parents: Coded in Categories Presumably "Outside" the Big Five Domain

| Country | U.S. (Georgia) | Belgium | Holland | Surinam |
|---|---|---|---|---|
| Language | English | Flemish | Dutch | Surinam/Dutch |
| Age of children | 4–12 | 3–12 | 3–12 | 6–10 |
| Categories (%) | | | | |
| VI. Independence | 1.1 | 3.5 | 3.7 | 2.5 |
| VII. Mature for Age | 1.5 | 2.4 | 3.1 | 1.7 |
| VIII. Illness/Health | 0.7 | 0.6 | 0.9 | 0.7 |
| IX. Rhythmicity | 0.2 | 0.9 | 1.0 | 2.0 |
| X. Gender-Appropriate/ Physical Attractiveness | 2.2 | 0.9 | 1.3 | 1.2 |
| XI. School Performance | 3.1 | 4.0 | 3.2 | 7.1 |
| XII. Contact Comfort | 0.4 | 1.7 | 1.1 | 0.9 |
| XIII. Family Relationships | 3.3 | 4.3 | 3.6 | 3.8 |
| XIV. Ambiguous | 5.0 | 4.5 | 5.4 | 4.1 |

the system are better utilized when older children are described, whereas the percentages of descriptors coded in other categories diminish with age. Increasing proportions have been found for categories III (Conscientiousness) and IV (Emotional Stability/Instability) for all samples. Decreasing proportions were found for I+ (Extroversion) and for II– (Disagreeableness). In all samples the percentages obtained for girls and boys are remarkably similar.

Generally, as can be seen from Tables 2.2 through 2.4, the concordance in proportions over categories (between the four different samples) is very high, though there are also some clear differences, notably in the subcategories (Table 2.4). A maximum difference of about 7% was found for subcategory Ic, Activity/Pace, with Georgian (United States) parents mentioning activity characteristics (see Table 2.1, Ic, for some examples) more frequently than Dutch and Belgian parents.

As indicated above, the characteristics mentioned by the parents were also coded as High, Low, or Neutral on the dimensions presumably underlying the categories (see + and – signs in Table 2.1). High and Low can also be termed positive and negative since on most, if not all, dimensions the positive pole is accommodating the more desirable behavioral characteristics. One should be careful, however, not to identify too quickly the plus pole with positive evaluation and the minus pole with negative evaluation, because cross-cultural value differences probably exist for some dimensions (e.g., for Extroversion/Introver-

**Table 2.4.** For the Three Largest Samples the Proportions of Child Descriptors Given by Parents, over the Subcategories of the First Five Main Categories of the Coding Scheme (Specification of Table 2.2)

| Country | | | U.S. (Georgia) | Belgium | Holland |
|---|---|---|---|---|---|
| Categories (%) | | | | | |
| I | | | | | |
| | A | Sociability | 17.9 | 14.7 | 16.6 |
| | B | Dominance/Leadership | 2.3 | 6.1 | 6.6 |
| | C | Activity/Pace | 12.0 | 6.2 | 4.7 |
| II | | | | | |
| | A | Helpfulness | 13.4 | 10.9 | 9.6 |
| | B | Manageability | 6.7 | 7.9 | 9.0 |
| | C | Honesty/Sincerity | 0.8 | 0.6 | 0.5 |
| III | | | | | |
| | A | Carefulness | 2.6 | 4.7 | 3.4 |
| | B | Dependability | 0.2 | 0.5 | 0.3 |
| | C | Diligence | 3.5 | 3.2 | 3.0 |
| IV | | | | | |
| | A | Emotional reactivity | 4.4 | 6.7 | 7.4 |
| | B | Self-confidence | 1.1 | 2.1 | 2.6 |
| | C | Anxiety/Fearfulness | 0.4 | 0.6 | 0.6 |
| V | | | | | |
| | A | Openness to experience | 4.8 | 3.8 | 3.7 |
| | B | Interested in . . . | 6.4 | 6.5 | 5.4 |
| | C | Intelligence | 5.8 | 2.7 | 3.4 |

sion). Children described as highly active (Ic+) are often considered by their parents and teachers as too active, impulsive, and difficult to manage. Also, mildly critical remarks regarding the child's behavior are equally coded on the minus side of the categories.

For all categories separately, and for the total of all characteristics together, the percentages of "negative," "neutral," and "positive" characteristics were computed. Across all samples, about 30% of the characteristics mentioned by the parents were coded on the negative side of the presumed dimensions underlying the categories.

However, the categories differ widely in the proportions of "negative" characteristics. Category IV (Emotional Stability/Instability) received the most. About 75% of all characteristics mentioned by parents and coded in this category are referring to emotional instability and neurotic behavior. On the other extreme is category V (Openness to Experience); only about 5% of all characteristics coded in this category were evaluated by the coders as "negative."

# Discussion

Collecting and analyzing free parental descriptions of child characteristics in different countries and languages has thus produced remarkably similar outcomes. When samples are large enough, groups of parents collectively mention characteristics, 70–80% of which can be categorized in Big-Five related categories and subcategories. The proportions each category receives from independent coders are remarkably similar between countries and languages, between fathers and mothers, and for boys and girls. Presently, the effect of the socioeconomic status of the parents is being analyzed.

Although we expect to find more cross-cultural differences once the Chinese, Greek, and Polish samples have been fully coded, we also expect that the free-language descriptions by parents will continue to show cross-cultural and cross-language concordances large enough to move to next phases of this project, with instruments that are not identical but still comparable over languages and cultures.

The large differences in proportions over categories within each sample partly reflect the conceptual span of the categories: The broader one makes a category, the more characteristics the category will receive by the coders. An alternative explanation, that some categories have a greater number of adjectives available in the language to denote specific behavioral characteristics, is less plausible.

First, only a minority of the trait descriptions given by the parents contain adjectives, and, second, Havill, Allen, and Halverson (1994) found that the frequency of category use does not correspond to the availability of adjectives in American English.

As to the first argument, when parents give free descriptions of their children, they use sentences made up of articles, pronouns, verb forms, nouns, adverbs, and also adjectives. Because the number of different sentences one can make is practically without limits, the proportions as given in Tables 2.2 through 2.4 must reflect conceptual width or span, as well as saliency of the behavioral characteristics for parents, rather than the availability of the number of personality relevant words in a language.

It is already clear that important differences in content of descriptions have to do with the age of the children described. Some samples not discussed in this chapter have included very young children (Harkness and Super, personal communication), and the preliminary results suggest an abundance of category I and II descriptors for infants and toddlers. In category III, the proportions of descriptors suddenly increase when the children go to school, and so on. That sort of difference is certainly not dependent on either width of categories or availability of word types in the language but merely on the saliency and relevance of the behavioral characteristics (for parents) and on the developmental differentiation of the stage children are in.

It is expected that a representative process of selection from the collections of descriptors will result in somewhat different selections for each age level. The history of rating scale construction for use in childhood shows the need for such age-graded versions.

Both exploratory and confirmatory factor-analysis procedures will be used in the empirical analyses. This may finally result in a new type of temperament and personality scales for childhood, comparable across the participating countries in respect to their origin in parental free descriptions. How much the factorial structure underlying these scales will resemble the FFM is difficult to predict, but preliminary coding reported here gives some clues indicating that these instruments may be more similar to the FFM than instruments now in use, in particular for older children. From the initial results presented here, it is already clear that a FFM-inspired category system is at the very least a good heuristic for classifying elements of free parental descriptions of child characteristics. The fact that between 70% and 80% of these elements can be coded in a FFM-inspired category system facilitates the search for the possible antecedents of the Big Five in childhood.

Once the new questionnaires are ready, a fifth phase of this project is foreseen: testing the validity and the usefulness of the new instruments, both for clinical use in individual cases and for research purposes.

What can we anticipate from the results of this project when we compare our new scales to existing procedures for assessing temperament and personality in childhood? Martin et al. (1994) have demonstrated that in studies using the Thomas–Chess and Carey questionnaires for parents, five major factors appear to replicate across studies. They labeled these five factors as Activity Level, Negative Emotionality and Irritability, Task Persistence (including focused attention and distractibility), Adaptability/ Agreeableness, and Approach/Withdrawal. In our FFM-inspired category system (see Table 2.1) this means I(c), IV, III, II, and I(a).

The fact that FFM category V was not assessed in the Thomas–Chess tradition needs a short historical explanation. First, in the 20 or more centuries of thinking and writing about the four classic temperaments, cognitive characteristics have never played a prominent role. Second, in the personality theories by 20th-century theorists such as Cattell and Eysenck, cognitive differences between people were left to the psychologists working on intelligence and intelligence tests. The assessment of personality characteristics developed separately from the assessment of intelligence. Only in the last two decades has attention been directed at the interplay between emotions and cognitions, and the artificial conceptual boundaries between the two domains are now rapidly disappearing. One of the great advantages of the FFM is that it abandons this dichotomy.

In the specific case of the New York Longitudinal Study by Thomas and Chess, another explanation is that their initial psychiatric focus on problem behavior in infants and toddlers made the assessment of cognitive capacities and curiosity less obvious. The fact that Task Persistence/Focused Attention prove to be replicable factors in their questionnaires probably relates more to FFM factor III than to V, but this awaits further empirical study of the developmental antecedents of the Big Five.

Van Lieshout and Haselager (1994) have demonstrated that principal component analyses of a large sample of sorts by parents and teachers of the Dutch version of the California Child Q-sort (CCQ; Block, 1961/1978; J.H. Block & J. Block, 1980) produced a best solution of seven factors, the first five resembling the adult Big Five. A sixth factor was labeled Motor Activity (compare with the study by Martin et al., 1994, mentioned earlier) and a seventh Dependency (compare with category VI in our coding scheme). A similar study by John and his colleagues, analyzing the CCQ sorts for a sample of young adolescent Pittsburgh boys, came with comparable results (John, Caspi, Robins, Moffitt, & Stouthamer-Loeber, 1994; Robins, John, & Caspi, 1994).

The domain of phenomena covered in the CCQ consists of a large set of statements chosen by the Blocks and aimed at the comprehensive description of the wide range of affective, cognitive, and social attributes that manifest themselves in the behavior and personality of children and adolescents between the ages of 3 and 18. The Blocks had no knowledge of the FFM when generating these statements (just as the parents in our study have no knowledge of the FFM). Also, Jack Block himself sees little value in the FFM (Block, 1995), making the emergence of the FFM in the CCQ all the more remarkable.

Our group is aware of the danger of a FFM bias and has taken precautions not to be overinfluenced by it. Different kinds of factor analysis will be employed to see how robust the clustering of items is over methods. We do not expect that more variance will be explained by the replicable factors than is commonly the case. Even if some of the childhood factors found resemble some of the factors of the adult FFM, at least as far as important *facets* of the Big Five are concerned, proof of empirical continuity can only come from longitudinal studies. In such studies the factor scores obtained with our instruments in childhood can be correlated with those obtained in adulthood, using good

FFM assessment techniques. Until those longitudinal data are available, the resemblances in structure, however plausible, will only be hypothetical.

## Acknowledgments

The authors wish to thank their research teams for their contribution at every phase of this project: Anne Marie Slotboom and Eric Elphick (The Netherlands), Kathy Allen and Hilary Rose (U.S.), Filip de Fruyt and Veerle Buyst (Belgium). The Surinamese data were collected and coded by Gaytrie Kartaram and Jo-Ann Calor. Support for the U.S. part of the project came from National Institute of Mental Health Grant No. MH 34899 to Charles Halverson. The Belgian part is supported by Grant No. 0ZF-0112792 from the Research Council of the University of Ghent awarded to I. Mervielde. The Dutch part is supported by the Leiden section of the Institute for the Study of Education and Development.

## Notes

1. We note that these nine scales do not appear, nor do the second-level clusters, when items rather than scales are clustered. See Martin, Wisenbaker, and Huttunen (1994) for a discussion of this issue. This point is also discussed later in our text.

2. The English-language coding manual and the coding instructions are available from any of the authors. Thu• far, other language versions are available in Chinese, Dutch, German, Greek, French, and Polish.

3. In Greece this work is done by Elias Besevegis, Vasilis Pavlopoulos, and Sophia Mouroussakis of the University of Athens; in Poland by Slawomir Jarmuz of Wroclaw University and by Magdalena Marszal of the Polish Academy of Sciences; in Germany by Alois Angleitner of the University of Bielefeld; in French-speaking Belgium by Christiane Vandenplas of the University of Louvain; and in China by Zhang Yuging of Peking University.

4. No examples are given for the neutral descriptors in each category.

## References

Angleitner, A. & Ostendorf, F. (1994). Temperament and the Big Five Factors of personality. In C. F. Halverson, G. A. Kohnstamm, & R. P. Martin (Eds.), *The developing structure of temperament and personality from infancy to adulthood* (pp. 69–90). Hillsdale, NJ: Erlbaum.

Bates, J. E., Freeland, C. A. B., & Lounsbury, M. L. (1979). Measurement of infant difficulties. *Child Development, 50,* 794–803.

Berry, J. W. (1980). Introduction to methodology. In H. C. Triandis & J. W. Berry (Eds.), *Handbook of cross-cultural psychology* (Vol. 2, pp. 2–28). Boston: Allyn & Bacon.

Block, J. (1978). *The Q-sort method in personality assessment and psychiatric research* (rev. ed.). Palo Alto, CA: Consulting Psychologists Press. (Original work published 1961)

Block, J. (1995). A contrarian view of the five-factor approach to personality description. *Psychological Bulletin, 117,* 187–215.

Block, J. H., & Block J. (1980). The role of ego-control and ego-resiliency in the organization of behavior. In W. A. Collins, (Ed.), Development of cognition, affect, and social relations. *Minnesota symposia on child psychology* (Vol. 13, pp. 39–101). Hillsdale, NJ: Erlbaum.

Brislin, R. W. (1983). Cross-cultural research in psychology. In M. R. Rosenzweig & L. W. Porter (Eds.), *Annual review of psychology* (pp. 363–400). Palo Alto, CA: Annual Reviews.

Carey, W. B., & McDevitt, S. C. (1978). Revision of the Infant Temperament Questionnaire. *Pediatrics, 61,* 735–739.

Cavior, N., & Dokecki, P. B. (1973). Physical attractiveness, perceived attitude similarity, and academic achievement as contributors to interpersonal attraction among adolescents. *Developmental Psychology, 9,* 44–54.

Church, A. T., & Katigbak, M. S. (1988). The emic strategy in the identification and assessment of personality dimensions in a non-western culture: Rationale, steps and a Philippine illustration. *Journal of Cross-Cultural Psychology, 18,* 143–164.

Church, A. T., & Katigbak, M. S. (1989). Internal, external and self-reward structure of personality in non-Western culture: An investigation of cross-language and cross-cultural generalizability. *Journal of Personality and Social Psychology, 57,* 857–872.

Costa, P. T., & McCrae, R. R. (1988). From catalog to classification: Murray's needs and the Five-Factor Model. *Journal of Personality and Social Psychology, 55,* 258–265.

Digman, J. M. (1963). Principal dimensions of child personality as inferred from teachers' judgments. *Child Development, 34,* 43–60.

Digman, J. M. (1990). Personality structure: Emergence of the Five-Factor Model. In M. R. Rosenzweig & L. W. Porter (Eds.), *Annual review of psychology* (Vol. 41, pp. 417–440). Palo Alto, CA: Annual Reviews.

Digman, J. M., & Inouye, J. (1986). Further specification of the five robust factors of personality. *Journal of Personality and Social Psychology, 50,* 116–123.

Eysenck, H. J., & Eysenck, S. B. G. (1975). *Manual of the Eysenck Personality Questionnaire.* Loughton, Essex: Hodder & Stoughton.

Goldberg, L. R. (1993). The structure of phenotypic personality traits. *American Psychologist, 48*(1), 26–34.

Halverson, C. F., Kohnstamm, G. A., & Martin, R. P. (Eds.). (1994). *Development of the structure of temperament and personality from infancy to adulthood.* Hillsdale, NJ: Erlbaum.

Hartup, W. (1983). Peer relations. In P. H. Mussen (Series Ed.) & E. M. Hetherington (Vol. Ed.), *Handbook of child psychology* (Vol. 4, pp. 103–196). New York: Wiley.

Havill, V. L., Allen, K., & Halverson, C. F. (1994). Parents' use of Big Five categories in their natural language descriptions of children. In C. F. Halverson, G. A. Kohnstamm & R. P. Martin (Eds.), *Development of the structure of temperament and personality from infancy to adulthood* (pp. 371–386). Hillsdale, NJ: Erlbaum.

John, O. P. (1990a). The "Big Five" factor taxonomy: Dimensions of personality in the natural language and in questionnaires. In L. A. Pervin (Ed.), *Handbook of personality: Theory and research* (pp. 66–100). New York: Guilford Press.

John, O. P. (1990b). Towards a taxonomy of personality descriptors. In D. M. Buss & N. Cantor (Eds.), *Personality psychology: Recent trends and emerging directions* (pp. 261–271). New York: Springer-Verlag.

John, O. P., Caspi, A., Robins, R. W., Moffitt, T. E., & Stouthamer-Loeber, M. (1994). The "little five": Exploring the nomological network of the Five-Factor Model of personality in adolescent boys. *Child Development, 65,* 160–178.

Kohnstamm, G. A. (1989). Cross-cultural and sex differences. In G. A. Kohnstamm, J. E. Bates, & M. K. Rothbart (Eds.), *Temperament in childhood* (pp. 483–508). Chichester, England: Wiley.

Konstamm, G. A., Mervielde, I., Besevegis, E., & Halverson, C. F., Jr. (in press). Tracing the Big Five in parents' free descriptions of their children. *European Journal of Personality.*

Kohnstamm, G. A., Halverson, C. F., & Mervielde, I. (Eds.). (in press). *Lexical analyses of child personality across cultures.* Hillsdale, NJ: Erlbaum.

Langlois, J. H., & Downs, A. C. (1979). Peer relations as a function of physical attractiveness; The eye of the beholder or behavioral reality? *Child Development, 50,* 409–418.

Lanning, K. (1994). Dimensionality of observer ratings on the California adult Q-set. *Journal of Personality and Social Psychology, 67,* 151–160.

Malpass, R. S., & Poortinga, Y. H. (1986). Strategies for design and analysis. In W. J. Lonner & J. W. Berry (Eds.), *Field methods in cross-cultural research* (pp. 47–86). Beverly Hills, CA: Sage.

Martin, R. P., Wisenbaker, J., & Huttunen, M. (1994). Review of factor analytic studies of temperament measures based on the Thomas–Chess structural model: Implications for the Big Five. In C. F. Halverson, G. A. Kohnstamm, & R. P. Martin (Eds.), *The developing structure of temperament and personality from infancy to adulthood* (pp. 157–172). Hillsdale, NJ: Erlbaum.

McDevitt, S. C., & Carey, W. B. (1978). The measurement of temperament in 3- to 7-year-old children. *Journal of Child Psychology and Psychiatry, 19,* 245–253.

Mervielde, I. (1994). A Five-Factor Model classification of teachers' constructs on individual differences among children aged four to twelve. In C. F. Halverson, G. A. Kohnstamm & R. P. Martin (Eds.), *The developing structure of temperament and personality from infancy to adulthood* (pp. 387–398). Hillsdale, NJ: Erlbaum.

Ritter, J. M., Casey, R. J., & Langlois, J. H. (1991). Adults' responses to infants varying in appearance of age and attractiveness. *Child Development, 62,* 68–82.

Robins, R. W., John, O. P., & Caspi, A. (1994). Major dimensions of personality in early adolescence: The Big Five and beyond. In C. F. Halverson, G. A. Kohnstamm, & R. P. Martin (Eds.), *The developing structure of temperament and personality from infancy to adulthood* (pp. 267–292). Hillsdale, NJ: Erlbaum.

Shwalb, B. J., Shwalb, D. W., & Shoji, J. (1994). Structure and dimensions of maternal perceptions of Japanese infant temperament. *Developmental Psychology, 30,* 131–141.

Strelau, J. (1983). *Temperament, personality, activity.* London: Academic Press.

Super, C. M., & Harkness, S. (1986). Temperament, development, and culture. In R. Plomin & J. Dunn (Eds.), *The study of temperament: Changes, continuities and challenges* (pp. 131–149). Hillsdale, NJ: Erlbaum.

Thomas, A., & Chess, S. (1977). *Temperament and development.* New York: Brunner/Mazel.

Van Lieshout, C. F. M., & Haselager, G. J. T. (1994). The Big Five personality factors in Q-sort descriptions of children and adolescents. In C. F. Halverson, G. A. Kohnstamm, & R. P. Martin (Eds.), *The developing structure of temperament and personality from infancy to adulthood* (pp. 293–318). Hillsdale, NJ: Erlbaum.

Williams, J. E., & Best, D. L. (1990). *Sex and psyche: Gender and self viewed cross-culturally.* Newbury Park, CA: Sage.

Windle, M., & Lerner, R. M. (1986). Reassessing the dimensions of temperamental individuality across the life-span: The Revised Dimensions of Temperament Survey (DOTS-R). *Journal of Adolescent Research, 1,* 213–230.

Yang, K., & Bond, M. H. (1990). Exploring implicit personality theories with indigenous and imported constructs: The Chinese case. *Journal of Personality and Social Psychology, 58,* 1087–1095.

Yik, M. S. M., & Bond, M. H. (1993). Exploring the dimensions of Chinese person perception with indigenous and imported constructs: Creating a culturally balanced scale. *International Journal of Psychology, 28,* 75–95.

CHAPTER 3

# Processes of Generalization in Parental Reasoning

Jaan Valsiner
Gorjana Litvinovic

Parenting is a complex, real-life phenomenon, which can be looked at from many levels of analysis. It entails specific episodes of conduct that are generated prospectively, as the conditions that make up everyday situations unfold. Parenting is a multiple-criteria problem-solving practice guided by oversocialized affective–mental framing brought into it by the parents. Hence it can be viewed as a social role-related personal form of conduct, closely intertwined with all the superstitions and experiences of the adult society. It is strongly influenced by the cultural communication processes between the parents and different ideologically interested social institutions and persons (see Lightfoot & Valsiner, 1992).

Here we approach parenting as a cultural phenomenon by focusing on the parent as a self-constructing individual who develops within a broader social world while continuously being challenged by the necessity to resolve real-life situations. We wish to focus on the real-time reasoning *processes* that on the one hand are triggered by immediate interpretations of concrete situational necessities and, on the other, are guided by cultural expectations. This focus fits well with the general directions in co-constructivist thought in developmental psychology (Valsiner, 1989b, 1994), and the present chapter is an effort to analyze parental reasoning processes from that viewpoint.

The chapter is divided into two sections. In the first section, we describe our understanding of the relationship between the individual and the collective cultural aspects of psychological functioning as these relate to the construction and expression of parental roles. The second section focuses on the actual mechanisms—within the individual and in microprocess—that operate at the intersection between individual and collective cultural contents. As generalized statements are the stuff of culture—at least the part of it that consists of behavior-regulating norms—we focus on the coordination of inductive and deductive processes (i.e., those processes that juxtapose and coordinate immediate experience and previous knowledge). We try to point out how cultural novelty can be created in this process within the individual. Relating cultural novelty to the relationship between what is individual and what is collective illustrates the social origin of individual parents' ideas and actions as well as the individual origin of collective cultural constructs about parenting.

## The Relationship between Personal and Collective Aspects of the Parenting Culture

### Culture in Parental Reasoning Processes

Culture is not one of psychology's "independent variables" but an organizational semiotic resource characteristic of all human species (Valsiner, 1989a). When brought into the domain of parenting, culture does not "determine" (or "cause") one or another form of conduct or reasoning but serves as the main semiotic vehicle to organize both the conduct and reasoning of the actors in the role of parents. Parenting is simply the process of resolution of real-life problems, necessitated by the situation at hand, based on the culturally organized content and constraints as those function within the specific parent's self. In this sense, parenting is a reflection of the particular parent's idiosyncrasy, which developed through one's culture in the form of the rich input of heterogeneous social suggestions over the person's life course. Not only the person but also his or her culturally organized world is *unitas multiplex*—as pointed out by William Stern in the beginning of this century (Stern, 1906, 1911). Contemporary psychology, despite episodic reminders that approximate in nature the emphasis given by Stern (Allport, 1937; Franck, 1986; Grossmann, 1986), has largely refused to address the fundamental issues of the heterogeneous structural organization of psychological systems.

Just like any other event that might take place in an organized system, parental reasoning feeds forward into the development of this system, in smaller or greater ways (depending on the centrality of the issue at hand, on the flexibility of the system at that moment, etc.). Arising from the present state of the individual's psychological system, feeding on the input from the immediate situation, and proactively tending toward a needed solution, parental reasoning represents the parenting role of the individual's functioning in the personal future. On another scale, this psychological future-oriented construction also feeds into the reorganization of the cultural system. In order to understand what this means in terms of culture construction, we must look at the relationship of the individual and his or her cultural world.

## Parenting and Culture: A Case of Constructive Multidirectionality

The flow of events in psycho-social reality (i.e., those events that both constitute and construct this reality) cannot be taken to consist of one clearly uniform dynamic. Although parts of the total system of human culture and individual minds are undeniably interdependent, it is a matter of phenomenological reality that the individual (intrapersonal) dynamic constitutes a separate field from the external (extrapersonal) dynamic. Any given person has direct access only to one's intrapersonal psychological phenomena and indirect (mediated through extrospection and communication) access to others' psychological worlds. A person can explain others' psychological processes only through comparing his or her observations of others with his or her lived-through personal experiences (via *Einfühlung*; Lipps, 1923, and coordination of "subjective" and "objective" inductions; Morgan, 1894). Semiotic mediation of the extrospective investigation plays a central role in such explanations. Based on the intrapersonally constructed personal understanding of the world, the semiotic devices narrow the realm of possible interpretations of the next extrospectively available experience. It is through such selectivity, made possible by semiotic means (primarily, but not exclusively, language used in speech) (Bühler, 1934/1965; Vygotsky, 1934), that the social world provides its canalizing input into the development of personal knowledge. The cultural interpretive schemata lead persons' construction of their knowledge, so that "the ontology of the world . . . is framed by the epistemology of humans" (Eckensberger, 1992, p. 8).

Nevertheless, the social and personal realms—as different, yet interdependent as those are—constitute two qualitatively different levels of human functioning, governed by different particular forms of organization. Whereas the level of the external dynamic comprises social processes at various levels (from dyads to small social groups, to social institutions and societies), the internal dynamic comprises the person's psychological processes—the private phenomenological field of personal awareness, the processes that take place within this field and in relation to it, and the structures that serve it.

By "structures that serve" the private phenomenological field of awareness, we mean the set of relatively permanent constraints that an individual person bears, and that enable this person both to think and delimit (or canalize) the patterns of his or her thought. These constraints are personal reconstructions of social expectations that have come into being in the constructive process of internalization (Lawrence & Valsiner, 1993). As *re*constructions, these personal–cultural constraints include features that go beyond the collective cultural social expectations. This novelty–constructive nature of the internalization process fits the co-constructivist axiom of bidirectional culture transmission in social communication (Valsiner, 1989b, 1994).

Whereas one can think of social reality as a rather fluid and heterogeneous unity, in spite of the separability of various foci within it, individual personal reality is particularistic: There are as many separate phenomenological fields as there are living individuals. All these individual phenomenological fields are undergoing transformation within irreversible time, and in conjunction with the person–environment semiotically mediated relationships. Hence the definitive methodological alley for psychological research as an epistemological enterprise with an empirical component is that of individual life-course psychography, or comparative analysis of personal life courses (see Stern, 1911, p. 18). The individual longitudinal case study method allows us to explain the dynamic of personal phenomenological fields (see Valsiner, 1986).

Without doubt, there is communication and mutual influence going on between the individuals and groups of individuals, but this does not change the fundamental nature of lack of access to the individual's phenomenological field by anybody else. It is the communication and mutual influences of the individuals that synthesize at a supraindividual level into social phenomena, which may then go on to construct higher-order social phenomena (Sherif, 1936). These ontological levels acquire laws of process of their own (e.g., the rules by which a social group operates are not mere replications of those of a person; or rules that regulate social institutions are not those of small groups), yet—from an individual's point of view—there exists only individual awareness. In other words, while individual psychological events can only be experienced from "within," collective social and/or cultural events can also be experienced only from "within"—because the personal phenomenological field is the only domain within which human beings have immediate access to psychological phenomena. Because that personal phenomenological field is culturally guided via the internalization–externalization process, it is appropriate to consider it structured in the form of *personal culture* (see Valsiner, 1989b). That personal culture is interdependent with its external counterpart—the *collective culture*.

## Dynamics of Culture: Social Roles and Internalization–Externalization

Attending to the individual parent who is constructing one's role on the basis of collective cultural notions about parenting, we see a multitude of within- and across-level connections that frame a constantly ongoing dynamic of mutual influence. This influence is not direct but filtered through the "borders" between the individuals—first, in their construction of their social roles (Oliveira & Rossetti-Ferreira, 1995), and second, and related, by their meaning systems. Furthermore, it is boundedly indeterministic (Valsiner, 1987): The mutual influences take the form of mutual constraints, which enable the adaptation process to solve the tasks. The socially constructed constraints (norms or roles) guide further conduct of the constructing persons in the direction of collective culturally accepted task solutions. Yet the constraints are not passively followed but constantly remade so as to take the person- and context-appropriate features of any particular setting into account.

Nowhere is that general feature of human development more visible than in the case of parenting. The individual parent is self-constructed through his or her personal history. In a real-time sense, this corresponds to ontogeny and the events within it that have been relevant for the construction of the parent's role identity and propensities for action within parenting situations. The personal history of the parent may be taken in another sense. Diachronically, this history consists of the sequences of construction of various symbolic elements and complexes in social groups and institutions within which the person—now in the parent's role—has found himself or herself (e.g., family, the school, the tribe, the gender-related activities, and the profession). That is, elements of the parenting culture that the particular person we are observing has internally reconstructed have their origins in the sphere of social experiences.

These collective cultural forms, however, have a history that encompasses both the individual and the collective levels. At the collective level, these forms become encoded and endure in various structures, which are either shared (e.g., the organizational principles for social groups, scripts for various activities, and language) or equally accessible to all with sufficient knowledge base (e.g., books, works of art, useful artifacts, cultural knowledge in the form of proverbs, and games). The actual real-life implementation of these cultural forms takes place through the activity of individuals, who have become innovating carriers of such cultural knowledge (accumulated and reorganized during their ontogeny) but also who, at every moment, receive new information from their environment (i.e., who are in a constant active dialogue with their social and physical environment).

The role of persons as innovating carriers of the collective culture is crucial for the constant modification of the cultural forms. The forms of cultural constraints reappear in every interactive situation in a new light, depending on the participants in the interaction, the relationships between them, and the constraints of the specific situation. They are reworked to a certain extent in the situation and may be reconstructed in the minds of the participating individuals.

In a longer-term historical perspective, with an eye on the collective level, one would not expect to see each and every personal reconstruction of cultural forms feeding back somehow into the shared corpus of cultural forms. In fact, the whole set of existing cultural forms that organize a certain area of social task-related conduct (e.g., parenting) may be heterogeneous and redundant and may extend beyond the needs of all persons at the given historical period. Hideo Kojima (in press) has coined the term "ethnopsychological pool of ideas" (EPI) for that collectively shared heterogeneous set of cultural forms of parenting. Based on his historical analyses of parent-oriented texts in Japan over two centuries, Kojima (1988, 1990, 1991) has demonstrated the relative conservatism in the EPI along the historical changes in the macrosocietal structure of Japan.

Despite the richness and relative continuity of EPI in a given society, it is not just likely but logically obvious that specific general changes in a society can lead to the widespread acceptance of specific reconstructions of certain cultural forms, or the creation or introduction of new ones. The EPI is not a closed, heterogeneous set but a semiopen pool within which novel collective cultural forms can emerge (and previously present ones become extinct). We cannot imagine this history, however, to be monolithic. It depends on the social stratification and heterogenization of society.

Collective culture is constantly being reconstructed by communication between different social units (groups, institutions, persons with public fetish roles, etc.) in a society. As various groups in society communicate mutually and share living conditions from different perspectives, varying also the reception of potentially culture-changing events and the production and reception of particular shared reconstructions of such events, we expect a differential construction of certain cultural forms by various subgroups in the population. Cultural history at the collective level consists of a network of strands that show the various forms being created and changed differentially in different social groups, with possible synthesis at higher levels of abstraction and at later times. Going back to the individual level, this history applies to the symbolic psychological structures of any individual person we observe at a particular moment, as well as to any situation in which forms of culture are applied. In these cases, we are looking at the apex of a bunch of cultural strands that have situationally been brought together.

For example, when examining the psychological structure of a person, we might see a number of coexisting cultural forms, each of which originates in interactions of that person with different collective "cultural strand contexts." Looking at a situation, we may isolate cultural forms whose history in collective culture might be traced, and which are brought together at this moment and in this situation in a novel way. Through the synthesis and reconstruction of cultural forms in the process of personal internalization, and by way of externalization of these forms by self to others in situations of social interaction, followed by the externalized result becoming a trigger for further internalization, the personal culture constantly produces new versions of the collective cultural forms. This notion rests on Baldwin's concept of circular reaction. Thus, the person—for instance, a parent we are observing—comes to represent in an innovative way the collective culture. "Represent" here has two meanings: re-present the content of the culture to oneself (constructive internalization) and be a representative of the culture (reconstructive externalization). In the latter sense, the personal history of a single person is the history of the collective cultural forms that are *re*presented in his or her intrapsychological symbolic system in a novel way, which is personally idiosyncratic but yet continuous with the collective culture.

The person, therefore, develops within a collective culture, constructing the contents of his or her mind on the basis of offerings from the social world but also on the basis of whatever is already existent as preserved in the personal life history in the form of internalized semiotic means that operate as constraining devices. At the same time, the person acts as environment for others, directly or through products of his or her activity. It is the domain of activities that shows relative interpersonal overlap and hence can be considered "shared" in the sense of extrospectively accessible perception and participant observation (see Rogoff, 1990). Individual, dyadic, and group thoughts and interactions all reflect the shared aspects of our psychological constructions. Yet, beyond sharing the expectable ways of relating with the environment, human beings create meaningfulness in their worlds via personal symbolic construction.

It is only the symbolic, constructed, semiotic forms that constitute culture. Those shared symbolic aspects of our psychological makeup, and the patterns of interaction between us that result from these shared aspects, constitute the living culture of the time. The living culture, thus, is composed of sediments of the past (i.e., that which is shared, in the sense of isomorphism of individual psychologies, and which was constructed during ontogeny) as well as a constant future-oriented constructive process, which takes place in the context of interaction between individuals. Of course, the active culture of the time also includes other material (i.e., products of the externalization of symbol-constructive processes of other times). These are the diachronic forms in culture. They participate in co-constructive interactions with living persons, the results of which are unilaterally internalized. In brief, the development of culture—its transmission, change, and the introduction of novelty—depends on (although not only on) the psychological processes involved in the internalization, externalization, and reconstruction of its symbolic content.

## The Active Culture of Parenting

The active culture of parenting is borne at any one time by individual people (both parents and nonparents) in the form of their parallel personal constructions of conceptions, ideas, and attitudes about parenting and childrearing in general and also in the form of those symbolic constraints on thought and action that are not directly related to parenting but affect the shaping of parental behaviors. The active culture of parenting at this time also comprises such products as may be used to inform people of the functions of parenting or to aid them in these functions. These products may be books on children and parenting, objects meant for child care and amusement, and so on, as well as messages and objects that, although not specificallly meant for parents and children, lend themselves to interpretations that affect the functions of parenting. The latter point is important from the present co-constructionist perspective: Even if certain cultural messages are not targeted at parents, they may still be interpreted *as if* they were. The forms of the active culture of parenting are results of personal and collective histories. The culture of parenting may also be described as a living culture. In that sense, it exists within the reality of individual persons' functioning in relation to parenting as a constantly emergent process. It comprises acts of parenting motivated by and based on real-life situations and is shaped by the individual psychological constraints of the actors in these situations. Most important, the very process of situation assessment and acting within it feeds back into the individual's symbolic constructions about such situations and parenting in general. The content of the feedback, furthermore, depends on the context of the social situation, including the externalized elements of others' symbolic constructions. In other words, *culture construction depends on the processes taking place constantly between and within individuals and in constantly unique environmental settings* (granted by the irreversibility of time and unpredictability of events within that).

It is exactly here that culture-construc*ted* and culture-construc*tive* mental processes overlap with those traditionally viewed in culture-free terms: mental, affective, cognitive, and reasoning processes. Focusing on the real-time process of the reconstruction of cultural constraints, we are now interested in the way that the laws of reasoning, which are generally not thought of as being culture related and are certainly couched within the individual, relate to the cultural context of parenting. From that angle, the traditions of the so-called cognitive revolution in modern-day psychology have not moved the discipline closer to psychological reality (Valsiner, 1991). It is only with the increased focus on cultural psychology in its different versions (Cole, 1990; Eckensberger, 1992; Shweder, 1990) that limitations of the cognitive approach are slowly being overcome.

In case of parental reasoning, then, we are telling a story within a story. The meta-level, or the bigger story, pertains to the parent–collective culture dynamic. The story within is that of the constructive microprocess, the quirks of parental reasoning that participate in the construction of both parent and culture. In our further discussion of reasoning, we concentrate on a reconciliation of its "fuzzy" nature ("inconsistent," "irrational," "illogical") and its de facto constructive nature. The questions are: How are solutions (temporary) and, by possible extension, constraints (more or less permanent) constructed in the midst of a process that often seems to be so unruly? When are these solutions novel, or "successful," in terms of bringing about change in the system?

# Parental Reasoning:
## Coordination of the General and the Specific

### Existing Research on Parental Reasoning

Parental reasoning has been studied from a variety of viewpoints. Several features make parental reasoning a better model for general analysis of reasoning processes than any laboratory or even real-life so-called cognitive problem-solving tasks. First, contrary to the usual interest of researchers in business-type problem-solving tasks, parental reasoning represents a case of high emotional involvement of the reasoner in the long-term outcomes of the problem solving (e.g., child guidance; see LeVine, 1974). Second, parenting tasks are necessarily ill defined—as every parental problem-solving effort is prospectively oriented and takes place within constantly changing circumstances of child–parent–environment relationships. Finally, much of the parental reasoning is oriented not toward production of future outcomes but toward avoidance of a potential detrimental state of affairs (e.g., accidents; Valsiner, 1985).

As Goodnow & Collins (1990) show, the study of this topic has dealt with the nature of parental ideas as well as the sources and consequences of these ideas (Sigel, 1985a; Sigel, McGillicuddy-DeLisi, & Goodnow, 1992). Parental reasoning has been studied mostly on the basis of "worry domains" of the parents, which in themselves reflect the historical changes in a collective culture (Alwin, 1990). For instance, the widespread interest in the issues of parents' reasoning about how children could be disciplined is built on a long collective cultural history (see overview by Peisner, 1989). Or, likewise, issues of "toilet training," "handling of troublesome adolescents," or "gender-role socialization," and many other practical-looking ideological constructs, can constitute specific collective culturally constructed domains of social preoccupation. Finally, the issue of integrating "expert advice" with parents' everyday concerns can be viewed as a socially constructed domain of preoccupation (Harkness, Super, & Keefer, 1992; Whiting, 1974). In general, the following simple social mechanism generates the empirical research on parental reasoning: from socially constructed content domains of adults' preoccupation with childrearing issues with the presence of the belief (also socially constructed) in the necessity of utilizing "expert knowledge," and as there exists a social group that symbolically represents and monopolizes the given expertise (e.g., "child psychologists," rather than "medicine men" or priests), research in selected fashionable topics in the areas of parental preoccupation domains follows.

Not surprisingly, as a consequence of the collective cultural canalization of empirical research activities, the mass of research findings in the area of parenting constitutes a rather disorganized field of mostly applied-oriented specific studies. Among the concepts that Goodnow and Collins (1990) used in order to organize that field, sources of parental ideas and their consequences are relevant in the present context as anchor points to locate the present approach. Although the *consequences* of parental ideas, such as their impact on the socialization of children or on the parent's own identity (the latter, by the way, has not been investigated to any significant extent), are doubtless of crucial social importance, and also necessarily enter any theoretical discussion of the broader context of parental reasoning as links in the historical construction of parenting models, we will not discuss these here. Likewise, we shall not deal with the *sources* of individual parental ideas in the sense of pinpointing their structural predecessors in the form of cultural patterns. We are interested in the reasoning process per se, the constructive process within the person that relevantly (and potentially permanently) alters the content of existing internalized ideas, may be traceable to various sources, and has immediate consequences in terms of decisions for action in concrete situations, on the one side, and novel ideas or new forms or corollaries of old ones, on the other. We view parental reasoning, thus, as a sort of dynamic transition point between source and consequence, where the "sources" are reconstructed and "consequences" fed with the outcome of the reconstruction (which also feed back into the sources).

The process aspect of parental psychological functioning is, of course, not overlooked in the literature (Holden & Ritchie, 1988; Pickering, 1991; Stratton, 1988). Yet, there exists no persisting focus on the study of the ongoing parental reasoning processes that would be similar to classic approaches to problem solving (Duncker, 1945) and their later elaborations, which pay attention to the dynamic and generative aspects of the process (Ericsson & Simon, 1980; Toda, 1976, 1983). In those few efforts that do exist to view the dynamics of parental reasoning, the issue of multilevel semiotic organization of parents' conceptual sphere has received attention.

## Hierarchical Organization of Reasoning

The notion of hierarchical organization of psychological processes is no news to any developmental psychologist who considers the general "orthogenetic principle" of Heinz Werner (1957) in a serious way. Yet in nondevelopmental cognitive psychology the emphasis on the hierarchical coordination of abstract and concrete levels of reasoning is only slowly being accepted (see Smith, Langston, & Nisbett, 1992). Any perspective that attempts to explain the ongoing reasoning process (rather than merely "measure" the quality of its outcomes) needs to start from an inherently developmental basis of a microgenetic orientation (Draguns, 1984). In the course of development by differentiation, hierarchical integration of the developing system indicates the emergence of greater flexibility of the system. Likewise, the whole issue of the development of higher psychological functions (see Van der Veer & Valsiner, 1991) concerns the emergence of hierarchical control systems in the ontogeny of the self.

In the case of parents (as adults), the notion of the hierarchical organization of their parental reasoning should not be surprising to anybody. Thus, Sigel (1985b) emphasizes the hierarchical organization of parental beliefs and implies the coordination of semiotic means of different levels of generality in the reasoning process. The organization of parental beliefs is already a product of the constructive reasoning process, and by focusing primarily upon it we bypass the constructive process itself. In a similar vein, Sameroff and Feil (1985) introduce conceptual levels in parents' reflection upon their actions and emphasize the intricate relation of general conceptual categorizations of a child and the framing of the interpretations of the child's actions:

> The parent who has had a successful experience with his or her child assigns positive labels, for example, the good child, the pretty child, or the bright child. Once labels are assigned, however, they are thought to belong to the object. Just as the young preoperational child thinks that the label "cup" belongs to a particular object in the same way as its color or shape, so the "labeling" parent thinks that the child is "the good child" in the same way that he has blue eyes or brown hair. This device can be very adaptive, for when the good child acts badly, such as crying too much, breaking a few dishes, or throwing a tantrum, the parent will still think of the child as the good one. On the other hand, this device can be very maladaptive as in the case where the parent, because of the negative early experiences he or she may have had with the child, comes to label the child as difficult, bad, or ugly. Even though infants may outgrow the behavior that caused them to be labeled as difficult in the first place, the perceptions and reactions of the parent restricted to the categorical level will continue to be dominated by the original label. (Sameroff & Feil, 1985, p. 87)

The generalizing, constructive, and stereotyping functions of human semiotic mediation are, of course, general features of our mental functioning (Rommetveit, 1979). However, the process of parental coordination of categorizing and immediate (action) experiences provides a relevant elaboration of that point—the inductive process in parental reasoning (reflection on specific experiences with the child) can lead to the establishment of a generalized concept (e.g., "good child"), which subsequently operates as a general premise in the deductive reasoning process. In that function, it allows the parental reasoning to create specific accounts of the child that remain pointedly "blind" to selected aspects of reality and may even lead to exaggerated new generalizations (see Pollner & McDonald-Wikler, 1985). More important, it is exactly at the intersection of the construction and use of general concepts where the individual psychological construction and collective cultural suggestions (e.g., in the form of "cultural models"; see Harkness & Super, 1992; Holland & Quinn, 1987; Reid, 1989) meet. The collective cultural "folk models" provide actively reasoning parents with socially suggested direction in the construction of their general categorizations of the child's characteristics. Cultural models operate at the foundation of the parental construction of their understanding of the child, suggesting certain general categorizations (rather than others) and narrowing down the many ways in which these categorizations can be linked with direct experience with children. They do not determine the exact process of parental reasoning but channel it in collective culturally desirable directions.

## Unity of Deductive and Inductive Processes in Parental Reasoning

Human reasoning is a process of mental construction on the basis of human semiotic capabilities, which in their turn have evolved in the course of cultural history (Vygotsky & Luria, 1930). There are two, mutually opposite, component constructive processes that can be posited to exist in the human reasoning process—the deductive process (which involves the construction of specific novel ideas on the basis of general believed premises and conventional derivation rules) and the *inductive process* (which entails generalization of ideas based on specific lived-through experiences of the reasoner). Reflections of these processes (albeit without the constructive role attributed to them here) can be found in modern cognitive psychology under the labels of "rule-based" and "instance-based" reasoning (Smith et al., 1992). In the *process of coordination* of inductive and deductive processes, we find the key to understanding the natural "fuzziness" of human reasoning. The ongoing reasoning process entails both inductive efforts (based on remembered instances of previous experiences) and episodic abandonment of those in favor of some general meaning or constructed abstract reasoning rule—only to return to the specifics in a subsequent inductive effort. We argue that novelty in human reasoning can emerge as a result of opposition between the deductive and inductive processes (via "goodness of misfit"; see Valsiner & Cairns, 1992). Under specifiable conditions of their coordination, either novel generalizations are constructed (and used) or deductions are created that go "beyond the information (immediately) given."

In traditional cognitive psychology, deductive and inductive reasoning processes usually have been viewed either in the context of research on the logic of reasoning (e.g., research utilizing "syllogistic reasoning tasks") or as a part of "inductive logic" (e.g., efforts to study laypersons' utlization of statistical inference techniques). For analytic purposes (and those of experimentation), the two processes are usually separated from each other, and viewed as independent (even if at times interfering; see Luria, 1976) entities. However, this separation of these two processes eliminates the actual reasoning process (in which both of these processes are integrated and coproduce novelty) from psychologists' focus.

The novelty construction in reasoning takes place both in the realm of *symbolic content* (i.e., reasoning rules are not "empty" processes) and in the domain of *symbolic constraints* (i.e., following certain rules or guidelines, which guide the form of reasoning). The reasoning process thus involves coordination of a twofold kind: between deductive and inductive lines of reasoning on the one hand and (within each line) integrating the symbolic form and content into one flow of semiotically encoded product.

What does the focus on the coordination of inductive and deductive processes in real-time, real-life reasoning mean for the construction of parenting in individual lives as well as in cultural groups? We believe that it provides a better understanding of the component of indeterminacy in constructive processes. Instead of simply stating that constructive processes within and between individuals are indeterminate, we are trying now to point out a source of the indeterminacy. This particular source of indeterminacy lies in the nature of reasoning processes within individuals, but carries over to interindividual levels, as these processes are externalized. Of course, there are additional sources of indeterminacy to be sought at the levels of psychological externalization, social interaction, information diffusion, and so on, and none of them is less important in terms of outcome than the one we are describing.

In concrete terms, the reasoning always proceeds at some intermediate level of abstractness–concreteness, with possibilities for generalization and specification constantly available. Every moment in the reasoning process depends on prior knowledge, and as this knowledge is often self-contradicting and not employed in a consisent manner, the outcome of the process is not deducible from what we might in principle know about the momentary knowledge base of the thinker (because that knowledge base exists in a heterogeneous and hierarchically organized form).

## Forms of Coordination of Deductive and Inductive Processes

Inductive and deductive reasoning processes cannot be separated from each other. Efforts to use "purely" inductive processes will necessarily remain inconsequential, as George Miller (1990) has pointed out:

The impossibility of proving a general statement on the basis of a finite number of positive instances had long been recognized. . . . That is to say, the "inductive leap" from a finite set of examples to a universal generalization can land almost anywhere. It should not have been surprising, therefore, when cognitive scientists realized that different people can draw very different conclusions after observing the same set of instances—that the consequences of experience are as much constructed by as imposed on the learner. (p. 11)

Example 1 represents exactly this indeterminate nature of a "purely" inductive "leap":

**Example 1.** Inductively driven reasoning process in a dialogue (a possible way in which parents might interact about their experiences with children)

PARENT 1: You know, last week John played with a vase, let it fall on the floor, and it broke into pieces.

PARENT 2: I know what you mean—Mary has done that many times with our coffee mugs—thank goodness those do not break. Those *children are such innocent playful creatures.*

PARENT 1: Well . . . you know . . . it is not so simple. The other day John took a paper napkin from the dinner table and brought it to the burning candle, proceeding to make a small fire on his plate. . . . We had to put out the fire!

PARENT 2: How inventive! Mary has not done anything like that . . . but she explores her world, indeed, very actively. *Children are adventurous, and come up with new and surprising actions.*

PARENT 1: Adventurous . . . hmm . . . yeah—just yesterday we caught John in the bathroom; he was about to throw our Minnie, our dear little family cat, into the toilet! Those *children can be cruel* to animals, and *they are such little devils who come up with nasty ideas. Parents must always control them.*

Example 1 illustrates a case in which the inductive reasoning processes of both parents in this invented dialogue dominate the deductive ones. Of course, our point is that no "purely" inductive generalization exists—if we see generalization based on induction, it resorts to the use of some (usually implicit) general meanings (or cultural models). As the parents were chatting about their particular children (John and Mary) and comparing specific instances of their conduct, they obviously inductively (on the basis of concrete examples, i.e., data) *inferred certain general statements about children* (i.e., what children in general "are like" or what they "can" do or be). However, the deductive line of reasoning entered the ongoing dialogue in the form of implicit assumptions about the ways the induction is to be made. For example, there is an underlying general premise (among others in the same reasoning step) that "those who let things fall on the floor playfully are innocent creatures," and this is in turn based on a combination of a number of cultural assumptions about actions, human traits, and values placed on traits and outcomes of actions. A specific instance of conduct is being generalized by introducing a general meaning (or belief) into the discourse. A general statement about children is either directly imported (from proverbial knowledge, child-care manuals, grandmother's sayings, what my neighbor said the other day, etc.) or constructed on the spot, but always on the basis of the playoff between a concrete event brought up at that specific moment to serve some purpose in the dialogue and a set of preexisting general beliefs. Note also that there is a certain circularity involved. If we were to consider the reasoning process in timeless and nonutilitarian terms, much of what goes on would become illogical. Namely, a general statement imported at this moment on the basis of some implicit belief may easily play the role of implicit premise to this belief at some other time. Such dead-end circularity is surpassed when *meaning is reconstructed* within the process. Once such a general statement is imported or reconstructed, it can guide further discourse in accordance with the whole complex implied by the general meaning or belief (e.g., general belief that "children are innocent" can guide further interpretations by parents, differently from a belief that assumes that "children are little devils").

All generalizations of the described kind (i.e., inductively based but generically framed) go beyond the given particulars—*and are constructed exactly for that purpose.* Parental reasoning is oriented toward future encounters with children's novel conduct; hence, present-time generalizations are functional in the preparation of the adults for the (highly unpredictable) future. Such generalizations are not "correct" in any sense because in the case of dynamic constructive processes that take place in irreversible time, criteria for "correctness" (or "falseness") of any generalization are in principle indeterminable (see Valsiner, 1992, on open-endedness of development).

The indeterminacy of generalization determines the quality of culture construction in several ways. First, there is a resulting variability of reception, understanding, and application of cultural knowledge. Second, conflicting meanings within the same corpus of knowledge may exist. A good example is conflicting opinions expressed by proverbs within the same language, such as "A spanking comes straight from heaven" versus "A good houselord doesn't beat his animals" (implicitly, "let alone his children," but also possibly, "this doesn't apply to children"). These proverbs exist as shared expressions of experience (not necessarily with a uniformly shared meaning) and have gained sustained circulation thanks to the nature of reality, which is not always singularly patterned, and also to the inclusion of value positions in the reasoning process, which is clearly illustrated in the above expressions. The value positions are included arbitrarily and feed into the deductive support of the reasoning process at times when such statements are generated. Furthermore, in every situation in which such pearls of wisdom are pronounced as a confirmatory seal on reality (the current and concrete one or the general, abstract one—the subjective confirmation might work both ways, again bespeaking the reversibility of general and specific in our understanding), they are made applicable to the concrete situation by an "inductive leap," which is aided by the offering of patterns toward which the leap may be made. A third result of the indeterminacy of generalization in culture construction is that the implicit categorization of reality that is established is not necessarily clear. This speaks to the assumption that culture is composed of something like schemata or patterns that are handed down in quantums or tidy packages (successfully or unsuccessfully). In fact, the packaging is nothing like tidy, although the labels might appear to be so.

Let us look at an example of a deductively driven process in parental reasoning. Example 2 can be viewed as a continuation of Example 1, only now both parents complement each other's narrative by deriving concrete conclusions from previously constructed major premises.

**Example 2.** Deductively driven reasoning processes in a dialogue

PARENT 1: *There is so much cruelty in children.* I often see John chasing our cat and worry that he might do worse things to her. What could be done to make him behave gently toward Minnie?

PARENT 2: Oh, don't worry, he is just a little boy, *and little boys are adventurous*, they like new experiences. If I were you, I would not worry, *boys need to conquer the world*, and chasing animals and experimenting with objects *is their natural way*, and *a need for all males.* John is a little boy and is not , therefore, any different. But what should I do with Mary. My dear little girl is only interested in boyish ways of playing with toys. She gets into fights with boys in the playground . . . is that what being in day care produces? *Girls should be different.* So, I decided to buy her some of the toys which were my favorites when I was a little girl; maybe they'll catch on.

Again, we have underlined the general statements (about "cruelty" being a characteristic of children, hence applicable to John; the differential beliefs about boys and girls). In this example, the "figure-ground" relationship of the two processes is reversed—the deductive process is in the foreground (and leads the talk about specifics in the parental discourse), while the inductive process remains implicitly in the background yet supports the foreground. Any general statement or deduction thereof would not, in fact, make any sense unless it was related to a parallel inductive inference from experience with the object of interest. For example, the statement that John is like other boys (in a certain aspect) would not be a meaningful part of a dialogue unless it leaned on the inductively inferred idea that John often did exactly that sort of thing that all boys are purported to do, or at least that he shows an inclination to do them (where the deduced "truth" in conjunction with an inductive leap toward the obvious kinds of thing to be expected of John leads to a proactive and essentially novel question about possible preventive measures). It is also possible that the deduced statement about a specific case (e.g., Mary should be like all girls in some respect) is not met with a confirmatory inductive generalization about Mary's usual behavior. This is the case in our example. Again, the parents' understanding of their own statements is contextualized by the parallel drawing upon personal experience in numerous concrete situations, with inductive generalization from these, and the importation into the current dialogue of general beliefs that each parent has internalized from an ethnopsychological pool of ideas and reconstructed for themselves. In the case of either inductive confirmation or disconfirmation of deduced statements, the meaning of the outcome is colored by values and affective attitudes held by the parent and both is seen in light of ongoing intentional activity (immediate or longer-term projects and expectations of them) and serves as feedback information in guiding such activity.

Deductive reasoning, in order to be adequate to the cognitive function of human self-regulation, cannot remain "pure" because the experiences of living human beings are constantly changing:

> Deductive logic is used to argue from initial premises through intermediate steps to some final conclusion that is implied by the premises. By *modus ponens*, for example, one is allowed to argue that, given *P* and *If P, then Q,*

it follows that $Q$. But when attempts are made to formulate actual situations in these terms, they may fail. For example . . . if Mary believes *If I look in the cupboard, I will see a box of Cheerios* and *I am looking in the cupboard*, then by *modus ponens* she should also believe *I see a box of Cheerios*. But if, in fact, Elizabeth finished the Cheerios yesterday and the box is now gone, Mary should not conclude that she is seeing a box of Cheerios that isn't there! Instead, she should revise her premises. Commonsense reasoning follows different principles from the rules of deductive argument. (Miller, 1990, p. 10)

This passage illustrates that a syllogism-like formulation in reasoning that actually states something about real-life contents is in fact based on experience and not on logical necessity (e.g., "I know that the Cheerios were there yesterday"), and the premises are therefore open to revision: Thus a deductive form passes into an inductive form of reasoning, with times overlapping. Namely, the same sequence of statements is analyzable from both standpoints, depending on stress in analysis. The overlap, or intermingling of the processes, is a place where the construction of new forms of reasoning might take place (see Cole, 1992; Valsiner, 1993).

However, a more important point illustrated in both of our examples, as well as the quote from Miller, is the *proactivity of real-life reasoning*. The purpose of the *if . . . then* statement is not to ascertain a universally true law about cupboards and Cheerios, even within a limited context (such as my cupboard at this moment), but to plan and monitor one's action. The syllogistic form, a logically correct one, too, is a necessary tool in the organization of our everyday thinking, but the deductive inference is never its pure result or a result in itself. It cannot be a pure result because with the moment of its emergence it becomes contextualized and gains meaning from the particular context in the given situation (situation in the mind, so to speak). Although it is a product of syllogism, it is also meaningfully divorced from syllogism by the meaning it has gained from the context into which it has emerged. Also, we say that it is not a result in itself because it feeds into a future-oriented process of regulation of conduct. The recontextualized result is not simply produced to stand out without use; it is produced for and immediately picked up by other ongoing thought processes. Everyday reasoning, therefore, is driven by purpose, and although it involves forms of both syllogistic deduction and inductive inclusion, it takes place within the frame of an irreversible real-time contextualized process in which the two "types" of reasoning are not just intermingled but continuously interact in indeterministic ways, potentially creating new forms.

## Forms of Coordination: Recombinatorial and Synthetic

The reasoning process proceeds in irreversible time in its microgenesis; hence, it is its constant immediate future orientation that makes it possible for moves between inductive and deductive orientations to take place. In case of *both* inductive and deductive orientations, novelty can be created within the given microconstructive process. It takes the form of either construction (or importation) of an encoded general meaning, which then produces specific expectations (if the person operates in the deductive orientation), or reconstruction of some personal experience of the past in the present (if in the inductive mode). In the ongoing flow of reasoning, the two orientations flexibly switch between each other and become coordinated in ways that allow for novel sense to be generated. Both the imported semiotic devices and the memories of previous personal experiences coact in the ongoing reorganization of the given present new experience, either by way of a recombination of signs and experiences or by synthesizing new semiotic devices in conjunction with the given situation. In both cases novelty emerges, yet in the first case it is based on the richness of lived-through personal experiences and the pool of semiotic devices; in the second case on the synthesizing role of the human psychological system.

In the case of *recombinatorial coordination* of the inductive and deductive orientations, we can observe novelty emerging from the specific supports that each orientation provides the other. Yet the emerging novelty preserves the context—it is merely a novel combination of previously known parts. Given the heterogeneity and richness of the EPI of parenting, very often this form of coordination is sufficient for the given situation. An analogy with language use is fitting here. When necessary, a person can express oneself by way of a novel recombination of words in an utterance and yet not produce a completely novel structure of the utterance or a neologism in lexicon. It has recently been suggested (Siegfried, 1993) that psychology's explanatory efforts be enriched by making better use of the richness and heterogeneity of the common language terms. If that project for psychology's revitalization were to succeed, it would amount to a recombinatorial construction of novelty in the discipline.

The general process of reasoning in the recombinatorial form unfolds as a train of reasoning that is constructed on the basis of closed sets of general beliefs (or meanings) {A, B, C, D}, specific events {a, b, c, d}, and of relationships between the two sets {conjunction, implication}. By way of previously established constraints, for instance, implications "if a & b $\rightarrow$ A"; "if A $\rightarrow$ c", and "if c & d $\rightarrow$ D" have been established. Hence the reasoning process can proceed along a familar path, as in Example 3:

**Example 3:** A recombinatorial form of reasoning

| Event | Implication | Explanation |
|-------|-------------|-------------|
| a |  | Toddler looks at the cat |
| b |  | The child pulls cat's tail |
|  | a & b → A | The child is cruel |
|  | A → c | Child may hit the cat |
| c |  | Child does hit the cat |
| d |  | Cat screams and attacks child |
|  | c & d → D | Children learn lessons from life |
| b |  | Again pulls the tail |
| b |  | Continues |
|  | b & b → C | If that cat allows tail being pulled, the cat must be masochistic |

This artificial example shows how parent's reasoning can lead to a new recombinatorial form by lifting a previously (experientially) established constraint on the kinds of implications expected in this situation. However, the sets of beliefs, events, and relationships were not modified; their relationship merely came to include a recombined version (b & b → C).

The *synthetic type of coordination* entails the emergence of qualitatively new mental–affective phenomena in the process of coordination of the inductive and deductive processes. To follow along the lines of the formalistic example, here any one (or more) of the sets (of beliefs, events, or connectors) suddenly opens, and its elements are basically redefined. Novel forms may emerge in any of the sets in terms of paradigmatically new ideas, general or specific, and/or new forms of their connection. The coordination process here loses its simple "computable" nature and moves into the realm of emerging novelty of a Gestalt kind. In a situation of emotional turmoil, new meanings emerge in the personal as well as collective cultural realms. There may be periods in the course of this mental functioning during which the relationships between the deductive and inductive processes enter into a state of confusion (or a state that from the perspective of an external viewer looks like "confusion"), from which totally new solutions (innovations) emerge. Importantly, it may be exactly at times of maximally indeterminate states of psychological phenomena (which defy our well-established conventional classificatory schemes) that cognitive innovation is being made.

Undoubtedly, the focus on mental synthesis is a general one and pertains to all human mental processes (see Vygotsky, 1971, on its application to adults' understanding of literary texts). Still, the tasks of parenting are an increasingly challenging domain for the invention of synthetic-type reasoning forms because the target object—the child (and his or her relations with the immediate environment)—is constantly developing. The child's actions are likely to produce constantly novel challenges for the parent's reasoning processes. Hence, parental reasoning may be a very fitting phenomenological domain to study the processes of mental synthesis.

## General Conclusions

We have focused on how specific transitions between the inductive and deductive mental processes can take place at the interaction of collective culture and parental personal cultures. An important facet of the coordination of those processes is the irreversible nature of the time-flow within which all developmental processes take place (Valsiner, 1994). It is exactly because of the irreversibility of human experiences that the mental functioning of human beings entails the *constant construction of relative stability* in their understanding of their ongoing experiences and efforts to prepare themselves for the possible novelties of the future. This function is accomplished by semiotic encoding of the flow of personal experiences. Likewise, rules of thought—or indigenous "logic"—help to construct stability in the midst of uncertainty. However, all these constructed means can only create subjective present-state belief in relative certainty because the reality of existence is constantly fluid in its open systemic organization.

It is therefore not surprising that in recognizing the context dependency of psychological phenomena, our contemporary developmental psychology has entered a theoretical impasse that legitimizes discoveries of "context effects" of culture on human mental functioning and leads us to replace the search for general laws of psychological development with the empirical study of particulars. Instead, the "context dependency" of psychological phenomena needs to be addressed by explicating both the "context" involved and the forms of "dependency" (Valsiner & Benigni, 1986).

In explaining inductive and deductive processes in this chapter, we treated those two as constantly copresent (even if at times implicit) parts of a mental–affective system that is preemptively future-oriented and present-bound. It is obvious that our analysis is limited to the nuances of possible verbalizations (i.e., the products of externalization). Even with that limitation, it is still possible to demonstrate that reasoning entails movement between different forms of coordination (e.g., classical–logical–inductive and deductive–to dialectical and back; see also Haviland & Kramer, 1991), and that the interesting phenomena of reasoning that we often denigrate as "inconsistencies" are exactly the ways to keep our forward-oriented psychological system open to new adaptational challenges (Chapman, in press). The persistent inconsistency of human reasoning is its most powerful resource for the context-dependent life courses of persons whose lives entail much more than mere following of culturally constructed standards of "right" ways of thinking.

We tried to demonstrate in broadest terms how the microprocesses of parental reasoning entail a context-bound employment of personal and collective cultural resources, at the same time handling the forms and contents of these resources in ways that reconstruct them. The outcomes of their reconstruction are then employed in the solution of immediate real-life problems, as well as in a transformation of the personal systems of memories and beliefs. Ultimately, such innovations as those produced at the individual level will influence future social interactions with members of the same culture, and may in some cases and under certain conditions influence the very collective cultural pool of parenting ideas.

# References

Allport, G. W. (1937). The personalistic psychology of William Stern. *Character and Personality, 5,* 231–246.

Alwin, D. F. (1990). Historical changes in parental orientations to children. In P. A. Adler, P. Adler, & N. Mandell (Eds.), *Sociological studies of child development* (Vol. 3, pp. 65–86). Greenwich, CT: JAI Press.

Bühler, K. (1934/1965). *Sprachtheorie: Die Darstellungsfunktion der Sprache.* Stuttgart: Gustav Fischer. (Original work published 1934)

Chapman, M. (in press). Everyday reasoning and the revision of belief. In J. Puckett & H. W. Reese (Eds.), *Mechanisms of everyday cognition.* Hillsdale, NJ: Erlbaum.

Cole, M. (1990). Cultural psychology: A once and future discipline? In J. Berman (Ed.), *Nebraska Symposium on Motivation* (Vol. 37, pp. 279–336). Lincoln, NE: University of Nebraska Press.

Cole, M. (1992). Context, modularity, and the cultural constitution of development. In L. T. Winegar & J. Valsiner (Eds.), *Children's development within social context: Vol. 2. Research and methodology* (pp. 5–31). Hillsdale, NJ: Erlbaum.

Draguns, J. G. (1984). Microgenesis by any other name . . . In W. D. Froehlich,

G. Smith, J. Draguns, & U. Hentschel (Eds.), *Psychological processes in cognition and personality* (pp. 3–17). Washington, DC: Hemisphere.

Duncker, K. (1945). On problem solving. *Psychological Monographs, 58*(270), 1–113.

Eckensberger, L. H. (1992). Agency, action and culture: Three basic concepts for psychology, in general, and for cross-cultural psychology, in specific. *Arbeiten der Fachrichtung Psychologie, Universitat des Saarlandes,* No. 165.

Ericsson, K. A., & Simon, H. (1980). Verbal reports as data. *Psychological Review, 87*(3), 215–251.

Franck, I. (1986). Psychology as a science: Resolving the idiographic-nomothetic controversy. In J. Valsiner (Ed.), *The individual subject and scientific psychology* (pp. 17–36 ). New York: Plenum Press.

Goodnow, J. J., & Collins, W. A. (1990). *Development according to parents: The nature, sources, and consequences of parents' ideas.* Hove and London: Erlbaum.

Grossmann, K. E. (1986). From idiographic approaches to nomothetic hypotheses. In J. Valsiner (Ed.), *The individual subject and scientific psychology* (pp. 37–70). New York: Plenum Press.

Harkness, S., & Super, C. M. (1992). Parental ethnotheories in action. In I. E. Sigel, A. McGillicuddy, & J. J. Goodnow (Eds.), *Parental belief systems: The psychological consequences for children* (2nd ed., pp. 373–391). Hillsdale, NJ: Erlbaum.

Harkness, S., Super, C. M., & Keefer, C. H. (1992). Learning to be an American parent: How cultural models gain directive force. In R. G. D'Andrade & C. Strauss (Eds.), *Human motives and cultural models* (pp. 162–177). Cambridge, MA: Cambridge University Press.

Haviland, J. M., & Kramer, D. A. (1991). Affect–cognition relationships in adolescent diaries: The case of Anne Frank. *Human Development, 34,* 143–159.

Holden, G. H., & Ritchie, K. L. (1988). Child rearing and the dialectics of parental intelligence. In J. Valsiner (Ed.), *Child development within culturally structured environments: Vol. 1. Parental cognition and adult–child interaction* (pp. 30–59). Norwood, NJ: Ablex.

Holland, D. C., & Quinn, N. (Eds.). (1987). *Cultural models in language and thought.* Cambridge, MA: Cambridge University Press.

Kahneman, D., Slovic, P., & Tversky, A. (Eds.). (1982). *Judgement under uncertainty: heuristics and biases.* Cambridge, MA: Cambridge University Press.

Kojima, H. (1988). The role of belief–value systems related to child-rearing and education: The case of early modern to modern Japan. In D. Sinha & H. S. Kao (Eds.), *Social values and development* (pp. 227–253). New Delhi: Sage.

Kojima, H. (1990). Family life and child development in early modern Japan. *Zeitschrift für Sozialisationsforschung und Erziehungssoziologie, 10*(4), 314–326.

Kojima, H. (1991). Auto-régulation dans la façon traditionelle dont on élève les enfants au Japon. In C. Garnier (Ed.), *Le corps rassamblé* (pp. 276–290). Montreal: Éditions Agence d'Arc.

Kojima, H. (in press). Construction process of traditional child-rearing theories in Japan. In M. Lyra & J. Valsiner (Eds.), *Construction of psychological processes in interpersonal communication.* Norwood, NJ: Ablex.

Lawrence, J. A., & Valsiner, J. (1993). Social determinacy of human development: An analysis of the conceptual roots of the internalization process. *Human Development, 36,* 150–167.

LeVine, R. A. (1974). A cross-cultural perspective on parenting. In M. D. Fantini & R. Cardenas (Eds.), *Parenting in a multi-cultural society* (pp. 17–26). New York and London: Longman.

Lightfoot, C., & Valsiner, J. (1992). Parental belief systems under influence: Social guidance of the construction of personal cultures. In I. Siegel, J. Goodnow, & A. McGillicuddy-DeLisi (Eds.), *Parental belief systems* (2nd ed., pp. 393–414). Hillsdale, NJ: Erlbaum.

Lipps, T. (1923). *Grundlegung der Asthetik* (8th ed.). Leipzig: Leopold Voss.

Luria, A. R. (1976). *Cognitive development.* Cambridge, MA: Harvard University Press.

Miller, G. A. (1990). On explanation. In D. N. Robinson & L. P. Mos (Eds.), *Annals of theoretical psychology* (Vol. 6, pp. 7–37). New York: Plenum Press.

Morgan, C. L. (1894). *Introduction to comparative psychology.* London: Walter Scott.

Nisbett, R., & Ross, L. (1980). *Human inference: Strategies and shortcomings of social judgement.* Englewood Cliffs, N.J: Prentice Hall.

Oliveira, Z. M. R., & Rossetti-Ferreira, M. C. (1995). Understanding the co-constructive nature of human development: role coordination in early peer interaction. In J. Valsiner & H.-G. W. Voss (Eds.), *The structure of learning processes.* Norwood, NJ: Ablex.

Peisner, E. S. (1989). To spare or not to spare the rod: A cultural–historical view of child discipline. In J. Valsiner (Ed.), *Child development in cultural context* (pp. 111–141). Toronto: Hogrefe & Huber.

Pickering, M. R. (1991). Guilt loops. *Canadian Journal of Psychiatry, 36,* 447–451.

Pollner, M., & McDonald-Wikler, L. (1985). The social construction of unreality: A case study of a family's attribution of competence to a severely retarded child. *Family Process, 24*(2), 241–254.

Reid, B. V. (1989). Socialization for moral reasoning: Maternal strategies of Samoans and Europeans in New Zealand. In J. Valsiner (Ed.), *Child development in cultural context* (pp. 193–220). Toronto: Hogrefe & Huber.

Reid, B. V., & Valsiner, J. (1986). Consistency, praise, and love: Folk theories of American parents. *Ethos, 14*(3), 282–304.

Rogoff, B. (1990). *Apprenticeship in thinking.* New York: Oxford University Press.

Rommetveit, R. (1979). On common codes and dynamic residuals in human communication. In R. Rommetveit & R. M. Blakar (Eds.), *Studies of language, thought, and verbal communication* (pp. 163–175). London: Academic Press.

Sameroff, A. J., & Feil, L. A. (1985). Parental concepts of development. In I. Sigel (Ed.), *Parental belief systems: The psychological consequences for children* (pp. 83–105). Hillsdale, NJ: Erlbaum.

Sherif, M. (1936). *Psychology of social norms.* New York: Harper & Brothers.

Shweder, R. (1990). Cultural psychology—what is it? In J. W. Stigler, R. A.

Shweder, & G. Herdt (Eds.), *Cultural psychology* (pp. 1–43). Cambridge, MA: Cambridge University Press.

Siegfried, J. (Ed.). (1993). *The role of common sense in psychology.* Norwood, NJ: Ablex.

Sigel, I. E. (Ed.). (1985a). *Parental belief systems: The psychological consequences for children.* Hillsdale, NJ: Erlbaum.

Sigel, I. E. (1985b). A conceptual analysis of beliefs. In I. E. Sigel (Ed.), *Parental belief systems: The psychological consequences for children* (pp. 345–371). Hillsdale, NJ: Erlbaum.

Sigel, I. E., McGillicuddy, A. V., & Goodnow, J. J. (Eds.). (1992). *Parental belief systems: The psychological consequences for children* (2nd ed.). Hillsdale, NJ: Erlbaum.

Smith, E. E., Langston, C., & Nisbett, R. E. (1992). The case for rules in reasoning. *Cognitive Science, 16,* 1–40.

Stern, W. (1906). *Person und Sache: System der philosophischen Weltanschauung.* Leipzig: J. A. Barth.

Stern, W. (1911). *Die Differentielle Psychologie in ihren methodischen Grundlagen.* Leipzig: J. A. Barth.

Stratton, P. (1988). Parents' conceptualization of children as the organizer of culturally structured environments. In J. Valsiner (Ed.), *Child development within culturally structured environments: Vol. 1. Parental cognition and adult-child interaction* (pp. 5–29). Norwood, NJ: Ablex.

Toda, M. (1976). The decision process: A perspective. *International Journal of General Systems, 3,* 79–88.

Toda, M. (1983). What happens at the moment of decision? Meta-decisions, emotions and volitions. In L. Sjöberg, T. Tyszka, & J. A. Wise (Eds.), *Human decision making* (pp. 257–284). Bodafors: Doxa.

Valsiner, J. (1985). Theoretical issues of child development and the problem of accident prevention. In T. Gärling & J. Valsiner (Eds.), *Children within environments: Towards a psychology of accident prevention* (pp. 13–36). New York: Plenum Press.

Valsiner, J. (1986). Between groups and individuals: Psychologists' and layper-sons' interpretations of correlational findings. In J. Valsiner (Ed.), *The individual subject and scientific psychology* (pp. 113–152). New York: Plenum Press.

Valsiner, J. (1987). *Culture and the development of children's action.* Chichester: Wiley.

Valsiner, J. (1989a). From group comparisons to knowledge: A lesson from cross-cultural psychology. In J. P. Forgas & J. M. Innes (Eds.), *Recent advances in social psychology: An international perspective* (pp. 501–510). Amsterdam: North-Holland.

Valsiner, J. (1989b). *Human development and culture.* Lexington, MA: D. C. Heath.

Valsiner, J. (1991). Construction of the mental: From the "cognitive revolution" to the study of development. *Theory and Psychology, 1*(4), 477–494.

Valsiner, J. (1992). Social organization of cognitive development: Internalization and externalization of constraint systems. In A. Demetriou, M. Shayer, & A. Efklides (Eds.), *Neo-Piagetian theories of cognitive development* (pp. 65–78). London: Routledge.

Valsiner, J. (1993). Making of the future: temporality and the constructive nature of human development. In G. Turkewitz & D. Devenney (Eds.), *Timing as initial condition of development* (pp. 13–40). Hillsdale, NJ: Erlbaum.

Valsiner, J. (1994). Bi-directional cumtural transmission and constructive sociogenesis. In R. Maier & W. de Graaf (Eds.), *Mechanisms of sociogenesis*. New York: Springer.

Valsiner, J., & Benigni, L. (1986). Naturalistic research and ecological thinking in the study of child development. *Developmental Review, 6,* 203–223.

Valsiner, J., & Cairns, R.B. (1992). Theoretical perspectives on conflict and development. In C. Shantz & W. W. Hartup (Eds.), *Conflict in child and adolescent development* (pp. 15–35). Cambridge, MA: Cambridge University Press.

Van der Veer, R., & Valsiner, J. (1991). *Understanding Vygotsky: A quest for synthesis.* Oxford: Basil Blackwell.

Vygotsky, L. S. (1934). *Myshlenie i rech.* Moscow-Leningrad: Gosudarstvennoe Sotsialno-eknomicheskoe Izdatel'stvo.

Vygotsky, L. S. (1971). *Psychology of art.* Cambridge, MA: MIT Press.

Vygotsky, L. S., & Luria, A. R. (1930). *Etiudy po istorii povedenia.* Moscow–Leningrad: Gosizdat.

Werner, H. (1957). The concept of development from a comparative and organismic point of view. In D. B. Harris (Ed.), *The concept of development* (pp. 125–147). Minneapolis: University of Minnesota Press.

Whiting, B. B. (1974). Folk wisdom and child rearing. *Merrill-Palmer Quarterly, 20,* 9–19.

Winegar, L. T., & Valsiner, J. (1992). Re-contextualizing context: Analysis of metadata and some further elaborations. In L. T. Winegar & J. Valsiner (Eds.), *Children's development within social context: Vol. 2. Research and methodology* (pp. 249–266). Hillsdale, NJ: Erlbaum.

# CHAPTER 4

# The Answer Depends on the Question

## A Conceptual and Methodological Analysis of a Parent Belief–Behavior Interview Regarding Children's Learning

Irving E. Sigel
Myung-In Kim

The purpose of this chapter is to share our experiences in the course of revising our earlier parent belief interview while planning a follow-up study. In the process of examining our previous interview data with parents of preschool children, we discovered how many opportunities we missed for getting a more in-depth understanding of the nature of parents' beliefs about children's learning and how this lack of knowledge stimulated another intense effort at reconstructing the interview because it is a basic research tool to study parents' cognitions—in our case, parents' beliefs.

Through the reanalyses of the interviews on a case-by-case basis we discovered that there were alternative ways to create an interview and obtain data that would enrich our understanding of the relationship between parents' beliefs and their teaching strategies. Lest the reader think this is a bit premature as an introduction to the larger model, we think that the way in which we have constructed and analyzed the interview will be instructive because we shall show how concept and method intersect in the creation of research instruments in ways not often considered by developmental psychologists and perhaps even anthropologists. Sharing this experience by providing data to demonstrate what we have found will be informative and, we hope, will start a dialogue focusing on some of the conceptual and methodological problems facing all of us engaged in this type of research. (See McGillicuddy-DeLisi, 1982a, 1982b; McGillicuddy-DeLisi & Sigel 1982, 1995; Sigel, 1982; Sigel, Stinson, & Flaugher, 1991; Sigel, Stinson, & Kim, 1993; Stinson, 1989, for details of the general findings from earlier studies, as well as the more recent studies.)

## A Conceptual Approach to Beliefs

We work on the assumption that all beliefs and/or theories parents have about the socialization of their children are anchored in a cultural context and function with certain levels of automaticity, or, in Polanyi's (1958) terms, tacit understanding and tacit knowledge. Whatever other labels are used for beliefs (e.g., ideas, attributions, or cognitions), each serves the common function of guiding the behavior and actions of parents toward their children (Goodnow & Collins, 1990; Harkness & Super, 1992; McGillicuddy-DeLisi, 1992; Miller, 1988). In addition to the phenomenal label sharing a common meaning, the psychosocial-cultural significance of any ethnotheory or world view shares the common purpose, namely, coming to understand how these beliefs, cognitions, or ideas influence the course of children's development.

## The Need for Empirical Confirmation of the Effects of Beliefs

One of the major challenges for those interested in the study of beliefs is to sharpen the belief concept so that it can be operational to use as a basis for collecting empirical data. Over the years, researchers in this field have not offered precise definitions to allow for valid and reliable assessment. Rather, the term "belief" is often just stated, with the assumption that the term is consensual for all English speakers. Therefore, the meaning is shared. Thus, for most writers, developmental psychologists use the term "belief" interchangeably with the terms "opinion," "attitude," and the like. Goodnow and Collins are exceptions. They avoid the term because of its surplus meaning and offer *parent ideas* as their construct. However, theirs is not a common position. The loose usage is more typical and it makes it difficult to devise consensual measures because the criteria for labeling a statement a "belief" are unclear. Similarly, the creation of interviews and probes would not have a criterial definition allowing for adequate theorizing and testing (Miller, 1988; Sigel, 1986, 1992). Many of the reasons for the difficulties in this type of research have been discussed in the literature. General conceptual issues regarding definition and measurement have been addressed by Goodnow (1988) and Goodnow and Collins (1990), attitudes and attitude measurement by Holden and Edwards (1989), belief and behavior linkages by Sigel (1992), parent beliefs by Miller (1988), values by Kohn (1977), and ecological factors on parenting by Bronfenbrenner (1979) and Luster and Okagaki (1993).

We have opted for a belief model because we have operated on the assumption that cognition and affect are inexorably bound and cannot be disentangled. Our formulation of the *belief* construct derives from the proposition that beliefs serve a generic function encompassing cognitive and affective aspects. Belief is defined as "*knowledge in the sense that the individual knows that what he (or she) espouses is true or probably true, and evidence may or may not be deemed necessary; or if evidence is used, it forms a basis for the belief but is not the belief itself*" (Sigel, 1985, p. 348).[1]

Beliefs are anchored in and ensconced in a schema that includes affect, intentionality, and value, which in their totality guide parent actions.[2] Beliefs are mental representations that function as a source of influence on behavior because they are conceptualized as the mediational means that encompass all facets of childrearing (e.g., parent goals, teaching and management interactions, or standards by which to evaluate children's performance). Focusing on the belief schema as fundamental, we view our approach as broader than many of the current studies and yet not as comprehensive as we would like. Part of the reason for this state of affairs is that the completed model as described in McGillicuddy-DeLisi and Sigel (1995) emerged as a consequence of our experiences to be described in this chapter. It evolved as we reflected on our data and findings in previous studies (McGillicuddy-DeLisi, 1980a, 1980b, 1982a, 1982b, 1985; Sigel, 1982, 1985, 1992; Sigel et al., 1991). Thus the belief schema has not been tested in its totality.

Part of the schema, however, has been carried out and will be reported in this chapter. Two particular aspects of the belief schema we shall address are (1) whether parents' beliefs elicited in the interview will be differentiated by the targeted probe, and (2) the degree to which the beliefs reported in the interview transcend knowledge domains or are influenced by the domain in question. Our argument is that parents may hold beliefs about children's learning that are particular to knowledge domains. Knowledge domains are delineated according to the epistemology of the classifier. Piaget (1971) has identified three knowledge domains of interest to us: *physical knowledge, social knowledge,* and *moral knowledge.* We used four knowledge domains, three from Piaget's notions and one we developed: *physical knowledge, social/interpersonal knowledge, moral knowledge,* and *self/intrapersonal knowledge.* We defined each domain as follows: *physical knowledge,* which refers to the physical universe of space, time, and distance, as well as ways for determining physical dimensionality; *social/interpersonal knowledge,* which refers to knowledge of social rules (i.e., aggression) dealing with social conflict; *moral knowledge,* which refers to matters of right and wrong (i.e., cheating and stealing); and *self/intrapersonal knowledge,* which refers to how the child comes to know about his or her inner feelings and emotional state.

Our focus is on parents' beliefs about how children come to know about their world. We asked the question: "Do parents believe that what children learn about their world depends on the knowledge domain?" For example, some parents may believe that children learn about the physical world through experimentation and exploration, whereas they may learn about right and wrong by being told what is right and what is wrong and being discouraged from experimentation or exploration. The difference may be due to the belief that physical knowledge is objective and "out there," to be discovered, whereas moral behavior is rooted in religious texts and may not be subject to change or exception.

Belief schemata are organized within boundaries, which may vary in permeability from tight and impermeable to loose and permeable. The degree of permeability or the degree to which a belief is held strongly or weakly may be a reflection of the parents' emotional and cognitive (rational) commitment to a belief. However, the permeability of belief(s) boundaries may differ among those sharing a common belief. For some, social or moral beliefs are relative, whereas for others they are absolute. Note how abortion debates among the committed and tightly bounded differ from those debates among the committed but not so tightly bounded. Thus, one group can justify abortion under conditions of health and welfare of the mother, or rape, or incest, while the others are absolute in their objections with no exceptions. Integral to our system is the fundamental premise that beliefs, however organized and held by individuals, define their world view and influence their actions. This is one way individuals maintain a cultural identity. To the degree that cultures enable and/or allow individuals to construct and/or transform cultural patterns of thought and action to meet their own idiosyncratic wishes, desires, and values, individuals will differ from each other. However, the degree of individuation is usually defined implicitly and/or explicitly by other cultural members or institutions.

In sum, beliefs are mental constructions imbued with cultural and personal meaning; while structurally similar, they may vary in content. The study of parents' beliefs poses challenging conceptual and methodological issues that still need to be addressed in spite of the considerable energy and talent devoted to this most complex field of research (Nisbett & Wilson, 1977). The prime concern revolves around such seemingly simple questions as the following: Can respondents articulate their beliefs relative to any issue? How complete a report is it? Can parents articulate their beliefs about the complex task of childrearing? Can they show the relationships between their beliefs and their actions as a source of influence on their children? Is the belief model a construction of the researcher and not a shared reality defining parents' relationships with their children? For example, are parents aware that they have beliefs about children's learning as they might have beliefs about politics? Or, do parents believe that their beliefs have an influence on their childrearing practices and can they demonstrate the kind of influence they have on the developing child?

## Background of the Research Program

The model evolved from our previous research efforts in which a belief interview was the prime source of parents' beliefs about children's learning (McGillicuddy-DeLisi, 1982a, 1982b; Sigel et al., 1991, 1993). The results from those studies, while informing us of the basic significance of parents' beliefs as a source of influence on parents' interactions with their children around cognitive tasks, also revealed how much more information we still needed to increase our understanding of how beliefs function. We had a sense that our interview procedures would be one source of difficulty because we missed probing the parents' responses for greater detail and also for connections to their behaviors.

Anyone studying parents' beliefs, ideas, ethnotheories, or root metaphors shares the same kind of conceptual and methodological concerns. The problem is how to assess any of these types of cognitions. The goals of these investigators are similar. They each wish to obtain valid, reliable, and contextual-based information. Because beliefs cannot be determined from observation, other than on a highly inferential basis, investigators are forced to use some type of self-report methods such as interviews, questionnaires, or sorting strategies that presume comparable and valid data. Each procedure has its strengths and weaknesses. Questionnaires usually limit the depth to which information can be given and are also decontextualized (Holden & Edwards, 1989). Sorting tasks share some of the same problems. Items used in "objective" measures are selected by the investigator and, hence, as our focus group informants told us in no uncertain terms, the items in these objective-type instruments reflect what the investigator is interested in and deems important. Thus, the respondent is revealing feelings and attitudes about the research ideas, which may or may not represent the issues of interest or meaningfulness to the parent. As one respondent told us when she was given a questionnaire, "These questions ask me to tell you how much I agree or disagree with you. There is no room for me to tell you what my views are. I would not have asked the questions you have asked."

The-face-to face interview is a method that can avoid some of this criticism. However, as we shall show in the course of our discussion, interviews have their own set of methodological difficulties which need to be addressed. It is our contention that our data are instructive and may provide some caveats and suggestions to those planning to use face-to-face interviews within particular settings.

Although many investigators have reported their experiences with interviews on beliefs (Goodnow & Collins, 1990; Mishler, 1986; Nisbett & Wilson, 1977), few have reported the type of analysis we report describing how we have constructed, used, and coded interviews addressing parents' reports of their beliefs as to how children learn: issues such as (1) targeting the content—child management, expectations and goals of children's development, sources of intellectual stimulation, and solving practical problems; (2) format hypothetical vignette, descriptive retelling of an actual event, and nature of probes; (3) framing the questions (closed or open or prestructured); (4) level of acceptance—minimal request for elaboration or more active interrogation; and (5) acceptance of parents' reconstructions or requests for historical accuracy. The material described in this chapter links our discussion to those of other investigators who have investigated parents' beliefs (as the general label, or ethnotheories) (Goodnow & Collins, 1990; Harkness & Super 1992; McGillicuddy-DeLisi, 1992; Miller, 1988). It is this common theme that has the potential for binding research in developmental, clinical, and social psychology; anthropology; and sociology, among other disciplines.

Each of these questions must be dealt with in order to maximize the authenticity, reliability, and stability of reported beliefs. Ironically, although much work has been done addressing similar questions by social psychologists, survey researchers, and public opinion researchers, their influence has not seeped into the developmental research literature.

*Basis for Selecting a Research Tool*

We begin with the proposition that the choice and construction of a research tool should be closely linked to the theory being studied. Choice of a procedure should not be one of convenience but should have a logical and psychological relationship to the question being studied. We elected to work with an interview because we were, and still are, interested in the respondent's construction of his or her beliefs, their degree of generality, and their predictive potential to parent behaviors.

# Description of Belief–Behavior Distancing Model

Over the past 15 years at Educational Testing Service, we conducted a series of studies exploring the relationships between parents' beliefs about children and their teaching strategies, which in turn are sources of influence on the development of representational competence. Thus, the flow of influence is from parents' beliefs, which are expressed in parents' teaching behaviors. It is the confluence of these sets of influence that contributes to children's understanding of representational material. We developed an interactive model based on the proposition that children's competencies to understand symbolic material are the outcome of social experiences that first occur within the family. Parents are the primary teachers and socialization agents of their children; they introduce the children to the physical, social, and cultural worlds in a variety of ways. The activities parents provide, the books they read to their children, the television programs they allow their children to watch, and, of course, the kinds of conversations they have with their children—in effect the total verbal/symbolic environment in the early years particularly—have a strong effect on parents and their children. The model is bidirectional because in part parental activities also evolve from parents' experiences with their children. As indicated earlier, parents' experiences with their children, while structured by their beliefs about how their children learn, are also affected by the way children respond to their actions. The parents may come to alter their beliefs as they interact with their children and their children's peers, and in this way they learn about their own children's individual characteristics relative to their peers. Our basic hypothesis is that parents' actions have a direct influence on children's intellectual and social understanding because it is through their direct and/or indirect communication patterns that beliefs are expressed. It is these parental expressions that let children know what parents believe. In fact, the child would have to infer what the parent believes because beliefs are

**Table 4.1.** Types of Distancing Behaviors Categorized by Levels

| High-level distancing | Medium-level distancing | Low-level distancing |
| --- | --- | --- |
| Evaluate consequence | Reproduce | Label |
| Evaluate competence | Describe similarities | Produce information |
| Evaluate affect | Describe differences | Describe, define |
| Evaluate effort and/or performance | Infer similarities | Describe—interpretation |
| Evaluate necessary and/or sufficient | Symmetrical classifying | Demonstrate |
| Infer cause–effect | Asymmetrical classifying | Observe |
| Infer affect | Enumerating | |
| Generalize | Synthesizing within classifying | |
| Transform | | |
| Plan | | |
| Confirm a plan | | |
| Conclude | | |
| Propose alternatives | | |
| Resolve conflict | | |
| Sequence | | |

covert. The only way beliefs are known to the child is through parental actions and activities. It is the consequences of all these direct engagements between parent and child that are the sources of influence on children's development of representational competence (McGillicuddy-DeLisi & Sigel, 1982; Sigel, 1982; Sigel & McGillicuddy-DeLisi, 1984; Sigel, McGillicuddy-DeLisi, & Johnson, 1980; Sigel et al., 1991, 1993; Stinson, 1989).

The specific class of verbal behaviors we have targeted as central to our model has been labeled "distancing behaviors." These are actions or teaching strategies that place demands on children to create temporal, spatial, and/or psychological mental distance between themselves and some person, object, or event. (See Table 4.1 for a list of these distancing behaviors.) The hypothesized outcome of the distancing engagement is the development of *representational competence*, which is the ability to comprehend the meanings of symbols and signs and to transform experiential events into mental events (Sigel, 1991). We have found that distancing behaviors do influence symbolic thought and representational competence among young children (Sigel, 1982; Sigel et al., 1991).

What brings us to examine our interview in some detail is that the level of prediction of parents' beliefs to their distancing strategies was lower than we had anticipated. Because we did not find the strong relationships we had expected, two questions immediately arose: (1) Was it a conceptual problem; namely, is it simplistic to think that one would find a one-to-one correspondence between beliefs and behaviors and that is why the correlations between beliefs and behavior are low; or (2) is the reason for the low correlations due to the type of interview and distancing behavior we used or were our data analyses too simplistic? Because we found that the distancing behaviors did correlate reasonably well with children's representational competence, we decided to reassess the data collection procedures and began with the parent belief interview.

In our earlier studies with preschool children we developed an interview that we discovered had limitations which could be corrected in subsequent studies (McGillicuddy-DeLisi, 1982a, 1982b; Sigel et al., 1980). In that study we elected to use vignettes to provide a standardized set of items focusing on the topics we identified as typical for children of that particular age. They dealt with such topics as the child's fears, emotional outbursts, questions about unusual physical events, and understanding time. These were detailed descriptions of situations familiar to most parents. The choices were made after considerable pretesting with parents who were asked to tell us the particular activities in which they found themselves frequently engaging with their children. The parents were asked what they would do to facilitate the children's learning. Then they were asked how the strategy of choice would help the children learn about that particular activity or topic. Finally, they were asked how they believed children learn that particular topic. An example of this early type of vignette and the probes used is presented in Table 4.2. Note how detailed the vignette is. The probes did not have a consistent target, nor were the items within each knowledge domain evenly distributed throughout the interview because at that time we did not believe they would yield distinctive beliefs. We used them to get a general sample of parent–child teaching–learning interactions. Of course, we know better now.

A detailed categorization of parents' beliefs was constructed using parents' responses to each of the probes. In this way we mapped the belief terrain of parents. Ten belief categories were identified and were reliably coded (see Table 4.3). However, correlations between each of the belief categories and parents' distancing strategies were not robust with one exception. Parents who believe that children learn by negative reinforcement tended to use didactic authoritative strategies (low-level distancing or rational authoritative techniques). (See McGillicuddy-De-Lisi, 1982a, 1982b, and Sigel, 1985, for a detailed discussion of these findings.)

In a subsequent review of the findings, Sigel suggested that the reason for the difficulty was that there may be two levels of beliefs: a core belief, which is general, and a specific belief, which is the rationale for a particular strategy. A core belief might be a belief that reflective thinking is the way children come to understand how to solve problems. Such a belief may be just an abstract statement with no specific operational behavior tied to it. But when asked what type of distancing strategy the parent would use to exemplify this belief, he or she may provide different strategies depending on the problem. When presented with a physical knowledge problem, the parent could elect to use a high-level distancing strategy because he or she believes this is the way children will solve such problems. On the other hand, if the issue is a moral one the parent might believe that children learn morality when the parents employ rational authoritative strategies because that is how the child will come to know right from wrong. (See Sigel, 1986, 1992, for a discussion of these arguments for possible methods when constructing research belief interviews.)

We worked with these ideas in reassessing the interviews and found that these approaches could answer some of the questions we had about the predictability of belief interviews. In addition, parents' beliefs seem to be consistent within domains of knowledge but different among the domains. For example, parents tended to offer different beliefs when

**Table 4.2.** Example of Vignette with Probes from Parent Belief Construction/Communication Interview

Karen and her father had earlier planned to go to the movies. It was getting late and Karen was still not ready. Father knew that Karen should be getting dressed now

Construction probes

1. (a) Does a _____-year-old understand time?

    (If necessary, the following probe may be used.)[a]

        Does a child know about an hour, tomorrow, a year?

   (b) How does a _____-year-old eventually come to understand about time?

2. (a) Do _____-year-olds plan what they want to do ahead of time?

    (If necessary, the following probe may be used.)[a]

        For example, does a _____-year-old plan that "For now I will watch TV and then I'm going to the movies"?

   (b) How does a child become able to plan?

[a]These probes are to be used only if the parent requests clarification or indicates that they do not understand the original questions.

they were dealing with a child learning about his or her feelings as compared to learning about some physical knowledge fact (e.g., about flotation or image reflection, as in a mirror). However, as we indicated previously, we did not work with those ideas in mind; rather, we aggregated responses across domains.

We were able to develop a new set of interviews in a subsequent follow-up study 5 years later, working with a subset of families from the original group.

In the follow-up study we set out to address the same questions but working with older children. We were interested in testing the distancing model with the expectation that the parents' beliefs would influence their distancing behavior which in turn would influence the child's representational competence. Thus we could catalogue the parents' beliefs, their distancing behaviors, and the child's representational

**Table 4.3.** Definitions of Parental Beliefs

| Parental belief | Definitions |
|---|---|
| Accumulation (ACC) | The child learns through practice and additive experiences. |
| Activity (ACT) | The child learns by doing, through hands-on experience. |
| Cognitive processes (CP) | The child learns through thinking and reasoning, considering options, drawing inferences, and weighing consequences. |
| Direct instruction (DI) | The child learns from being told what to do, from explanations or advice. |
| Experimentation (EXM) | The child learns by trying out alternate solutions in problem solving, trial, and error. |
| Exposure (EXP) | The child learns through imitation and modeling. |
| Manipulation of the environment (ME) | The child learns through adult structuring of activities and learning tasks. |
| Negative feedback (NF) | The child learns through being punished or criticized for behavior. |
| Positive feedback (PF) | The child learns through experiencing success, approval, and support. |
| Self-regulation (SR) | The child learns through figuring out own solutions. |

competence, and in so doing we would see whether the model was consistent over time.

The specific objectives were threefold: (1) to identify parents' beliefs regarding children's acquisition of knowledge, (2) to identify the methods parents use to teach their children, and (3) to examine how these strategies influence the child's cognitive functioning as expressed in representational competence.

The procedures we used were comparable in form, but not in content, with the initial study. The changes were made to make each of the tasks age appropriate. For the interview we changed the content of the vignettes, shortened them, and reduced the number of details to avoid making the situation so specific that the parent had to comply with the details of the vignettes rather than focus on the centrality of the theme. We also made sure that three vignettes were created for each of the four knowledge domains: physical, social, moral, and intrapersonal. Finally, we made sure that each probe had a specific target to get at the parents' beliefs underlying the strategy they used to deal with the issue in the vignette. For example, the second probe targeted the parents' belief regarding the way their child generally learned about that topic. The final probe targeted the parents' belief about how most children learn about that topic. Each probe moved from the specific situation with a particular child. The second belief probe focused on the general characteristics of each parent's own child and the third focused on what we thought might reveal each parent's social or cultural belief. Our concern was influenced by those investigators who reported that the way a probe is targeted and structured affects the kind of response that is elicited (see Table 4.4). For example, Holden and Edwards (1988), in their review of the parent attitude research, report that responses of parents differ depending on whether the item is framed in the third person, for example, "Children should _____," or in the first person, "my child _____." However, to our knowledge, this issue has not been addressed in parent interviews except in the context of public opinion surveys. Theoretically, its importance rests on our assumption from cognitive theory that holds that a probe can target a particular representational schema. For example, focusing specifically on the individual child in a particular context may elicit a specific representation of the particular child as an actor in that scene, whereas using the third person (e.g., "the child") might arouse a more abstract representation reflecting perhaps a view of the child's learning relative to some general cultural norm or belief.

This is an important topic and may be one reason why parents' beliefs have a relatively low correlation with their teaching strategies

(Miller, 1988). Finally, there is the question of the substantive content in the probe. In part this issue is consistent with that raised by Holden and Edwards, who pose the question of who the child is in the question. This concern is even more cogently stated by Goodnow and Collins (1990), when they write:

> A further issue to be faced in choosing measures involves the target of questioning. Shall we ask for ideas about children generally, typical children of a particular age group, "ideal" children, or the parent's own child? These different possible targets vary in the concreteness of the referent (although in getting ideas about children generally, one may actually be getting parents' perceptions of their own child). They may vary also in the effects of experience. Ideas about one's own child, for instance, are likely to show the effects of experience more strongly than ideas about "ideal" children or even "typical" children. In addition, the connections among the several judgements and types of judgement may vary from one family member to another. (p. 156)

**Table 4.4.** Revised Vignette with Probes

| Time | |
|---|---|
| It is 9 o'clock on a Saturday morning and [child] has just called his or her pen pal in California. [Child] is surprised and perplexed to discover that the friend is still sound asleep. You want to help him or her understand the principles on which time zones are based. | |
| Distancing strategy: | What would you do or say to help [child] learn the principles on which time zones are based? |
| | What words or actions would you use? |
| Belief probes: | |
| Probe 1 (Specific): | *How* do you think [your strategy] will help [child] learn the principles on which time zones are based? |
| | Knowing *how* [child] learns, *how* do you think [your strategy] will help him or her learn the principles on which time zones are based? |
| Probe 2 (Child in General): | How do you think [child's name] will eventually learn the principles on which time zones are based? |
| Probe 3 (Child in General): | How do you think most children eventually learn the principles on which time zones are based? |

Each of the targeted probes taps the same situation but differs in level of specificity. Following the strategy probe, we asked our first belief probe targeted at the specific situation, followed by the second probe targeted at how their child learns that subject matter in general. We followed this by a third probe which targeted children in general. Theoretically, the belief should be consistent across all probe conditions.[3] If, on the other hand, differences are found among these probes, it is evident that the content and the target of the probe item make a difference.

### Results from Analyses of Targeted Probes

We turn now to a report of the findings from our reexamination of the data to show the relationship between the type of probes to self-reported teaching strategies and teaching behaviors. We shall also examine the relationships between the answers given to questions with each targeted probe within each of the knowledge domains. Furthermore, the relationship between parental beliefs, self-reported teaching behaviors, observed parental teaching behaviors, and children's academic achievement will be examined to determine the relationship to the knowledge domain of the questions presented to the parent (Sigel, 1992).

### Research Measures and Procedures

The data used in this project were obtained from a sample studied in 1985–1986.[4] A matched sample of 78 families (40 with a communication-handicapped child and 38 with a non-communication-handicapped child) agreed to participate in the follow-up study. The families were intact, with testable children, and matched on family size, birth order of the target child, and gender. The children were between the ages of 8 years, 6 months and 14 years, 5 months (mean age of 11 years, 4 months). Fifty-one of the children were male and 27 were female. The families were white and middle-class, of different religious and ethnic backgrounds.

## Measures and Procedures

### Beliefs and Strategies

The *Manual for Parent Belief Construction/Communication Strategy Interview* (Sigel, Flaugher, Redman, Sander, & Stinson, 1986) was developed for this second phase of the study to assess the relationship between parental beliefs and teaching strategies on children's cognitive development. The parent interviews were conducted separately by a research assistant and were recorded on audiotape. The interview was coded on the spot by the interviewer. A second assistant listened to the audiotape at a later time and coded the parents' responses independently. An average agreement of 94% was obtained for each behavioral and belief category.[5]

In addition to coding each vignette and each probe for the parents, the strategies and belief categories were coded in terms of beliefs and distancing strategy categories as listed in Table 4.5.

The interview belief data were subjected to a confirmatory factor analysis to test the homogeneity of the four knowledge domains. A varimax rotation of the data revealed that these domains could be reduced to three[6]. Moral and social knowledge loaded on one factor, whereas physical and intrapersonal knowledge completed the set of categories we used.

To get at the overt behavior of the parent teaching his or her child, we videotaped each parent and child dyad while they were engaged in a teaching task in which the parent was instructed to teach the child how to tie various types of knots—a structured task equivalent to the paper-folding task in the earlier studies (Sigel, 1982). Parent–child interactions were videotaped through a one-way mirror and a portion of the tape (6 minutes sampled over a 10-minute observation ) was later coded according to the types of teaching strategies used (Sigel, Flaugher, LaValva, Redman, & Sander, 1987) (see Table 4.1).

While their parents were being interviewed, the children were administered a series of subtests from Woodcock and Johnson's (1978) Psycho-educational Battery (WJPB). This was given to measure the children's general cognitive ability; mathematics, reading, and verbal achievement; and reasoning skills—in effect, academic achievement. The WJPB was used as a proxy for a test of the children's representational skills, especially mathematics, which involves nonlinguistic notations.

**Table 4.5.** Beliefs and Teaching Strategies Addressed

| Belief | Teaching Strategy |
|---|---|
| Cognitive processing | High-level MOD |
| Direct instruction | Medium MOD |
| | Low-level MOD |
| | Structuring |

## Data Used for Analyses

There are four major belief categories: *cognitive processing, direct instruction, positive reinforcement,* and *negative reinforcement.* We used two of the four categories, cognitive processing and direct instruction because they consisted of the majority of the beliefs reported and were central to the distancing theory. Cognitive processing refers to parents' beliefs that children learn by using their imagination, figuring things out on their own, weighing the consequences, comparing, reconstructing, proposing alternatives, evaluating, inferring, synthesizing, anticipating, empathizing, or speculating. Direct instruction refers to parents' beliefs that a child learns from being given instructions, explanations, advice, or explicit guidance.

The basis for defining distancing strategies is in terms of mental operational demands (MODs)[7] (see Table 4.1). The name of the label reflects the mental operation targeted. This depends on the linguistic structure of the utterance of the parent.[8]

For this chapter, only three types of distancing strategies are used. Again, these are the strategies that represent the most important categories in terms of theory and the most frequently used teaching strategies.

### High-Level Mental Operational Demand (HMOD)

These can be statements or questions that require the child to engage in mental operations such as inferential reasoning, anticipating outcomes, reconstructing the past, and generating hypotheses. All of these are abstractions without the dependence on concrete manipulanda, but they employ mental operations, make inferences, and engage in hypothetical reasoning.

### Medium-Level Mental Operational Demand (MMOD)

These are cognitive demands that activate representational thinking but still depend on some observational evidence. The process activated involves specific information (somewhat concrete, somewhat focused) to produce a response.

### Low-Level Mental Operational Demand (LMOD)

These are mental operational demands that make minimal demands for the child to disengage from the concrete here and now. The demands are in the form of closed questions or definitive statements, which require more associative responding as compared to representational thought.

## Structuring

Although not a distancing strategy, structuring is an important category because it reflects the parent's control in defining the task with the presumed intention of facilitating or channeling the child's performance. Structuring can be explanations or demonstrations given to move the task along and/or set rules on an activity. Structuring can also be any utterance that is aimed at managing the child's behavior, whether or not it is task related.

The beliefs and strategies used in this analysis represent the most important theoretical categories in terms of the theory and they are also the most frequently reported in the interview with the parents (on average, more than 50% for each belief category and the distancing strategies, except for structuring, which is 80% of teaching categories reported).

## *Specific Hypotheses for These Analyses*

Although in general the beliefs reported in the interview are expected to relate to the teaching strategies reported in the interview, as well as those observed in the teaching situation, we developed specific hypotheses to test our theory.

On the assumption that parents' beliefs and behaviors coexist in a coherent world view of children's learning, we would expect parents' beliefs to be comparable across knowledge domains. Beliefs are representations and should be generic; therefore they transcend specific knowledge domains.

We had no theoretical basis for specific hypotheses as to how each targeted probe would play out. We shall just leave it at that for now and report the diverse relations among the probes. We would also expect that particular teaching strategies would be contingent upon the parents' belief. Thus, for the interview from which self-reports were obtained, we would expect cognitive processing beliefs to be related to distancing strategies, whereas direct instruction would be related to direct authoritative or rational authoritative strategies. A belief in cognitive processing would be expressed in distancing strategies at any level, with direct instruction expressed in direct or rational authoritative strategies.

The next issue is whether what parents say they will do is what they in fact will do. Here we would expect parents' stated beliefs and practices to relate to the use of the distancing strategies. Beliefs in cognitive processing, as well as self-reports of distancing in the interview, should relate to the higher two levels of MODs. We make this assertion because the theory holds that belief in cognitive processes relates to distancing strategies, which should enable the child to develop greater autonomy and responsibility by having the opportunity to think and reason on his or her own relative to his or her developmental level. However, the LMODs and structuring strategies are authoritarian and directive, allowing for few mental self-determined constructions and reconstructions of experiences. Rather, the parent is controlling the direction of the child's intellectual performance. In the next section we turn to a presentation of our correlation analyses to test the hypotheses of this study as well as describe the outcome for each of the probe questions.

# Results

## *Correlations among the Three Belief Probe Questions on the Interview*

When parents' beliefs in cognitive processing or direct instruction are aggregated across parent gender and knowledge domains, the strongest correlations are between parents' responses to their own child's general learning pattern and how children generally learn as listed in Table 4.6.

However, these general correlations inform us only about the degree to which the beliefs presented in response to the different probes yield different patterns of relationships irrespective of the gender of the parent and the target of the probe.

## *Relationships between Beliefs and Self-Reported Teaching Strategies for Mothers and Fathers*

Beliefs in cognitive processing should be positively related to distancing strategies and negatively related to both rational authoritative and direct authoritative strategies. Direct instruction, on the other hand, should be negatively related to distancing strategies and positively related to rational and direct authoritative strategies. Furthermore, if the target and the knowledge domain truly do not affect the parental responses in the interview, the correlations between all the beliefs and behaviors should not differ significantly in magnitude or direction. The expected pattern of correlations based on the distancing model was generally found, with cognitive processing related positively to reports of distancing strategies and direct instruction related positively to direct authoritative strategies. The correlations between the different probes and domains also varied.

Table 4.7 shows the correlations between mothers' beliefs in cognitive processing and self-reported teaching behaviors for each of the target probes. The relationships are as expected, with beliefs in cognitive processing being significant only for the two general contexts—one's own child and children in general self-reports. The relationships obtained for mothers' total beliefs scores are all positive as

**Table 4.6.** Correlations among the Parents' Beliefs

| Belief | Target Probe 1–Specific × Target Probe 2–Child in general | Target Probe 1–Specific × Target Probe 3–Child in general | Probe 2–Child in general × Probe 3–Child in general |
|---|---|---|---|
| | Mothers | | |
| Cognitive processing | | | |
| Total Score | .41** | .34* | .68*** |
| Knowledge domains | | | |
| Physical | .46** | .26 | .53*** |
| Intrapersonal | .13 | .22 | .81*** |
| Moral–social | .16 | .14 | .63*** |
| Direct instruction | | | |
| Total Score | .22 | .38** | .77*** |
| Knowledge domains | | | |
| Physical | .42** | .33* | .59*** |
| Intrapersonal | .07 | .04 | .75*** |
| Moral–social | −.06 | .27* | .65*** |
| | Fathers | | |
| Cognitive processing | | | |
| Total score | .48** | .43** | .89*** |
| Knowledge domains | | | |
| Physical | .32* | .34* | .83*** |
| Intrapersonal | .30* | .29* | .86*** |
| Moral–social | .50** | .47** | .71*** |
| Direct instruction | | | |
| Total Score | .40** | .33* | .66*** |
| Knowledge domains | | | |
| Physical | .31* | .30* | .78*** |
| Intrapersonal | .34* | .34* | .79*** |
| Moral–social | .39** | .29* | .61*** |

*Note.* The correlations are one-tailed tests. $N = 40$.
*$p < .05$; **$p < .01$; ***$p < .001$.

expected. However, the magnitudes varied with the target of the probe. The specific situational is significantly higher than the other two references.

Examining the breakdown by knowledge domain we again discover that the findings based on total scores mask beliefs within domains. Beliefs in cognitive processing and direct instruction are as predicted for the specific situation but variable. Interestingly enough, mothers who believe in direct instruction are more consistent across contexts.

Analysis by domains reveals a consistent pattern for the specific situation. Belief in cognitive process as a way for children to learn is consistently negatively related to the use of direct authoritative strategies. Relationships for the other probes are not significant.

**Table 4.7.** Correlations between Mothers' Beliefs and Self-Reported Teaching Strategies

|  | Cognitive processing belief | | | Direct instruction belief | | |
|---|---|---|---|---|---|---|
|  | Probe 1 Specific | Probe 2 Child in general | Probe 3 Child in general | Probe 1 Specific | Probe 2 Child in general | Probe 3 Child in general |
| **Total interview** | | | | | | |
| Distancing | .72*** | .42** | .40** | −.60*** | −.32* | −.38** |
| Rational authoritative | .02 | −.06 | −.19 | .31* | .05 | .03 |
| Direct authoritative | −.60*** | −.26 | −.27* | .56*** | .35* | .51*** |
| **Knowledge domains** | | | | | | |
| **Physical** | | | | | | |
| Distancing | .77*** | .39* | −.22 | −.49** | −.13 | −.05 |
| Rational authoritative | .01 | −.06 | .05 | .18 | −.02 | −.20 |
| Direct authoritative | −.48** | −.36* | −.35* | .44** | .45** | .50** |
| **Intrapersonal** | | | | | | |
| Distancing | .61*** | .03 | .07 | −.50*** | −.21 | −.18 |
| Rational authoritative | −.03 | .18 | .04 | .27* | −.13 | −.06 |
| Direct authoritative | −.47** | .07 | −.07 | .32* | .11 | .16 |
| **Moral–social** | | | | | | |
| Distancing | .68*** | .05 | .14 | −.47** | −.18 | |
| Rational authoritative | .07 | .06 | −.09 | .30* | .25 | .31* |
| Direct authoritative | −.51*** | .26 | .08 | .58*** | .00 | .32* |

*Note.* The correlations are one-tailed tests. $N = 40$.
*$p < .05$; **$p < .01$; ***$p < .001$.

Relationships obtained for beliefs in direct instruction demonstrate consistent findings for the specific referent. The probes targeting one's own child and children in general are positively correlated.

The correlations between fathers' beliefs and self-reported teaching behaviors are presented in Table 4.8. First, looking at the aggregated interview responses, it is clear that distancing strategies are positively and significantly correlated with cognitive processing as expected, as are the relationships with direct instruction, but only for the response to the probe for the specific situation and one's own child. The strongest correlations are with the probe targeted at the specific situation. Beliefs in direct instruction are significantly correlated with direct authoritative teaching strategies for one's own child and for

**Table 4.8.** Correlations between Fathers' Beliefs and Self-Reported Teaching Strategies

| | Cognitive processing belief | | | Direct instruction belief | | |
|---|---|---|---|---|---|---|
| | Probe 1 Specific | Probe 2 Child in general | Probe 3 Child in general | Probe 1 Specific | Probe 2 Child in general | Probe 3 Child in general |
| Total interview | | | | | | |
| Distancing | .77*** | .30* | .17 | −.37*** | −.30* | −.18** |
| Rational authoritative | −.21 | −.21 | −.14 | .44** | −.04 | −.01 |
| Direct authoritative | −.17*** | −.08 | −.01 | .22 | .37* | .28* |
| Knowledge domains | | | | | | |
| Physical | | | | | | |
| Distancing | .43** | −.15 | −.27* | −.26 | −.17 | .10 |
| Rational authoritative | −.34** | −.16 | −.18 | .11 | −.18 | −.11 |
| Direct authoritative | −.02 | −.05 | .13 | .11 | .18 | .14 |
| Intrapersonal | | | | | | |
| Distancing | .63*** | .39** | .36* | −.29* | −.32* | −.28* |
| Rational authoritative | −.19 | −.19 | −.08 | .24 | .16 | .03 |
| Direct authoritative | −.08 | .05 | −.06 | .14 | .20 | .38** |
| Moral–social | | | | | | |
| Distancing | .76*** | .40*** | .21 | −.33* | −.17 | −.02 |
| Rational authoritative | −.23 | −.24 | −.18 | .52*** | .05 | .04 |
| Direct authoritative | −.36* | −.27* | −.18 | .38** | .42** | .27* |

*Note.* The correlations are one-tailed tests. $N = 40$.
*$p < .05$; **$p < .01$; ***$p < .001$.

children in general. Authoritative strategies are significantly correlated with direct instruction for one's own child and children in general.

Fathers' cognitive processing beliefs and their distancing behaviors continue to be highly related for the specific targeted probe for each of the domains. Beliefs elicited by targeting probes about one's own child and children in general show a positive relationship with distancing strategies. However, an inexplicable negative, but very low, correlation was found for fathers' responses for children in general. It seems that they believe they would use distancing for their own children but that children in general learn in some other way. Inspection of the table of correlations will reveal some of the other inconsistencies among the fathers. However, it is clear that the targeted probe does yield different responses.

In general, the expected pattern for the correlations between the beliefs and self-reported teaching strategies was found for both parents. As expected, the cognitive processing belief is directly related to distancing, whereas the more didactic strategies are associated with direct instruction.

## Relationships between Beliefs and Observed Distancing Strategies—MODs

In this section we examine the correlations between the parents' reports of what they say they would do in the hypothetical context with each probe and the teaching strategies they use in the teaching situation. The teaching strategies are coded more precisely because there were more verbalizations in the actual instructional situation than in the interview. HMODs reflect optimum distancing, whereas LMODs share more with a didactic authoritative approach. The conceptual model guiding the analysis of these data is the same as that guiding the interview. Beliefs in cognitive processing should be positively correlated with HMODs and negatively correlated with LMODs and structuring behaviors. Conversely, beliefs in direct instruction should be negatively correlated with HMODs and positively correlated with LMODs and structuring. And, if the different referents and domains are not important to these relationships, the correlations, broken down by referent and domain, should approximately be in the same magnitude and direction as the total score correlations.

The expected pattern of correlations between beliefs and observed behaviors was found for HMODs and structuring (but for mothers only). The overall pattern for fathers is not as clear. Most important, the referents and domains did affect the magnitude and sometimes even the direction of the correlations (see Table 4.8).

Table 4.9 presents the correlations between mothers' beliefs and their observed teaching behaviors. Discounting LMODs for the moment, all the correlations between cognitive processing and direct instruction belief categories and observed frequency of distancing are in the predicted direction. But unlike the correlations between beliefs and self-reported behaviors, the strongest of these relationships are with response to how one's own children learn and how children in general learn. Of these two, the child general probe yields the highest and most consistent correlations. For the children in general probe, belief in cognitive processing is significantly and positively correlated with HMODs and direct instruction is significantly and positively correlated with structuring in the total, intrapersonal, and moral–social domains. It should also be noted that the only significant relationship within the physical knowledge domain is between cognitive processing in the specific context and HMODs.

The fathers' correlations between beliefs and observed behaviors are given in Table 4.10. Again, ignoring the correlations with LMODs for now, the only significant correlation between cognitive process belief and HMODs is in the physical knowledge domain for the first

**Table 4.9.** Correlations between Mothers' Beliefs and and Observed Teaching Behaviors

|  | Cognitive processing belief | | | Direct instruction belief | | |
|---|---|---|---|---|---|---|
|  | Probe 1 Specific | Probe 2 Child in general | Probe 3 Child in general | Probe 1 Specific | Probe 2 Child in general | Probe 3 Child in general |
| **Total interview** | | | | | | |
| HMOD | .25 | .44** | .49** | −.22*** | .19 | −.18 |
| LMOD | −.06 | −.05 | .09 | −.11 | −.17 | −.32* |
| Structuring | −.25 | −.30* | −.48** | .27* | .28* | .36* |
| **Knowledge domains** | | | | | | |
| Physical | | | | | | |
| HMOD | .31* | .18 | −.03 | −.14 | −.16 | −.02 |
| LMOD | −.11 | .20 | .18 | .04 | −.20 | −.39** |
| Structuring | −.20 | −.10 | −.07 | .22 | .11 | .13 |
| Intrapersonal | | | | | | |
| HMOD | .05 | .25 | .38** | −.03 | −.02 | −.12 |
| LMOD | .08 | −.14 | −.03 | −.13 | −.13 | −.11 |
| Structuring | −.24 | −.11 | −.26 | .11 | .44** | .40** |
| Moral–social | | | | | | |
| HMOD | .23 | .33* | .38** | −.26 | −.21 | −.23 |
| LMOD | −.10 | −.08 | .07 | −.13 | −.07 | −.20 |
| Structuring | .18 | −.30* | −.42** | .22 | .17 | .27* |

*Note.* The correlations are one-tailed tests. $N = 40$.

*$p < .05$; **$p < .01$; ***$p < .001$.

construct. The only pattern of correlations consistent with the distancing model for direct instruction lies between situational and HMODs (all are negative and three of the four correlations are significant).

The pattern of the correlations between LMODs and the beliefs for mothers and fathers poses a dilemma. They do not follow the expected pattern of results, nor do they follow any discernible scheme. It is not clear why this category of observed behaviors correlated with beliefs in this way.

On the surface, these results may seem to provide very little evidence for the relationship between beliefs and actual behavior, but this is not entirely the case. (See Sigel, 1992, for a full discussion of the belief–behavior connection.) The knot-tying task used in this experiment had very little to do with the knowledge domains addressed in the vignettes. In a sense we had "stacked the deck against ourselves" because we did not use identical situations on the belief interview and the observed teaching situation. This was done to test how specific or universal each parental belief was. It was found that the beliefs about how children learn were dependent on the knowledge domain of the situation (Sigel, 1992). Thus, it was encouraging to see that the correlations between cognitive proc-

**Table 4.10.** Correlations between Fathers' Beliefs and Observed Teaching Behaviors

|  | Cognitive processing belief | | | Direct instruction belief | | |
|---|---|---|---|---|---|---|
|  | Probe 1 Specific | Probe 2 Child in general | Probe 3 Child in general | Probe 1 Specific | Probe 2 Child in general | Probe 3 Child in general |
| Total interview | | | | | | |
| HMOD | .24 | .08 | .06 | −.34$^*$ | −.06 | .10 |
| LMOD | .07 | .19 | .22 | .09 | −.17 | .01 |
| Structuring | .08 | −.06 | −.11 | .07 | .12 | .05 |
| Knowledge domains | | | | | | |
| Physical | | | | | | |
| HMOD | .30$^*$ | .10 | .05 | −.37$^*$ | −.18 | .06 |
| LMOD | .01 | .09 | .09 | .17 | .06 | .09 |
| Structuring | −.01 | .11 | .11 | .03 | −.10 | −.34$^*$ |
| Intrapersonal | | | | | | |
| HMOD | .11 | −.07 | −.10 | −.03 | .18 | .27* |
| LMOD | .04 | −.05 | −.02 | .07 | .05 | .07 |
| Structuring | −.08 | −.07 | −.12 | .04 | .22 | .38$^{**}$ |
| Moral–social | | | | | | |
| HMOD | .16 | .12 | .19 | −.27$^*$ | −.05 | −.14 |
| LMOD | .09 | .29$^*$ | .34$^*$ | −.01 | −.33$^*$ | −.14 |
| Structuring | .19 | −.10 | −.15 | .07 | .13 | .11 |

*Note.* The correlations are one-tailed tests. $N = 40$.
$^*p < .05$; $^{**}p < .01$; $^{***}p < .001$.

essing and direct instruction in the situational context for the physical knowledge domain were positive and significant for both mothers and fathers. Of the three domains, knot tying is the type of task that requires planning, analysis, and synthesis. These are processes parents include in their cognitive processing beliefs.

As for the three targeted probes, it is clear that the beliefs correlated with the observed behaviors differently. For mothers, the more general the target of the probe, the stronger the correlations with the observed behaviors. For fathers, the specific context had the most significant correlations related to it, but not the strongest ones. When the items are analyzed by knowledge domains, the parents' response to the probe targeting how children generally learn has the highest magnitude correlations with observed behavior directions whether cognitive processing or direct instruction (this illustrates that the domains have an effect on the correlations as well).

### Relationships between Beliefs and Children's Academic Achievement Scores

It was hypothesized that parental beliefs in cognitive processing would correlate positively with academic achievement, whereas beliefs in direct instruction would correlate negatively. The mothers' pattern of correlations did not match our expectations based on the distancing model. And once again, the referents and the domains proved to have an effect on these relationships. Table 4.11 shows mothers' correlations between their beliefs and their children's achievement scores.

The most consistent results for mothers are again when the probe refers to children in general. The correlations depicted in Table 4.11 reveal low-level relationships whether using probes targeted at children in general or at one's own child. It is worth noting that for the specific probe, cognitive processing beliefs correlated with the WJPB Brief scale score and only for Math and Brief scores in the physical knowledge domains.

None of the mothers' beliefs in direct instruction were significantly correlated with any of the academic achievement scores, regardless of the probe used to elicit them.

Table 4.12 presents the correlation of the fathers' beliefs and their child's academic achievement. Inspection of Table 4.12 shows a different pattern of relationships as a function of the targeted probes. When the probe focuses on the specific situation, fathers' beliefs in cognitive processing are consistent with how their own children generally learn, whereas in terms of reading achievement, the beliefs are related to how their children learn as well as children in general. When beliefs in direct instruction are reported, primarily negative relationships are observed in terms of the specific and situational. The pattern for cognitive processing beliefs offers correlations that show a somewhat disparate, yet not too discrepant, set of findings. The correlations, even when not significant for the cognitive processing beliefs, tend to be consistent with whichever probe is used. Again, the reader can inspect Table 4.12.

For direct instruction, the targeted probes tend not to differentiate the types of responses produced. It seems that they do not relate to any of the academic outcomes.

**Table 4.11.** Correlations between Mothers' Beliefs and Children's Academic Achievement

| | Cognitive processing belief | | | Direct instruction belief | | |
|---|---|---|---|---|---|---|
| | Probe 1 Specific | Probe 2 Child in general | Probe 3 Child in general | Probe 1 Specific | Probe 2 Child in general | Probe 3 Child in general |
| Total interview | | | | | | |
| WJPB Brief scale | −.07 | −.00 | .17 | −.05 | .07 | .03 |
| Math achievement | .03 | .14 | .31$^*$ | −.09 | −.09 | −.09 |
| Reading achievement | −.12 | .05 | .18 | .30* | −.13 | −.16 |
| Verbal ability | −.13 | −.22 | .03 | −.03 | .16 | −.01 |
| Reasoning ability | .01 | .05 | .06 | .01 | −.04 | −.03 |
| Knowledge domains | | | | | | |
| Physical | | | | | | |
| WJPB Brief scale | .28$^*$ | .00 | .17 | .02 | .09 | .04 |
| Math achievement | .27$^*$ | −.08 | .00 | −.07 | .01 | −.04 |
| Reading achievement | .04 | −.21 | −.16 | .21 | .08 | .00 |
| Verbal ability | .14 | .07 | .27$^*$ | .06 | .10 | −.05 |
| Reasoning ability | .13 | −.01 | −.32$^*$ | −.02 | .04 | .10 |
| Intrapersonal | | | | | | |
| WJPB Brief scale | −.25 | −.09 | −.18 | .16 | .12 | .10 |
| Math achievement | −.14 | .01 | .00 | .16 | −.04 | −.06 |
| Reading achievement | −.15 | .06 | .03 | .36* | −.11 | −.07 |
| Verbal ability | −.07 | −.31$^*$ | −.26 | .02 | .06 | .07 |
| Reasoning ability | −.07 | .17 | .03 | .22 | .08 | .05 |
| Moral–social | | | | | | |
| WJPB Brief scale | −.11 | .07 | .34* | −.19 | −.02 | −.05 |
| Math achievement | −.01 | .26 | .48** | −.18 | −.16 | −.10 |
| Reading achievement | −.13 | .16 | .34* | .15 | −.26 | −.26 |
| Verbal ability | −.26 | −.11 | .14 | −.11 | .18 | −.03 |
| Reasoning ability | −.01 | −.07 | .26 | −.10 | −.16 | −.18 |

*Note.* The correlations are one-tailed tests. $N = 40$.
$^*p < .05; ^{**}p < .01; ^{***}p < .001$.

The pattern of results continues to support our contention that the target of the interviewer's probe is an important factor influencing the nature of the response in terms of academic achievement.

## Conclusions

What can we make from this array of findings? First, as reported in a previous publication (Sigel, 1992), parental beliefs about the knowledge acquisition of children are contingent upon the context and the knowl-

**Table 4.12.** Correlations between Fathers' Beliefs and Children's Academic Achievement

| | Cognitive processing belief | | | Direct instruction belief | | |
|---|---|---|---|---|---|---|
| | Probe 1 Specific | Probe 2 Child in general | Probe 3 Child in general | Probe 1 Specific | Probe 2 Child in general | Probe 3 Child in general |
| Total interview | | | | | | |
| WJPB Brief scale | .07 | .23 | .19 | −.30* | −.08 | .00 |
| Math achievement | −.01 | .23 | .22 | −.17 | −.15 | .00 |
| Reading achievement | .10 | .41** | .32* | −.34* | −.19 | .02 |
| Verbal ability | .35* | .28* | .25 | −.39** | −.11 | −.14 |
| Reasoning ability | −.16 | .11 | .07 | −.09 | −.08 | .03 |
| Knowledge domains | | | | | | |
| Physical | | | | | | |
| WJPB Brief Scale | .20 | .20 | −.01 | −.33* | −.21 | .14 |
| Math achievement | .00 | .17 | .03 | −.28* | −.25 | .05 |
| Reading achievement | .04 | .16 | .04 | −.23 | −.06 | .05 |
| Verbal ability | .29* | .08 | −.07 | −.45** | −.10 | .07 |
| Reasoning ability | −.26 | −.04 | −.05 | .03 | −.02 | .02 |
| Intrapersonal | | | | | | |
| WJPB Brief scale | .22 | .28* | .29* | −.18 | −.06 | −.24 |
| Math achievement | .29* | .33* | .33* | −.17 | .03 | −.11 |
| Reading achievement | .11 | .46** | .39** | −.21 | −.06 | −.04 |
| Verbal ability | .37** | .22 | .22 | −.14 | −.11 | −.24 |
| Reasoning ability | −.04 | .15 | .21 | −.19 | −.06 | −.17 |
| Moral–social | | | | | | |
| WJPB Brief scale | −.14 | .07 | .10 | −.12 | .10 | .05 |
| Math achievement | −.20 | .06 | .08 | .05 | −.01 | .05 |
| Reading achievement | .07 | .27* | .18 | −.24 | −.18 | .02 |
| Verbal ability | .18 | .26 | .30* | −.22 | −.01 | −.08 |
| Reasoning ability | −.10 | .10 | −.03 | −.05 | −.05 | .17 |

*Note.* The correlations are one-tailed tests. $N = 40$.

*$p < .05$; **$p < .01$; ***$p < .001$.

edge domain addressed, as well as on the gender of the parent. The results presented in this chapter extend those findings by focusing on the probe types. The notion that the particular structure, content, and focus of probes yield different information is confirmed. At first blush it seems reasonable to hypothesize that parents' beliefs should be similar, irrespective of contextual referent of the probe (e.g., a particular situation or one's own child or children in general). Even though the referential context is similar, that is, asking how the child learns a specific math task, how one's own child in general learns math, or how children generally learn math, respondents produce different types of responses. The responses produced relate differentially to their self-reported behavior or their observed teaching interactions. Therefore, it seems safe to conclude that the probes do not elicit comparable responses and are not interchangeable. Rather, our findings demonstrate convincingly that the information obtained with each probe taps different mental representations of the event being discussed and thus leads to different responses.

It will be recalled that the first probe targeted the parent's belief relative to a particular hypothetical situation. The parent offers a strategy to deal with that situation and then responds to the request as to why he or she believes the strategy will help the child learn, regarding why he or she believes that strategy explains his or her behavior, as well as how he or she thinks her child would learn in that situation. Everything is very concrete, with descriptions of the details that define the task in that situation. The second probe refers to that same child without detailing the setting but merely identifying the content to be learned. It may be the case that the parent at this point shifts from a representation of the specific teaching task to another representation of his or her child's typical way of learning that type of problem. The parent may be "averaging" out how his or her child generally learns about that area. Now, instead of thinking about how the child learns a specific task (e.g., how to tell time), the parent detaches the child from that specific situation depicted in the vignette and considers the child's learning about time in a general sense. This is far different from the specific context and it is for this reason that we speculate that the parent may be thinking of the child in many situations responding to an image of the "typical." Next we come to the broader question of how children in general learn about time. The parent may now shift the perspective to a "norm" of how the average child learns and the particular child may or may not be comparable. The fact that we did not probe the basis for the parents' source of that belief was unfortunate because it leaves unanswered the cognitive or value basis of the belief in each of the three probe conditions.

There have been some studies that address the form of the question used in self-report measures and report similar differences in response as a function of probe focus. In the area of questionnaires, Becker and Krug (1965) criticized the use of third-person items on Schaefer and Bell's (1958) Parent Attitude Research Instrument (PARI). In their study they concluded that "the parent might respond [to the third-person items on the PARI] in terms of *cultural norms, professional opinion, empirical facts,* or *beliefs* about what is best for others, none of which may have anything to do with what the parent actually does with his own child" (Becker & Krug, 1965, p. 361). Holden and Edwards (1989), in their review of attitudinal research, found that about 75% of these questionnaires were written in the third person. In their opinion, this practice enhanced the ambiguity of the questionnaires, which has led to interpretation problems. Both articles recommended that the questions used in belief and attitude questionnaires should be written in the first person, but the test for the effectiveness of this recommendation has not, to our knowledge, been reported in the developmental literature other than in the context of our interview study. Our findings question the universality of recommending the use of the first person. It depends on the study.

Our results show that the referent of the question has a variety of different effects. Similar to what was found for the knowledge domains (Sigel, 1992), the more specific and closer the question is to the experience or task to be taught or learned, the stronger the relationship will be. This can be seen by the high-magnitude correlations between parental strategies reported in the situational context as compared with the less specific targeted own child and children in general (see Tables 4.7 and 4.8). However, correlations between responses in the specific situation and a learning task of the same type might have yielded closer correspondence between the response in the self-report context with the actual teaching situation. Or, it may be the case that general beliefs with a different task or measure are anticipated. Then a more "global" question gives better relationships. This point is illustrated by the stronger correlations between parental beliefs and parental observed behaviors (Tables 4.9 and 4.10), as well as child academic achievement measures (Tables 4.11 and 4.12), with the child and general constructs.

We would like to clarify an important issue as it will permeate subsequent discussion of the statistical significance of our data. The tendency among developmental psychologists is to accept the probability value of a correlation as the basis for accepting a hypothesis (e.g., paying more attention to the significance level than to its magnitude). Thus, a correlation of .40 with the proper $N$ ($p < .05$) is often considered to be as psychologically significant statistically as one of .75 with a similar "$p$" value. Yet we know that a correlation of .40 accounts for 16% of the variance in contrast to one of .75, which accounts for over 50%

of the variance. Little attention, if any, is paid to the coefficient of alienation, or statistical power analysis, both of which attend to the question of the unaccounted variance (Cohen & Cohen, 1983). To ignore differences in magnitude is misleading because it leads to an inflation of the significance of the findings. Paying attention to the magnitude of the correlations among the probe questions led us to a concern for the differential effects of the probe question.

In addition to the statistical concerns, we should point out some methodological limits of the current study because we focused only on those parental beliefs concerned with how children acquire knowledge in only three knowledge domains in a particular type of self-report. Differences might exist between the different types of self-report measures. In their review, Holden and Edwards (1989) cited only one methodological study that compared interviews with questionnaires. In studying mothers' attitudes toward permissiveness and punitiveness about sex and aggression with their preschool children, Sears (1965) found that correlations between the two self-report methods for individual variable ranged from .53 to .63 for 19 girls' mothers and .22 to .67 for 21 boys' mothers. Even though most of these correlations were relatively high (8 of 10 > .52), he found that the questionnaire and the interview correlated to observed child and maternal behaviors differently. He concluded that the questionnaire method was better at predicting observed maternal behavior, but a replication study was required due to the relatively small amount of observed mother–child behavior used within his study. Since 1965, no such replication study has been reported in the literature to our knowledge after an extensive search.

Sears (1965) highlights yet another area that needs to be addressed in the study of parental beliefs. The differences between mothers and fathers are noted in our discussion, but not whether parents' beliefs differ as a function of the child's gender. We have found that teaching strategies vary as a function of the child's gender (Sigel et al., 1991). It might be possible that parental beliefs are also specific to the gender of the child. Future research should attempt to tie this issue in with the other methodological issues presented in this chapter to help broaden our knowledge of the study of parental beliefs. Nevertheless, researchers should take a hard look at the instruments they use to assess parents' beliefs and ask the degree to which the reports are contingent upon the assessment procedures.

This brings us full circle to our initial questions relative to the significance of the target of the probe item on the types of responses respondents produce. Our findings provide sufficient evidence to justify paying particular attention to the relationship between the probe and the response. Built into the research protocol should be internal replications of probe types to ascertain whether they are yielding comparable or different information. If each probe yields different information, we can identify the limits of the findings. In spite of the small sample in our study, it should be obvious that our theory held up but differently, depending on the probes. It is the different responses to the probes that limit the generalizations from this study. Significant variabilities of responses to the different targets in the probe raise some questions that can be addressed. For example, what do the different parental responses reflect? Is the meaning of interview and/or questionnaire responses so dependent on the content of the probe that the findings are of limited use?

The answer to this question is "no." Rather, our findings signal three actions: (1) alter the methods of employing self-reports to take into account the limits of univocal questioning, (2) clarify the target of the question and develop a conceptual position of what responses are expected, and (3) use a multimethod approach so that greater reliabilities will emerge.

Let us conclude by addressing each of these questions so that our concerns will, it is hoped, lead to some methodological improvements.

At the outset we argue that although the issue appears as a methods question, it is, in fact, a conceptual issue. Methods are reflections of some theory, be it a theory of measurement or methods reflecting theory. In this case, selection of an interview is a conventional approach to obtaining belief information from respondents. The theory is reflected in the structure of the interview. Recall that we selected the interview in lieu of a questionnaire because the informants contended that questionnaires do not allow them to use their own voices in responding to the questions. Because an interview allowed for that, we elected to compromise and create a semistructured interview. What we discovered was that the interview was too superficial in the sense that we did not get at the rationales for answers to the three belief probes. Now we are in a position to resolve this issue and had we an opportunity to redo the interview, we would know how to proceed. It is on this level that these data offer guidelines for future research.

A second implication of our findings is that there was minimal dialogue and high standardized questioning reflecting a unidirectional communication, thereby not providing an opportunity for true discourse. In effect, our findings confirm Mishler's (1986) critique of the stimulus–response model. His critique is important, not only for us but also for any of the ethnographic interviews done in anthropology and developmental or clinical psychology. Elaborating on his thesis that interviews in effect are speech events, which he describes as a thematic progression involving turn taking and following conversational rules,

Mishler (1986) writes: "Defining interviews, as I do, marks a fundamental contrast between the standard anti-linguistic, stimulus response model and an alternative approach to interviewing as discourse between speakers" (p. 77). Space does not allow for a detailed discussion of Mishler's perspective, but it is an approach that can resolve some of the problems discussed in this chapter and perhaps help unravel some of the problems identified. It may be a direction in which to go for further use of interviews in research.

## Parental Beliefs and Parent Ethnotheory

We conclude this chapter by showing that studies of parental beliefs are relevant to the "content" of ethnotheory, and that the method of getting at parents' ethnotheories requires consideration of the research methods. Thus the proposition that "the answer depends on the question" should be of concern to researchers who are interested in what people believe about some things and how they see their actions expressing these beliefs. In this context we can put the question in the form of whose answer we are getting in our research on parental beliefs, ideas, values, or ethnotheories. So we begin with the question, "What does *ethno* mean in the context of theory?" Garfinkel (1974), who is said to have coined the term "ethnomethodology," has some thoughts on what *ethno* means. In response to the question of how he came to create the term "ethnomethodology," Garfinkel answered:

> "Ethno" seemed to refer, somehow or other, to the availability to a member of commonsense knowledge of his society as common-sense knowledge of the "whatever." If it were "ethnobotany" then it had to do somehow or other with his knowledge of and his grasp of what were for members adequate methods for dealing with botanical matters. Someone from another society like an anthropologist would recognize the matters as botanical matters. The member would employ ethnobotany as adequate grounds of inference and action in the conduct of his own affairs in the company of others like him. It was that plain, and the notion of "ethnomethodology" or the term "ethnomethodology" was taken in this sense. (pp. 16–17)

Using this term in the service of parent ethnotheories we can say that parent ethnotheory of child development refers to the commonsense knowledge that a parent has of his or her society. The ethnotheory construct seems to transcend the disciplinary orientation of the investigator. However, this seeming transcendence does mask the specific subset of "whatever" is subsumed under the rubric of commonsense knowledge. We argue that attitudes, beliefs, attributions, and parents' ideas and values are explicitly or implicitly part of the cultural common sense, tapping particular domains selected by the investigator The metaphors with which investigators choose to work are their inventions and organizations of whatever is their social reality.

If, in fact, our view is accepted, to wit, ethnotheory is a broadly based and somewhat ill-defined concept essentially analogous to the idea of world view, a *Weltanschaung,* or root metaphors (Pepper, 1942/1970).

The point of contact with ethnotheorists in this effort is the acceptance of a fundamental assumption that parental theories are essentially beliefs, not theories in the scientific sense but rather a set of beliefs that may or may not hang together because we now realize that these theories or beliefs can guide parents' actions in particular ways depending on the context that evokes action. All these phenomena, labeled by the social scientist beliefs, are cultural products of the social scientist and the respondents, especially when they are members of the same community. The commonality among group members is based on their sharing of a collective culture. The individual's beliefs evolve in the course of growing in a particular culture and developing beliefs about many matters; for example, religious, political, childrearing, family life, and sexuality, and the list can be extended to virtually all aspects of social and physical reality. Beliefs are integral to one's world view and are guides to most aspects of life because they are organized in a structural–functional system with varying degrees of extensity and boundedness. Extensity refers to the degree to which the common or collective beliefs are all-encompassing, expressed, for example, in the right-to-life movement, whose members not only oppose abortion but often hold Creationist views, oppose sex education, believe in absolute values, and the like. On the other hand, one can object to abortion and bound that belief to that sector only. In addition, the boundaries encapsulating individual beliefs or belief systems may vary in degree of permeability, that is, the degree to which the individual is open and receptive to new information. Permeability depends on the affective intensity with which the belief(s) boundary is maintained. The extensity and the boundedness dimensions will determine the stability or changeability of parents' beliefs in the face of children's development.

We also view our analyses of face-to-face interviews as a research tool contributing to ethnotheory research because the central topic of concern is the parents' constructions of their cognitions of their parental activity. To maximize the confidence in data obtained in such research requires bringing together the shared types of research experiences from the disciplines focusing on similar problems (e.g., anthropology, psychology, and sociology). The data we have presented in this chapter provide ample evidence that a research interview used by investigators in each of these disciplines shares common problems in getting valid and reliable data. We hope that some of our findings and concerns will be of value as investigators plan and carry out interviews in any setting. Our findings suggest caution when using the technique of hypothetical vignettes (a common procedure) and indicate one of the limiting aspects of using vignettes.

We believe that the future bodes well for interview procedures provided investigators develop adequate conceptualization of the structure and function of the interview, particularly the probes (Nisbett & Wilson, 1977).

The difficulties identified by these authors have not dampened interest in studies of parental socialization. There seems to be resilience among investigators evidenced by their consistent striving to generate new paradigms and models for study (Sigel, McGillicuddy-DeLisi, & Goodnow, 1992). There is still the belief that understanding parent and/or family socialization conceptions and practices is possible but requires vigilance as to innovative methods and theoretical insight. In fact, the sequelae for such understanding are expected to contribute to practical recommendations for some of the educational and social problems facing our society.

## Acknowledgments

Portions of the research presented in this chapter were supported by the National Institute of Child Health and Human Development Grant No. R01-HD10686 to Educational Testing Service, National Institute of Mental Health Grant No. R01-MH32301 to Educational Testing Service, and Bureau of Education of the Handicapped Grant No. G007902000 to Educational Testing Service.

Portions of this chapter were presented at the Seventh Australian Developmental Conference, July 7–10, 1992, University of Queensland, Brisbane, Queensland, Australia.

We would also like to thank Lauren K. Baier for her editorial comments, and Linda Kozelski for her thoughtful and thorough preparation of the manuscript for publication.

## Notes

1. In previous publications we developed the rationale for the use of the term belief as the construct of choice. For the purposes of this exposition,

that discussion is not necessary to follow those arguments. (See Sigel, 1985, 1992.)

2. The details of the belief as schema theory are discussed in detail in McGillicuddy-DeLisi and Sigel (1995).

3. The subjects for this study are a subset of a much larger sample examined during the first phase of this longitudinal project. The child in each of these families was between the ages of 3 years, 6 months and 7 years, 5 months (mean age of 4 years, 6 months), with a male to female ratio of 160:80. The number of children in each family, as well as the ordinal position and spacing between the child and his or her sibling(s) varied among the sample.

Half the children from Time I (*n* = 120) were diagnosed by a service outside Educational Testing Service (i.e., public school child study team, Project Child, speech and hearing clinics, and private speech therapists) as having a communication or language disorder (communication-handicapped group [CH]). To ensure that these CH children were testable, all were given an audiogram to confirm that they did not have any hearing difficulties or problems.

The other half of the Time I sample (*n* = 120) were families with children that did not have any known learning or communication handicap (non-communication-handicapped group [NCH]). These families were chosen to form the best possible contrast group for the CH families, based on six factors: (1) the child's sex, (2) the child's age, (3) the ordinal position of the child, (4) the sex of the sibling closest in age to the target child, (5) the number and spacing of the children in the family, and (6) the parent's educational level.

4. The Woodcock–Johnson Psycho-educational Battery was used to index representational competence.

5. Details of the coding procedures are available from the authors.

6. The factor loadings ranged from .72 to .94 for the physical knowledge domain (three items), .78 to .95 for the intrapersonal domain (three items), and .76 to .95 for the combined moral–social domain (five items). To obtain intensity indexes that reflect the strength of a parent's belief or use of a strategy overall and within domains, the frequencies of the coded responses were summed and divided by the total number of possible responses over the entire interview and for each domain converting the data to percent scores.

The frequency of medium-level distancing mental operational demands (MODs) was low for the observed teaching strategies, so they were combined with the high-level distancing MODs (they subsequently will be referred to as high-level MODs). The frequencies for the coded strategies were then converted to percentage scores by dividing them by their individual totals of coded observed behaviors.

7. The rationale for the coding is that the message as stated in the utterance serves to activate particular cognitive processes.

8. The parents' strategies reported in the interview did not provide the same detailed utterance as could be observed in the actual teaching situation. The teaching situation was an actual dialogue between parent and child, whereas the interview was an hypothetical interaction.

# References

Becker, W. C., & Krug, R. S. (1965). The parent attitude research instrument—A research review. *Child Development, 36,* 329–365.

Bronfenbrenner, U. (1979). *The ecology of human development: Experiments by nature and design.* Cambridge, MA: Harvard University Press.

Cohen, J., & Cohen, P. (1983). *Applied multiple regression/correlation analysis for the behavioral sciences* (2nd ed.). Hillsdale, NJ: Erlbaum.

Garfinkel, H. (1974). The origins of the term "ethnomethodology." In R. Turner (Ed.), *Ethnomethodology* (pp. 15–18). Baltimore: Penguin Books.

Goodnow, J. J. (1988). Parents' ideas, actions, and feelings: Models and methods from developmental and social psychology. *Child Development, 59,* 289–320.

Goodnow, J. J., & Collins, W. A. (1990). *Development according to parents: The nature, sources, and consequences of parents' ideas.* Hillsdale, NJ: Erlbaum.

Harkness, S., & Super, C. (1992). Parental ethnotheories in action. In I. E. Sigel, A. V. McGillicuddy-DeLisi, & J. J. Goodnow (Eds.), *Parental belief systems: The psychological consequences for children* (2nd ed., pp. 373–391). Hillsdale, NJ: Erlbaum.

Holden, G. W., & Edwards, L. A. (1989). Parent attitudes toward child rearing: Instruments, issues, and implications. *Psychological Bulletin, 106,* 29–58.

Kohn, M. L. (1977). *Class and conformity: A study in values* (2nd ed.). Homewood, IL: Dorsey Press.

Luster, T., & Okagaki, L. (1993). (Eds.). *Parenting: An ecological perspective.* Hillsdale, NJ: Earlbaum.

McGillicuddy-DeLisi, A. V. (1980a). Predicted strategies and success in children's resolution of interpersonal problems. *Journal of Applied Developmental Psychology, 1,* 175–187.

McGillicuddy-DeLisi, A. V. (1980b). The role of beliefs in the family as a system of mutual influences. *Family Relations, 29,* 317–323.

McGillicuddy-DeLisi, A. V. (1982a). Parental beliefs about developmental processes. *Human Development, 25,* 192–200.

McGillicuddy-DeLisi, A. V. (1982b). The relationship between parents' beliefs about development and family constellation, socioeconomic status, and parents' teaching strategies. In L. M. Laosa & I. E. Sigel (Eds.), *Families as learning environments for children* (pp. 261–299). New York: Plenum Press.

McGillicuddy-DeLisi, A. V. (1985). The relationship between parental beliefs and children's cognitive level. In I. E. Sigel (Ed.), *Parental belief systems: The psychological consequences for children* (pp. 7–24). Hillsdale, NJ: Erlbaum.

McGillicuddy-DeLisi, A. V. (1992). Parents' beliefs and children's personal–social development. In I. E. Sigel, A. V. McGillicuddy-DeLisi, & J. J. Goodnow (Eds.), *Parental belief systems: The psychological consequences for children* (2nd ed., pp. 115–142). Hillsdale, NJ: Erlbaum.

McGillicuddy-DeLisi, A. V., & Sigel, I. E. (1982). Family constellation and parental beliefs. In G. L. Fox (Ed.), *The childbearing decision: Fertility attitudes and behavior* (pp. 161–177). Beverly Hills, CA: Sage.

McGillicuddy-DeLisi, A. V., & Sigel, I. E. (1995). Parental beliefs. In M. H. Bornstein (Ed.), *Handbook of parenting: Vol. 3. Status and social conditions of parenting* (pp. 333–358). Hillsdale, NJ: Erlbaum.

Miller, S. A. (1988). Parents' beliefs about children's cognitive development. *Child Development, 59,* 259–285.

Mishler, E. G. (1986). *Research interviewing: Context or narrative.* Cambridge, MA: Harvard University Press.

Nisbett, R. E., & Wilson, T. D. (1977). Telling more than we can know: Verbal reports on mental processes. *Psychological Review, 84,* 231–259.

Pepper, S. C. (1970). *World hypotheses: A study in evidence.* Berkeley: University of California Press. (Original work published 1942)

Piaget, J. (1971). *Psychology and epistemology: Toward a theory of knowledge* (A. Rosin, Trans.). New York: Viking Press.

Polanyi, M. (1958). *Personal knowledge: Toward a post-critical philosophy.* Chicago: University of Chicago Press.

Schaefer, E. S., & Bell, R. Q. (1958). Development of a parental attitude research instrument. *Child Development, 29,* 339–361.

Sears, R. R. (1965). Comparison of interviews with questionnaires for measuring mothers' attitudes toward sex and aggression. *Journal of Personality and Social Psychology, 2,* 37–44.

Sigel, I. E. (1982). The relationship between parents' distancing strategies and the child's cognitive behavior. In L. M. Laosa & I. E. Sigel (Eds.), *Families as learning environments for children* (pp. 47–86). New York: Plenum Press.

Sigel, I. E. (1985). A conceptual analysis of beliefs. In I. E. Sigel (Ed.), *Parental belief systems: The psychological consequences for children* (pp. 345–371). Hillsdale, NJ: Erlbaum.

Sigel, I. E. (1986). Reflections on the belief–behavior connection: Lessons learned from a research program on parental belief systems and teaching strategies. In R. D. Ashmore & D. M. Brodzinsky (Eds.), *Thinking about the family: Views of parents and children* (pp. 35–65). Hillsdale, NJ: Erlbaum.

Sigel, I. E. (1991). Representational competence: Another type? In M. Chandler & M. Chapman (Eds.), *Criteria for competence: Controversies in the conceptualization and assessment of children's abilities* (pp. 189–207). Hillsdale, NJ: Erlbaum.

Sigel, I. E. (1992). The belief–behavior connection: A resolvable dilemma? In I. E. Sigel, A. V. McGillicuddy-DeLisi, & J. J. Goodnow (Eds.), *Parental belief systems: The psychological consequences for children* (pp. 433–456). Hillsdale, NJ: Erlbaum.

Sigel, I. E., Flaugher, J., LaValva, R., Redman, M., & Sander, J. (1987). *Manual for Parent–Child and Family Interaction Observation Schedule.* Princeton, NJ: Educational Testing Service.

Sigel, I. E., Flaugher, J., Redman, M., Sander, J., & Stinson, E. T. (1986). *Manual for Parent Belief Construction/Communication Strategy Interview.* Princeton, NJ: Educational Testing Service.

Sigel, I. E., & McGillicuddy-DeLisi, A. V. (1984). Parents as teachers of their children: A distancing behavior model. In A. D. Pellegrini & T. D. Yawkey (Eds.), *The development of oral and written language in social contexts* (pp. 71–92). Norwood, NJ: Ablex.

Sigel, I. E., McGillicuddy-DeLisi, A. V., & Goodnow, J. (Eds.). (1992). *Parental belief systems: The psychological consequences for children* (2nd ed.). Hillsdale, NJ: Erlbaum.

Sigel, I. E., McGillicuddy-DeLisi, A. V., & Johnson, J. E. (1980). *Parental distancing, beliefs and children's representational competence within the family context* (ETS RR 80–21). Princeton, NJ: Educational Testing Service.

Sigel, I. E., Stinson, E. T., & Flaugher, J. (1991). Socialization of representational competence in the family: The distancing paradigm. In L. Okagaki & R. J. Sternberg (Eds.), *Directors of development: Influences on the development of children's thinking* (pp. 121–144). Hillsdale, NJ: Erlbaum.

Sigel, I. E., Stinson, E., & Kim, M. (1993). Socialization of cognition: The distancing model. In R. Wozniak, & K. W. Fischer (Eds.), *Development in context: Acting and thinking in specific environments* (pp. 211–224). Hillsdale, NJ: Erlbaum.

Stinson, E. T. (1989). *Parental ideology: Implications for child academic achievement and self-concept.* Unpublished doctoral dissertation. Philadelphia: University of Pennsylvania.

Woodcock, R. W., & Johnson, M. B. (1978). *Psycho-educational Battery.* Hingham, MA: Teaching Resources.

## PART TWO

# THE NATURE AND ORIGINS OF PARENTS' CULTURAL BELIEF SYSTEMS

# CHAPTER 5

# Essential Contrasts
## Differences in Parental Ideas about Learners and Teaching in Tahiti and Nepal

Robert I. Levy

For any ethnographic study concerned with the relations of historical and communal forms, on the one hand, and the private lives and worlds of individuals, on the other, adult ideas and fantasies about children are centrally interesting. They illuminate much about adults' orientations, motivations, fears, and hopes more clearly, often, than do discussions of other areas of adult life. At the same time, they illuminate a governing aspect of the field of forces and forms that shape children's experience and influence much of their psychological development.

When adults' ideas about children in different sorts and segments of communities are compared with each other, other issues are highlighted. Thus, I assume that the dramatic contrasts in teaching and learning in the two very different kinds of communities I will portray are, in some aspects, *proper* to communities of their kinds. Those contrasts are, so to say, induced by their contexts. This assertion might lead us to expect that "similar types" of communities (similar in one or another set of contextual features) may well share similar features of parental conception and practice.

I shall be concerned in this chapter with the aged sociological and anthropological contrast between relatively simple communities (simple in ways that always need to be specified) and relatively complex ones. The two communities in which I have worked, Piri and Bhaktapur, have, as we shall shortly see, great contrasts in many dimensions of complexity.

## Some Methodological Qualifications

It is important to recall some of the frequent biases of most anthropological studies of child development before turning to this one, which shares many of them. Such studies have tended to be preoccupied with a *subset* of learning and development that was thought to be the precursor of those particular adult behaviors in which the anthropology of the time was interested. Those particular aspects of learning and development were interesting to the anthropologist because they were thought to support adult "social behavior" (this sort of learning has been called "socialization"), or else to provide problems for it (an aspect that was of interest to psychodynamically oriented anthropologists and should now be of interest for contemporary concerns with contesting and subaltern cultural forms). Anthropologists have not been interested in childhood experience in itself, experience of importance to the child as child, but rather as a precursor of some chosen things to come. Furthermore, as anthropologists have almost always been interested in the differential features that characterize the communities they have happened to study (those communities' particular history, social organization, economy, ecological setting, etc.) they have, in looking at children's learning, emphasized (as this present chapter does) variation and difference from other communities rather than possible universals or widely shared features in development.

Another problem for anthropologists studying learning and development has been how to theorize what they studied. Anthropologists have hesitated between using some one powerful borrowed theory (a theory usually based on particular cohorts of Western children) and using bits and pieces of assorted theories in a "clinical" approach to their observations in the field. There was a third choice, which was to try to generate a theory of learning and development specific to anthropological interests, methods, and materials. Some strong efforts were made in the 1930s and 1940s by "patterns of culture" theorists, among others, most notably, perhaps, Margaret Mead and Gregory Bateson.[1] But since then, there has been little development of a specifically anthropological theory of what might be called "anthropological learning."[2]

If one is concerned about the relation of childhood learning to the shapes of community and adult life, there is considerable circularity in our assertions. Working from both directions—childhood experience up and adult behaviors down—we should not be too surprised that they seem to fit. But our connections should be plausible, and the data we are observing rich and properly placed in context, and informed, ideally, by a strong "intuitive" sense of things. We need also to be aware that the specific way a particular element or aspect of learning enters into the ecology of adult mind so that it affects particular adult behaviors in particular contexts is a centrally important problem whose neglect may lead to naive accounts.[3]

## The Ethnographic Context:
## Simple Places and Complicated Ones

It is necessary here to introduce two different communities, sketching and simplifying the features that will serve as a context for the particular aspects of adult conception and childhood learning experience I am concerned with here.[4]

Piri, where I did my first ethnographic studies, was a very small Tahitian-speaking Polynesian village community, which, in the autumn of 1962, had 284 people living in 54 thatch-roofed houses whose walls were constructed of wooden planks and bamboo. Piri's economy was based primarily on fishing and horticulture. Its people lived their lives, for the most part, within the context of the village and its immediate surroundings. At the time of my work, a motor launch circled the island on which Piri was located two or three times a day, connecting its widely separated lagoon-side villages with each other and the port town. But in the youth of many of the village's people, they were able to go from one village to another only by walking over the intervening arms of the extinct volcano that had formed the island, or by laboriously paddling an outrigger canoe. The village's culture was a variety of the widespread Pacific Polynesian culture, modified by a missionary Christianity, which the islanders had been able to adapt to their purposes, and by French colonial political forms.

Bhaktapur, in Nepal, a country that had never been colonized by Europe, was a very different kind of place. Located in the Kathmandu Valley, Bhaktapur had once been the center of its own small city–state as well as the principal royal center of the valley's many towns and villages. Its culture was Newar, the 2,000-year-old, literate, high Asian culture of the Kathmandu Valley. Bhaktapur had been for at least 800 years, as it was still at the time of my study, a society and culture of enormous social and cultural complexity. Its 40,000 people, inhabiting for the most part four-story, brick-walled, tile-roofed houses, lived in an area of about one-third of a square mile, and thus in a remarkable density of more than 100,000 people per square mile. Their economic life was based on a complex and rich agricultural production that had—along with the valley's strategic position on trade routes between India and Tibet—facilitated, from the first centuries of the Common Era, the flourishing of a rich culture and civilization.

Bhaktapur's people are organized into some 340 clan-like heredi-tary units, organized in turn into 20 hierarchical levels. Clan and level determine much of the occupational life, public religious roles, patterns of interaction, and lifestyles of the men and women born into them. The city's religious life—one greatly different in extent, significance, and use from both Piri and the modern West—is central to its overall organization. The city has a pantheon of some 26 different deities (each bearing a different symbolic meaning and put to different personal and civic uses), intricately interrelated sacralized spatial divisions (each with *its* own differentiated meaning, associated with and determining the residence of clans and hierarchical groups, as well as much economic and ritual activity), and a complex and dense calendrical cycle of festivals and rituals that serve to interrelate pantheon, space, time, and status. Bhaktapur may be taken to be representative of a class of cities, for the most part long gone, that Redfield and Singer (1954) called "administrative–cultural" cities, "which carry forward, develop, and elaborate a long-established local culture or civilization. They are cities that convert the folk culture into its civilized dimension" (p. 57). Such cities strive toward cultural and social integration. They are nothing like the large heterogeneous communities usually associated with the term "city," which induce, in comparison, as Redfield and Singer put it, "different states of mind" in their members than those of the "administrative–cultural" ones.

How are people coordinated into the community orders of the different sorts of places represented by Piri and Bhaktapur? I have argued that in Piri, and in many places that were once like it in its smallness and isolation (an isolation not so much from other commu-nities but from other *kinds* of communities),[5] much community order is maintained by the detailed local construction of widely shared interpretations, classifications, values, and ways of attending to and organizing perceptions and behaviors—in short, by means of a set of commonly held convictions, an imperious common sense about the way the village world and village people are and should be. The small scale of the community and its relative isolation not only make such consen-sus possible, but make it possible for it to be effective as an instrument of communal integration. In a very small and stable community, people know who each individual is and how he or she should be acting. They respond dependably to deviations through techniques of face-threaten-ing disapproval that are painful and effective. An intense, structured, small theater of the everyday constantly defines and reconstructs local reality. This sociocultural reality has a hardness approximating physical reality, where any attempt to walk through a wall will dependably remind people that they must use doors.

In Bhaktapur, culturally shaped face-to-face orientations and integrations exist, of course, but in limited arenas of city life. The problem, and the essential difference from Piri, is in the relation of these integrations—adequate to household, family, and urban neighborhood—to the larger city. Bhaktapur as an urban whole is too big and too complex for the community-integrating devices that are useful to Piri's village order. The lives of its various component units are too differentiated one from the other and too secret, carefully hidden from the other units of the community. Beyond the household and village-like neighborhood, people in Bhaktapur must learn from, be affected by, and relate to a great variety of larger urban components, which demand proper behavior and orientations and constitute a larger highly integrated urban order. Having learned to attend to shifting and different urban realities, deprived of the useful certainties of Piri's kind of culturally specific common sense, people in Bhaktapur must be integrated into the greater order of their city in a different way than are the people of Piri into their small village. In Bhaktapur, a resource that is used in Piri only on very limited and special occasions is greatly elaborated. I have called this resource "marked symbolism," the kind of symbolism that calls attention to itself as belonging to one or another special realm other than the realm of "ordinary" life by virtue of its dramatically "extraordinary" spatial arenas, practitioners, doctrines, and forms. "Marked symbolism" must be differentiated from the "embedded symbolism" of "ordinary reality," which is a dominant integrative force in Piri, a symbolism that is hidden and naturalized as part of that reality. Extremely compelling and extraordinary marked symbolic resources, derived for the most part from South Asian Hinduism, are employed as a system of "messages" to organize and maintain a very large component of the urban life of Bhaktapur and forcibly to engage individuals with it. Status, space, pantheon, and time are intricately divided, bounded, and interrelated through such devices. These elements of the city's structure are brought together in rituals and festivals, coordinated for the city as a whole through its annual festival calender, and for families' internal purposes through a multitude of developmental rites of passage. The city's symbolic enactments combine in a complex ongoing performance that is esthetically fascinating, intellectually instructive, and emotionally compelling, to induce a sort of dance of civic order. If one knows a person's surname (the designator of his or her clan), his or her age and sex, the day of the lunar calendar (for some purposes, the solar calendar), and where the person lives in Bhaktapur, one has a good chance of knowing where he or she is, what he or she is doing, what he or she is learning or reaffirming, and something of what he or she is experiencing in his or her private thoughts and feelings.

The conditions of life in Bhaktapur are very different from Piri's. To return to the theme of this chapter, those different conditions provide the context of possibilities, constraints, and tasks generating each community's traditional informal and formal education and its "socializers'" governing assumptions.

# Learning by Oneself:
## Ideas about Teaching and Learning in Piri

In both Piri and Bhaktapur, in the course of lengthy sets of interviews exploring a wide range of subjects, I asked respondents about their own and their children's childhoods. How, in a bird's-eye view, do people in the village of Piri think children learn and, thus, how they must be taught? We may note that "how parents think about children" conflates at least two different matters. One—most characteristic of my statements about Piri—is an outside analyst's inference about some "idea" or "principle" underlying parental discussions, a principle that may not be overtly stated (or, indeed, statable) by respondents as a dictum or rule. The other meaning, more characteristic of Bhaktapur than of Piri, is an overt rule formulated by respondents themselves of the sort "children learn in such and such a way, and this is what must be done to teach them," a doctrine that may well have problematic relations to actual practices. The relative overtness or covertness of ideas and rules (as well as their relations to various practices) are issues of obvious importance for exactly what is really being learned and how it is being learned.

Using for present purposes a mixture of overtly stated doctrines, the contexts and patterns in which those doctrines are expressed, and observations of parent–child interactions, we may make certain assertions about elders' conceptions of children in Piri. Children, it is believed, learn to perform tasks, for the most part, by themselves, in accordance with the gradual maturational unfolding of their abilities. Differences in achievements among children are due to differences in their inner natures. No one teaches them very much. They learn by watching and by playful trial and error that the adults often find amusing but sometimes annoying. The trial and error takes place, usually, at the edges of adult arenas where the task to be learned is often going on. Sometimes it is necessary to correct children verbally in more complicated or dangerous tasks—"no, that is *wrong*, do it this way"—for the child captures adult corrective attention mainly when it makes what parents take to be one of a comparatively limited class of mistakes. The child will do whatever it needs to do when it is eventually "mature" enough. There is nothing much an adult can do to initiate or encourage an activity (as opposed to correcting one that is already well under way). And there is little an adult can do if a child "can" but does not "want" to do something. This does not mean that a child should be ignored. In Piri a miseducated child is one who is "overindulged" and "spoiled." Elders through "too much love" or through negligence have failed to correct the child's errors, and the child becomes too willful, uncooperative, and stubborn. But corrected or not, the child achieves mastery by itself. In a learning situation—as opposed to a simple direct command—to tell a child what to do (as opposed to the occasional what *not* to do), to tell anybody what to do, is intrusive and taken as a sign of unjustified adult mood-driven irritability and impatience.

When asked about the teaching of various specific skills, people say children learn to talk, crawl, walk, and control their sphincters "by themselves." "What do you do to get children to stop bed wetting?" I asked. "Nothing. They stop. There is no medicine. I don't tease them or yell. You can't yell because this is a child's nature. He doesn't know good behavior. He doesn't know he should go outside." People wait and express their culturally unjustified disapproval in various covert ways. When, finally, children are assumed to "know" what to do and how to do it, caretakers may shame them or threaten them for continuing some undesirable behavior. (These shamings and threatenings and other prevalent sanctions used in a particular community have their own local shapes and consequences; see Levy, 1973, p. 446ff.)

Other necessary skills, such as talking, crawling and walking, are similarly said to "just happen." "We don't instruct children in walking, we just let a child alone and he walks." Asked about horticultural techniques, a father says of his sons, "I just let them watch. When they are ready, they will do the work." Both teachers and learners emphasize the child's watching. Through watching and, apparently, the "internal rehearsal" of an activity, as well as through trial and error, the child eventually comes to understand it, and to know how to do it. One entailment of this sort of learning is that what the child watches is a complex activity that is embedded in a "real" context, not an activity artificially separated off as "learning" or "education."[6] Modernized urban Tahitians, who must teach more actively and must prepare children for new kinds of tasks, think of these ideas and practices as rural and old-fashioned village practices. As an urban Tahitian schoolteacher commented of village families, "In Papeete [the main urban center of the territory] people encourage weaning by putting bitter substances on their breasts. Here [in the village] they are helpless and let them nurse as long as they want to. In Papeete [in contrast to here] parents *teach* their children to walk. They *help* them talk correctly. They have to get them ready for school."

The old Tahitian stance toward children (still characteristic of distant villages like Piri) looked to European observers, as it does to modern urban Tahitians, like helpless "tolerance" or "indulgence," or "passivity," or "neglect." As the British missionary William Ellis remarked at the beginning of the 19th century, "They are too tender towards their children and do not exercise that discipline and control over them which the well-being of the child and the happiness of the parent requires" (1830, Vol. 1, p. 343).

Reminiscences of their own childhood by Tahitian men suggested the effects on children of these parental orientations. (Tahitian female respondents emphasized independent learning somewhat less, and credited their mothers with having taught them many of their necessary household tasks.) They insisted that they had learned how to do life's tasks by themselves, by watching and by thinking things out. And, although they noted that parents occasionally usefully pointed out mistakes, they generally perceived caretakers' interventions as unpleasant and unneeded interferences and intrusions, typically generated by bad moods in the caretakers rather by than any desire to be really helpful.

In the face of such guiding libertarian orientations, Piri's educators' instructional activities are often disguised. They include signals of disapproval and impatience submerged in the general doctrine of tolerance. The child is manipulated in subtle (and, as far as I was able to ascertain, generally quite unconscious) ways to control his willfulness and to make him, ideally, timid, so that his sense of independence is tempered by caution, by a sense of the limits of the effectiveness of that will that parents and others find difficult to deal with. Although he follows—he will say—his own thoughts and desires, those thoughts and desires, fortunately from the point of view of the life of the village, usually turn out to be mysteriously congruent with the needs of his small equalitarian community.

# Learning from Others:
## Ideas about Teaching and Learning in Bhaktapur

In the enormously complex, hierarchically organized city of Bhaktapur, discourse about teaching and learning is strikingly different from Piri's. In Bhaktapur, everything seems to have to be taught and learned, and the rules and techniques for teaching are quite overt and widely shared.

People talk like this: The speaker is a young man, a member of a merchants' caste, reminiscing about his own childhood. "Our brother or elder sister, or other older people in the house, they just got hold of our hands and they used to say, '*tāchi, tāchi*' ['walk' in 'children's language']. They would get hold of our legs, pulling step by step. They would teach us how to stand on the ground with two legs, and they would just put us near the wall, so that the child might stand with the help of the wall . . . and then the child learns standing, and he will gradually walk." Children, he says, have also to be taught urination, defecation, and eating. "We give a bowl to the child and we teach the child to eat."

The speaker is from a particular social level, but such accounts are given by everyone, by people whose lives and hereditary status as Brahmans, aristocrats, merchants, farmers, musicians, potters, butchers, untouchables, and so on differ greatly in many other respects. To take an example from the very bottom of the status system, an untouchable informant tells how babies are taught to crawl, walk, stand up, excrete, and eat. His parents, he says, taught the children to sit up by piling up blankets and placing children against them. Babies, he says, are taught to walk by parents holding their hands. Sometimes the elders hold a stick for the child to grasp to help it stand. Elders, he says, "make the children stand up, and say to their children, '*phātā, phātā*' ['walk, walk']." When the child starts to walk, he says, the parents tell the child, "Don't do it like that; you will fall down and be hurt. Be careful." If the parents are away working, which is common in low-status households, teaching is the responsibility of older siblings, if there are any, for someone has to teach the children. "The parents are very busy with their work and do not have much time to teach the child how to walk." If children have no one to teach them, "such children walk very late." But when teaching is adequate the children "learn to say '*phātā, phātā*,' and quickly start to walk. They learn how to walk earlier [than children without siblings] because they have many older sisters and brothers. They teach their baby brother or sister how to walk. 'Let us walk, darling,' the elder brother or sister says to the child, and makes the child walk."

A very high-status English-speaking informant makes the parents' responsibility explicit. He has given the usual extensive list of elders' tasks and techniques. I ask him why they have to teach such things as crawling and walking, for example. "If we did not teach him [he has been talking of his son], it would be hard for him to acquire the technique of walking and all this [sort of thing] . . . that is why we need to train him." He then goes on to talk of a child, a girl, who is slow in learning to talk because her parents did not teach her properly.

In Bhaktapur the untaught child would be incompetent not only in his or her physical skills but in his or her moral nature. As one man put it, "Unless parents control and educate children, children will have bad characters." And, another, "If father had not disciplined me I would be a thief, or have died in an accident." In Bhaktapur the "natural man" is not only inadequate in his skills but morally problematic. In Tahiti, the child who learns by itself "naturally" achieves both task and moral competence. If the child turns out to be "bad," there are various explanations, but not usually because of failure in his or her education.

In Bhaktapur this idea of a child's dependency for its development on the active participation of its superiors is gradually extended beyond the household to the extended family, to the city as a whole, and to the realm of the urban deities. There are, for example, certain deities who are necessary for the child's normal development and for his or her successful learning. There are also special deities and rituals for those who have problems in development and learning. These deities are not only necessary for the original phases of learning, but for the successful continuing performance of learned tasks, and their worship is a regular aspect of the annual religious cycle and of many rites of passage, as well as of ad hoc worship. The elaborate series of rites of passage that all people undergo has as one of its implications the progressive entry of the developing individual into wider and wider circles of dependency on progressively wider segments of the community beyond the household. The maturing boy or girl looks to these expanding segments for instruction in new kinds of moral and interpersonal responsibilities, for information about caste vocational and religious specialities, for information about proper behavior, and for instructions as to how to orient himself or herself to each of the various segments of the complex and community-integrating religious sphere.

## Differences in Parental Verbalization in Bhaktapur and Piri

As these excerpts indicate, in Bhaktapur verbalization by elders, and eventually by the child, is an important part of these accounts. This emphasis is ubiquitous. Here are some examples.

A farming woman asked about excretion control, answers this way: "'It is not right to urinate [freely]. . . . It is not right to defecate [freely],' the mother tells the child. 'Let us go out to defecate.'" Or, she goes on, "The child may come to say, 'I have to urinate.' Now he knows to tell us to take him out."

Asked about the teaching of eating, she begins, "I say, 'Eat rice,' [*hāpu*, children's language] grandmother will give you a plate.' Then he will take it and eat. Then he will learn. Then, holding a dish he will say, 'Let me have rice.' After he begins his third year [i.e., at his second birthday] he will know how to ask for rice."

A mid-caste man puts it, "They always used to repeat the same words, and they made us practice. When we were put in the latrine they used to say '*āchi yagu, āchi yagu*' ['defecate!' in children's language]. They used to teach the same words [repeatedly] and we learned very rapidly."

The untouchable respondent, whom I quoted earlier on standing and walking, says of urination control, "When the baby is 6 months the mother sits the baby on her feet [making a kind of seat] and says 'make *susu*' [urine, in children's language]. After a few months the child comes to understand what that means." And, "Teaching the child to eat rice, the mother says to the child, '*hamu ya, hamu ya*' ['eat, eat' in children's language]."

A very low-caste informant talking of how crawling is taught says, "A toy is placed on the ground, and the parents say, 'Come on, boy, take the toy.'" And on standing: "People stand the child against a wall, saying, 'Let us see, baby, if you can stand.'"

Proper language use, the child's ability to understand and to use verbal signals in relation to a task, is in Bhaktapur an overt component of mastery. The farming woman quoted previously, in an extended fantasy about the future of her baby boy, her first child, says, "When my darling has entered his second or third year he will know about urinating. He will know that it is not the proper thing to do to urinate. 'Mother, I need to urinate,' he will say. In his second year he will know our language. . . . Then when I say 'don't be dirty' he will understand." He will come to achieve not so much "self-control" as the ability to understand and respond to, to manipulate and be manipulated by, a mobile realm of discursive symbols. He is being taught to attend to the constructed set of directives and marked symbols that integrate the city.

People retrospectively associate their own development of mastery with language. Thus the man from a merchant's caste quoted earlier says, "They used to teach us how to say [it] when we needed to urinate. They used to teach us the words 'do *susu*.'" He stopped wetting the bed, he says, at 2 or 2½ as "after that, then I knew to say that I wanted to urinate. I learnt to say it." He adds another important point. If he then continued to wet the bed occasionally his elders would say, "You fool," in part because he should now have overcome bed wetting, but in part because he has failed to ask others for help.

In Bhaktapur, people believe that everything must be taught to children, and that there are proper techniques for so doing. Added to this conviction is the emphasis on talk of a certain sort, what we may call "instructional language." The child is being taught not only what the language says, but to attend to words, and word-like forms.

It may be useful at this point to provide a summary list of some features of instructional language that differ in Piri and in Bhaktapur:

1.  The use of directive discursive language (in contrast to talk to others about the child, or chit-chat and expressive noises directed to the child) is ubiquitous in Bhaktapur and rare in Piri.

2.  Tahitian parental directive verbal interventions when they do occur are largely negative: "Don't do this or that." Bhaktapurian interventions—prior to the time when the child is thought to have tentatively mastered an action—are ideally positive: "Do it like this."

3.  When negative interactions are used, as they are in Bhaktapur after some mastery is assumed, they are more likely in Bhaktapur than in Piri to be given an overtly moral form. "It is not right to do that," rather than "Don't do that."

4.  As several of the examples I have given indicate, in Bhaktapur, in contrast to Piri where there is no special children's language, Bhaktapurian talk to children is to a considerable degree in a special vocabulary. The first extensive English–Newari dictionary (compiled by a Newar: Manandhar, 1976)[7] lists a large number of words designated "child talk." It is not only their presence in large numbers in the dictionary that is interesting, but the fact that the lexicographer assumed that it was important to include such terms in the proper description of Newari vocabulary. It is important to note that these words are often not, in any obvious way, simpler than the standard terms they replace. For example, the word for meat is *lā* in adult language, *cici* in children's language. Milk, *duru*, is *tutu* in children's language. Cooked rice is *wā* in adult language, *hāpu* in children's language. That is, the different vocabulary seems motivated by something more than a simplified baby talk. A special children's vocabulary changing to a standard vocabulary as the young child matures is the earliest example of a pervasive and consequential "code switching" that characterizes social action in Bhaktapur. "Code" is being split from "content" and "message," and is made interesting in itself.

5.  In Bhaktapur, in contrast to Piri, the ability to use and understand talk is understood to be an essential part of training and a condition of task mastery.

## Some Developmental Consequences of Differences of Parental Ideas and Practices in Piri and Bhaktapur

I have noted some striking contrasts between Piri and Bhaktapur in elders' ideas about how children learn and develop and, therefore, how they have to be taught; in the use of positive techniques versus negative ones; in the relative quantities of learning embedded and disguised in the ordinary flow of community life versus the quantities separated out of that flow as a special activity; and in the playing down, on the one hand, and the massive emphasis, on the other, of parental use and children's mastery of "instructive talk" as essential tools in teaching. I have also emphasized the peculiarity in Bhaktapur of the use of a special children's vocabulary as a special "code" that will later be switched to a new one. I assume that these differences in elders' ideas and practices in the two places have different consequences for what children learn in each place, consequences of anthropological interest not so much in *how* they affect directly the way a particular skill is learned, but in their educational implications across a variety of specific concrete tasks for very general psychological orientations.[8]

### Piri

Piri's elders' conceptions of children's natures and their allied teaching practices are the result of the history and present realities of that village, and contribute through their educational effects to the further development of that history and the maintenance of those village realities. The effect of what is learned under the guidance of village conceptions of children on an individual's later behaviors and "inner being" are diffuse. I have been emphasizing contrasts in conception and practice between Piri and Bhaktapur, and we can now suggest briefly and very approximately some of the contrasting implications of those difference for such "psychological" forms as thinking, fantasy, self, and morality in the two places.

Local ideas about the outer world and the inner self are, of course, logically interrelated. The outer world, the environing village world of Piri, is mediated to learners (in comparison to Bhaktapur), principally through their observation of its culturally shaped but apparently "natural" non-verbal forms, which are woven into the basic given realities of the perceived environment, reinforced by "negative" comments (comments on error) from adults. The social dimensions of the outer world are (as I have argued in the sections on child development in Levy, 1973) mediated to learners through a large and diffuse network of elders, all of whom have very similar messages to impart. Social reality, as we have

earlier, seems to be given and a matter of perceptually based and
irresistible common sense. What Pirians perceive through their senses
as they scan their social and physical worlds is more or less "true" and
dependable, much truer than things mediated to them through verbal
messages, about which they are skeptical. (The word for "to know" in
Tahitian, as in much of Polynesia, is significantly the same as the word
for "to see." And the word for truth is the same as the word for "fixed,"
"unable to change its position.") Information conveyed through language is, unless supported and tested against the primary evidence of
sensory experience, mere hearsay or opinion or fantasy, and is suspect
to concrete and literal villagers. This is in contrast to Bhaktapur, where
language and language-like messages may well convey deeper truths
than does the perception of non-verbal forms.

The hardness of directly perceived, unchallengeable, fixed village
reality is a powerful force for the social stability of the village. The
potentially subversive and transformative power of analytic, logical,
discursive, and, in short, *verbal* thought is muted. People live in a world
where social and physical truths tend to coalesce, and where the fixity
of the social world is evident to the common sense of all sane and
competent observers. This conservative epistemic orientation ("what I
see is real and fixed") is supported by an orientation to the avoidance
of error, a carefulness which in the face of a problem produces a certain
apathy in any problematic encounter with the "outer world." Like the
weather, there is nothing to be done about it. Pirians' relatively early
self-sufficiency also contributes to a sort of closure of the desire for or
the sense of possibility of learning new things, and thus to a sort of
blunting of "intellectual curiosity."

One consequence of the orientation to the sensorially perceived
hardness of the phenomenal sources of their knowledge is an anxious
playing down of the extraordinary realities of the supernatural, of fantasy,
and of imagination (which all belong to what is called in Piri "the realm
of the night")—kinds of alternate realities which are central to Bhaktapur's
communal organization. In contrast to the primitivistic fantasies of
earlier Western concepts about simple pre-modern others, in Piri at least
(and the same was true for Tahiti as described at the time of European
discovery) people were uncomfortable in the presence of the supernatural, and made use of it in very limited, constricted ways, for limited social
purposes. Reality bound, avoiding dream-like and fanciful realms of
thought, people's thought (as illustrated in village discourse, and in
lengthy interviews with me) tended to be (in stark contrast to Bhaktapur)
concretely conveyed, unimaginative, unanalytical, accepting of the given,
and thus, in short, uncreative. This kind of thought worked well for the
social ordering and economic needs of tiny, and ecologically blessed, Piri.

Their learned sense of the nature of the world in which they must operate is reflected, in a complementary way, in Pirians' discourse about "self" and in the "structure" of those selves as modeled by an outside observer on the basis of local discourse and behavior.

In accordance with what they learn about themselves from the conditions of learning generated by the assumptions of their elders, learners come to believe or, better put, to *know*, that their own "inner nature"—their desires, values, capabilities—is relatively fixed at any given time in their life, although they expect it to change automatically and naturally in time (particularly as they reach each of the culturally defined stages of life). Their nature and behavior are not easily affected by others' willful pressures or by their own efforts at self-change or self-control. To "modern" eyes, Piri's villagers seem "fatalistic" and passive but, at the same time, optimistic about the consequences of their passivity.

The sense of a naturally developing "inner nature" is reflected in Piri in discourse about "self." The self (in contrast, as we shall see, with Bhaktapur) is not perceived as problematic or thought provoking. It is a given, something that one must work with, like the physically given state of one's body or one's gender. The ethnographer's question (after he or she has come to know them), "Who are you?" seems bizarre to them, in contrast to the Bhaktapurians who have often already asked themselves that question. Referring action, choices, and decisions to their comparatively unproblematic inner natures or selves, people as far as possible make decisions after their own lights or, when this is not possible, submit, most often ambivalently and tentatively, to some temporary community consensus.[9]

Insofar as learners in Piri come to believe that (1) success or failure is a function of their own being, and (2) that being is a fairly fixed natural entity, there are implications for their moral orientations. The moral problem for such actors is that when they perceive themselves or are perceived by others as having done something socially wrong, as they have simply grown into what they are, as they are doing the best they can with what they are, their failure is taken to be a deficiency in their *being*, like a physical deformity, and they are ashamed. Their sense of self and its relation to its surrounding mental and social world, in contrast to Bhaktapurian experience, does not *comparatively* predispose them to guilt.[10]

When the people of Piri, and Tahitian villagers in general, move into new situations—when they move to modern Tahiti, Europe, or America, or as the village changes around them—it takes a generation or two for the new worlds to affect their village-based sureness, and in the meantime, they appear to others as provincial, and intellectually constricted, simple, stubbornly closed off, simplistically old-fashioned or other-fashioned.

## Bhaktapur

Bhaktapur's elaborate programs for teaching add a superordinate stream of carefully staged instruction to children's direct learning from the ordinary forms of communal life. These instructions are consciously shaped techniques, made use of by highly regarded superiors. They are perceived as essential gifts to otherwise helpless learners, who have to learn to attend carefully to these clearly marked off aspects of their experience. Elders must teach and juniors must learn not at their own tempo but in accord with the schedule of others, a scheduling reflected in the traditional timing of educational rites of passage, marking the times at which a boy or girl must be able to deal with ever more complex tasks and social responsibilities. Where instructional knowledge is in competition with perceptual knowledge, the instructional knowledge is generally judged corrective and superior. It is often said to reveal secrets and that true understanding that allows the learner, often an initiate to new knowledge, to understand the truths his or her perceptions have veiled.

The system of instruction is mobile. New instructors take their turns as children grow older, and people learn different sorts of things, from different but always respected instructors (prototypically a *guru*) in different arenas of their lives. It is essential to note for what is being learned that these different arenas—in contrast with the often chaotic and contradictory or simply mutually irrelevant arenas of modern life—are understood to be all legitimate and coherently interrelated parts of a larger sociocultural unity, elements in a unified game, as, to a large degree, they are.

People's behavior in Bhaktapur suggests that these forms of learning have implications for many aspects of Bhaktapurian orientation and being. I can only suggest here some of their implications for aspects of self, morality, and thought, as accented in contrasts with Piri. Discourse about the self (and arguably the actual structuring of selves) reflects Bhaktapur's doctrinal emphasis on self-constituting external instruction from others—and from shifting others. Thus, when I asked a man in Bhaktapur, after interviewing him for several weeks, "Who are you?" he answers that he and his friends talk about that a good deal. He refers me to a remark of the god, Krishna, that a person is really "everything else." "To a great extent," my respondent goes on, "it seems that I [too] am everything other, because whenever I cook, I am a cook; whenever I love some girl, I am a lover; whenever I have a son or a daughter, I am a parent, I am a father; whenever I am with my father, I am a son; whenever I am alone with a friend, I am a friend; whenever I am with foes, I am an enemy." This is more elegantly put than the remarks on self of many others in Bhaktapur, but the remarks of others consistently tend to suggest, as this quotation does, that self is something that needs to be thought, talked and, perhaps, read about, that it is problematic—not a simple given in the world, and that it is in part at least, a shifting function of present significant relationships as well as of some now fixed past history.

Like discourse about self, moral discourse and orientations also differ from Piri's, in ways that are consonant with differences in teaching and learning and that reflect the problems of selfhood. The emphasis in childhood learning (and life in general) on hierarchical interdependency (allied to doctrines and teaching about the learner's responsibility and indebtedness to the people who have constituted him or her) tend to predisposes someone who has done something "wrong" to guilt, for he or she has through wrongdoing hurt people whom are held in high esteem, and without whose efforts he or she would be nothing.

Some of the most interesting implications of differences in teaching and learning between the two communities would seem to be manifested in aspects of thinking and its expression. The various and shifting sources of knowledge, the emphasis on language (and thus discursively formed thought), and the occasional conflicts and contradictions in different legitimate sources of knowledge all encourage or even require people in Bhaktapur to be discursively thoughtful, to make internal or external logical arguments. This thought is often abstract and analytical, innovative, and creative. Playing freely with the relations and contradictions of different kinds of information, discursive thought often moves beyond cultural doctrine and generates a potentially subversive skepticism, which is then in Bhaktapur brought under social control through a doubt-transcending commitment of faith to the city's integrative religious system. If the social order of Piri can be thought of as largely based on the interactive commonalties of the usually unchallenged common sense of its citizens, in Bhaktapur, where shifting, sophisticated, analytical, and deconstructive thought is common, special and forceful social forms—religious ones—have been developed to bind together such "sophisticated" people, whose solidarity is not and cannot be based on shared common sense about the naturalness of social forms.

Closely associated with the cognitive consequences of this complex calculus of truths and realities of various types, facilitated through not having been taught to limit oneself to a privileged realm of the concrete and the obvious, there is in Bhaktapur a flourishing of a realm of personal and cultural fantasy, of art and literature—attempts to grasp in an extra-discursive manner the ontological complexity of experience in the city. This realm, which is taken to have its own kind of truth, is also the realm of the city's integrative system of marked symbols.

Bhaktapurians having been taught to learn from human authorities, open to such learning, to learning new things, to learning the codes for the behavior proper in different contexts, to reading regulatory signs and signals, are quickly adaptable to life in other societies and cultures, whose rules for proper behavior they quickly grasp and (with the exception of a few taboos) follow. They appear to urbane observers in such places as "sophisticated." And, whatever the losses for their ancient culture, it has been a relatively easy personal move for many of them to an engagement with modern education, advanced study in foreign universities, and active participation in Nepal's modernization.

# Conclusion

The consequences of parental ideas and fantasies about children in Piri and Bhaktapur provide plenty of problems for learners and for their communities; their outcomes are not in any simplistic way directly and unproblematically "functional." Yet by and large they work well in the ordering of Piri's tiny and relatively homogeneous community, on the one hand, and for Bhaktapur's large and very heterogeneous one, on the other. They seem to be essential to those orders. Somehow, one is not surprised by them. They are what one might expect to find in such places. If this is so, we must ask where those ideas and techniques derive from. Some would seem to be direct implications of the forms, structures, and constraints provided by the two contexts. For example, if a family lives in a house with many rooms and stories, a parent must be able to talk a great deal to children who are out of sight, the child must be able to respond dependably, and a great deal of verbal information must be exchanged. Such direct and necessary educational responses to significant features of a particular context are relatively simple and passive, and necessary if the life of the community is to go on at all. But other educational responses (such as Piri's way of controlling aggression by vague threats that "nature" will dependably punish erring children through painful "accidents," rather than through the use of aggression-reinforcing parental punishments; Levy, 1973, Chap. 13) must have been actively arrived at through some long process of trial and error, like so much other useful local knowledge, and worked into local tradition.

These consequences of both the direct implications of context and of useful historical adaptive inventions interact with a wide set of random contingencies, freely creative innovations, accidents, compromises, and stupidities that have lead to the formation of pedagogical traditions in Piri, Bhaktapur, and everywhere else—that is, to the formation of very consequential parental ideas and fantasies about children.

## Notes

1. These are best (and most abstractly) theorized in Gregory Bateson's approaches to learning in his *Steps to an Ecology of Mind* (1972). See particularly the section "Form and Pathology in Relationship." This approach is concretely illustrated in *Balinese Character* (Bateson & Mead, 1942).

2. I have discussed the formally related problem of a specifically anthropological psychiatric theory in an earlier chapter (Levy, 1992).

3. I have discussed Tahitian learning in relation to the complex of controls on aggression in a Tahitian village in an earlier chapter (Levy, 1977).

4. I have described the two communities for the purposes of a general "person-centered ethnography" in two earlier books (Levy, 1973, 1990) and in various articles. Much has changed in the two places since the time of my studies.

5. Those small communities in premodern Melanesia that were embedded in an integrated set of relations with communities of very different languages and cultures generated different forms of community life and "states of mind," characteristically "Melanesian" in many ways, from those small Polynesian communities whose relations were with very similar communities.

6. Some of the comparative effects of such embeddedness in contrast to teaching and learning structured as a separated-off and self-conscious activity are discussed in Levy (1976).

7. This dictionary was later published in a shortened and edited form (Vergati, 1986), which I have not had a chance to compare with the draft.

8. This distinction is related to Gregory Bateson's (1972) ideas about "primary" and "secondary" learning.

9. The implications of this individuality for the delicate task of village leadership is examined in Levy (1973, Chap. 6).

10. See Levy (1973, Chap. 10) for a fuller discussion of "moral behavior" in Piri.

## References

Bateson, G. (1972). *Steps to an ecology of mind.* New York: Ballantine.
Bateson, G., & Mead, M. (1942). *Balinese character.* New York: New York Academy of Sciences.

Ellis, W. (1830). *Polynesian researches* (2 vols.). London: Fisher, Son, & Jackson.

Levy, R. I. (1977). Tahitian gentleness and redundant controls. In A. Montague (Ed.), *The socialization of aggression.* New York: Oxford University Press.

Levy, R. I. (1973). *Tahitians: Mind and experience in the Society Islands.* Chicago: University of Chicago Press.

Levy, R. I. (1976). A conjunctive pattern in middle class informal and formal education. In T. Schwartz (Ed.), *Socialization as cultural communication.* Berkeley: University of California Press.

Levy, R. I. (1990). *Mesocosm: Hinduism and the organization of a traditional Newar city in Nepal.* Berkeley: University of California Press.

Levy, R. I. (1992). A prologue to a psychiatric anthropology. In T. Schwartz, G. White, & C. Lutz (Eds.), *New directions in psychological anthropology.* New York: Cambridge University Press.

Manandhar, T. (1976). *A brief Newari–English dictionary.* Unpublished manuscript, Summer Institute of Linguistics and Institute of Nepal and Asian Studies, Kirtipur, Nepal.

Redfield, R., & Singer, M. (1954). The cultural roles of cities. *Economic Development and Change, 2*(1), 53–73.

Vergati, A. (Ed.). (1986). *Newari–English dictionary.*

CHAPTER 6

# *How Do Children Develop Knowledge?*
## *Beliefs of Tanzanian and American Mothers*

Ann V. McGillicuddy-De Lisi
Subha Subramanian

It was a student from Tanzania . . . who, while chatting about his boyhood, made this statement: "Strange as it may seem, I know more about my childhood now than I ever did. It's hard to believe, but through all these years of moving up through school, managing to do well in one State examination after another, I've felt that the little African boy I used to be has long since disappeared. In secondary school, and particularly now here at Makerere (University in Uganda) where we wear white shirts and speak English all the time, I've been saying to myself, 'Yes, that little boy who herded the goats and skipped down the hill to carry messages for my father is no more; he's gone, completely gone.' But now, you will be glad to hear, I know that isn't so. The little boy I used to be is part of me still, an important part. Many of the ways I now think and look at things that go on around me I can trace back in one way or another to my experiences as that African child."—Fox (1967, p. iv)

This Tanzanian young man tells us that the way he thinks and looks at the world can be traced back to his experiences as an African child. The way he speaks of his world view as connected to his childhood experiences exemplifies our view of the relation of the adult's beliefs to the culture. Beliefs—the way we see the world, what we know to be true—are derived from our experiences as a child and as an adult in a community, in a particular cultural context that has its own history, a history that is shared by all the members of the culture and yet is uniquely connected to each child who develops in that culture. Like the African child inside the adult college student, far removed in time and space from the hills and people of his past, the culture is part of the individual, still, even if the individual never thinks of it as so, or feels that it is part of himself or herself. In this chapter, we will consider parental beliefs about the nature of the child and beliefs about the way children acquire knowledge as one aspect of the "ways one now thinks and looks at things" that is connected to experiences that occur within two different cultural contexts.

These beliefs about the nature of the child and about developmental processes responsible for children's acquisition of knowledge are conceptualized as cognitive and are a result of the individual's own constructions. This approach to beliefs is derived from George Kelly's (1955) theory of personal constructs. Within this framework, individuals form ideas about the nature of the world on the basis of their experiences with people and objects. These constructs are used to interpret events and actions of the self and other people, and to predict future actions. Beliefs are organized so that there is some psychological consistency among them. Beliefs about the nature of the child and developmental processes are predominantly cognitive and are held as fundamental truths by the individual, although values and affect are related to these beliefs (see McGillicuddy-De Lisi & Sigel, 1995).

## The Relation of Belief to Culture

There have been many different views of the relation between culture and individual offered by anthropologists, sociologists, and ethnographers. More recently, social scientists have addressed the more specific question of the relation between culture and beliefs about children. Given the proposition that beliefs about children are constructed on the basis of experience, beliefs necessarily vary with the culture in which such experiences occur. There are at least three ways in which beliefs are related to culture, with the result that both the content and the functioning of beliefs are viewed as inextricable from culture.

For example, specific content of beliefs about developmental timetables, how children develop, and about customs of child care may be adopted ready-made from the culture (Goodnow, 1988). Within this perspective, ideas about children exist externally from the individual and become internalized as the person is socialized in the manner depicted in Figure 6.1. These beliefs are adopted in the manner described as foreclosure in Marcia's (1980) formulation of the develop-

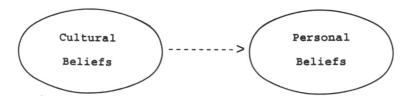

**FIGURE 6.1.** Beliefs copied directly from the culture.

ment of identity. There is little reflection, questioning, or consideration of alternatives. A static process of internalization provides a means for incorporating specific information about children into belief systems, although it is presumed within a constructivist approach that some level of internal organization occurs, integrating old and newly learned information, for example. The internalization of beliefs through socialization leads to specific content that is shared by members of a particular culture who have each been exposed to that content and is not shared by individuals who are socialized into different cultures. This specific content consists of information about children that is presumed to be true, but if these beliefs do not provide an adequate basis for childrearing, as might occur as the culture changes or when special childrearing problems arise in the course of parenting, the content of these beliefs will diminish in usefulness and parenting may become more stressful and difficult.

Lamb and Sternberg (1992) suggest a second perspective on the belief–culture relation that also results in variability in beliefs between cultures and similarities in beliefs within cultures. They propose that social organizations (aspects of cultures) develop within the context of particular human ecologies. Variations in beliefs about children across cultural groups exist to the extent that ecologies and social systems vary. Within this perspective, the culture (or some aspect of the culture) creates particular types of experiences that then lead to beliefs about the nature of the child and development. This process, in which experiences embedded within the culture lead to beliefs of the individual, is depicted in Figure 6.2.

LeVine's (1988) analysis of the relation between parental beliefs and the socioeconomic structure of the society is consistent with this approach. High fertility and careful attention to practices that maximize infant survival are related to the value of child labor in food production in agrarian but not urban–industrial societies. Morelli and Tronick (1991) similarly linked the ways in which farming and foraging communities function to the manner in which child care and beliefs about child development have evolved. Whiting's (1980) notion that constraints imposed by the way of life across different cultures create different parenting styles and different settings for the child is also consistent with this view. In essence, the culture frames the experiences of the members of the culture, and the resulting beliefs therefore reflect the culture. The content of the beliefs varies between cultures (e.g., advantages of multiple caregiving for developmental outcomes in the case of foragers but not farmers) but the functioning is similar across cultures in the sense that the sociocultural system shapes the beliefs (see also Bornstein, Tal, & Tamis-LeMonda, 1991). This process is assumed to operate across cultures and independently of the content of beliefs that parents accept as true about children and their development.

A third view of the relation between culture and beliefs is illustrated by Harkness and Super's (1992a) assertion that beliefs are instantiations of the culture. We do not interpret this to mean that beliefs are derived from the culture, as implied by the first two ap-

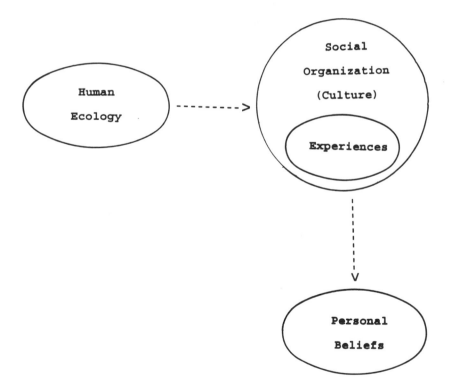

**FIGURE 6.2.** Beliefs shaped by experiences that occur within a particular cultural context.

proaches, but that beliefs *are* the culture. Beliefs cannot be dissociated from the culture, even in an attempt to examine their general content and functioning. The definition of culture in this sense is derived from Blount's (1982) concept of culture as knowledge. The totality of knowledge of the people comprising a society is the culture. The relation of beliefs to culture is transactional, as evidenced by Lightfoot and Valsiner's (1992) description of effects emerging in the course of interactions that occur within a *system* rather than a linear view of culture affecting parents. The system in this case is the individual within the culture, both giving and taking meaning from the culture. The intertwining and indissociability of belief and culture are depicted in Figure 6.3. In this view, beliefs are neither appropriated (copied) nor shaped by particular experiences. Beliefs are constructed through the exchange of social meanings among peoples as individuals integrate personal experiences with their participation in the parenting role suggested by the culture at a particular point in history. Beliefs are constructed out of the transaction of the individual with the social meanings or knowledge that is the culture.

We accept each of these approaches to the culture–belief connection as valid and propose that (1) the specific content of some beliefs

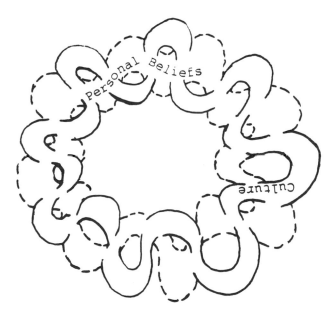

**FIGURE 6.3.** Cultural knowledge and personal beliefs are intertwined and indissociable.

are adopted without transformation directly from the culture; (2) the culture frames experiences that each individual has as a child, as a member of a family and community, and as a parent, and these experiences shape beliefs about children and development; and (3) in the course of transactions between changing individuals and changing cultures, personal and cultural knowledge about children is constructed. Beliefs are therefore the result of at least three processes. Each presumes an intimate connection between the personal knowledge characterized as child development beliefs and the knowledge that is characterized as cultural information. The result of these processes is variation in beliefs between cultures.

In addition, both the individual and the culture are the product of their histories. Each of these histories is significant in the formation of beliefs, as indicated by the Tanzanian college student's insight that his world view can be "traced back in one way or another to my experiences as that African child." The personal history of the individual implies that the intersection between individual and culture has an idiosyncratic effect on beliefs. That is, some points of the intersection with culture are unique and unshared among individuals. Hence, beliefs are personal. On the other hand, there are general shared meanings in the knowledge that is the culture, creating a commonality among the beliefs of individuals that is derived from the knowledge that is historical and greater than that held by a single member of the culture. As a result, the cultural context of beliefs is shared by members of the culture and yet the connection of belief to the culture is personal and unique for each individual.

This sociohistorical aspect of the culture maintains its significance within each of the three ways that culture and personal beliefs intersect (i.e., copied from culture, constructed from experiences that were framed by the culture, and coconstructed through transactions with the culture), in part because developmental niches in which caregiving occurs (see Super and Harkness's [1986] discussion of the developmental niche) evolve in the sociohistorical context of the culture. The beliefs that parents construct in their present lives reflect the experiences of generations before them, as well as their own personal history within the present (construed) culture. Hence it is observed that immigration does not lead to displacement of beliefs from the culture of origin, nor does it lead to a mixing of old and new (Okagaki & Sternberg, 1993; Pomerleau, Malcuit, & Sabatier, 1991). Rather, new models that are consistent with views of development from the culture of origin are observed as parents adapt to new pressures within the framework of cultural and personal histories.

Consideration of sociohistorical factors should not be limited to the study of beliefs of immigrant groups or beliefs of peoples in cultures undergoing rapid and intense change, however. LeVine (1980) suggests that all cultures are disappearing. Each culture requires and reflects adaptations that parents make in beliefs and customs, as individuals both create and adjust to these disappearing cultures. When cultures are studied in relation to parents' ideas about children, the importance of the sociohistorical aspect of the culture is apparent because the culture through which beliefs were constructed has disappeared except as it is observed in those beliefs and practices. The individual and the society can only be understood through consideration of both the culture that was the basis of current knowledge and the culture that is the current knowledge.

For example, LeVine and LeVine (1988) report that Gusii parents of Kenya have adapted their ideas and practices in response to changes such as commercial development, educational reform, and waged employment that have occurred in Kenya. The adaptations reflect the historical social structure, however, which included reliance on and training of child caregivers. Caregiving functions have been transformed as many people now work in the towns and villages for wages, but the framework of shared rearing among kinship groups and child caregivers remains as the starting point for such changes in child care. Similarly, Harkness and Super (1992c) examined trends in child care in a Kipsigis community that is shifting from rural pastoralism to waged employment, increasing emphasis on formal schooling and establishing urban residences. They, too, found that cultural continuities were apparent in the adaptations parents make in both beliefs and practices, although Western cultural ideas of childhood and extrafamilial child care are becoming more apparent as family life has been altered. The employment, schooling, and residential changes in groups such as the Gusii and Kipsigis are similar, but the adaptations that parents make are tied to the history of those groups as much as to the currently occurring changes in their lives.

The importance of the cultural history to the beliefs that organize views of the child is not limited to those cultures that are undergoing major shifts in industrialization, urbanization, education, and so on. Harkness, Super, and Keefer's (1992) analysis of American parenthood revealed that parents in three cohorts living in suburbs of Boston reconstructed historical schemas representing parenthood and family life in terms of the present environment and cultural models. Thus, parents' beliefs about the nature of the child and of child development processes are tied to their sociocultural origins in a general sense and to the current cultural setting in a more specific sense.

As a result of these considerations, we shall examine mothers' beliefs while keeping in mind the current setting and the sociohistorical milieu in which ideas about children developed. We have focused on mothers' beliefs about the processes that are responsible for children's knowledge acquisition in two samples that are very different in cultural history and similar in their advantaged positions within their own societies and in their educational goals for their children. The mothers' beliefs in various developmental processes were examined in relation to ideologies and childrearing customs that have been reported within each culture by various sources, such as anthropological observations, analyses of popular media presentations, ethnographic methods, and so forth. The goal was to explore the meaning of beliefs about children and child development for these mothers within the context of the culture in which the beliefs operate.

## The Research Settings

Mothers' beliefs about children's cognitive development were studied in two different settings that have been described in detail as part of a previous study (McGillicuddy-De Lisi & Subramanian, 1994). One sample consisted of 75 mothers of public elementary school children in a suburban community in the northeastern part of the United States (population about 25,000). Each family had at least one child between 5 and 12 years old who was enrolled in public elementary school. School districts in the state were classified into 1 of 10 categories on the basis of socioeconomic indices of resident citizens. Education, income, occupational status, urbanization, household density, unemployment, and percentage below poverty level were used to define the categories. The school district of the participant families was in the highest category. Nearly all children in the community attended school (there were a small number in home school) and advancement to the secondary level was nearly universal. There were no entrance exams.

All the mothers were white and all but one of the mothers were married. All but one of the children lived with a mother, father, and siblings, most often in a single-family dwelling. Twenty-nine of the mothers worked outside the home in a skilled or professional position. Child care was provided by a nonrelative in these cases, either in the child's home or in a neighborhood home or in a community child-care facility. None of the participant mothers had been born in the community, which is known as an area for young and middle-level executives moving upward through three international companies located in and around the community. Nearly all mothers had a college degree (mean years of education was 16.0) and the mothers were an average of 39.8

years old. The mean number of children in the American families was 2.7, above average for the United States in general. The fathers' average level of education was 17.3 years.

The other sample consisted of 71 mothers from Dar es Salaam, the largest city in Tanzania (population about 4 million). Tanzania is ethnically heterogeneous, with more than 120 tribes, many of which are historically connected with tribes in the other East African countries of Kenya and Uganda. Most of these groups were farmers or herders, practiced polygyny, had patrilineal social structures, and valued children highly, although there was much variability. These ways of life still predominate in the countryside, although urban Tanzanians such as residents of Dar es Salaam are more likely to be monogamous, have smaller families, and have more mothers who are unmarried. Both the rural and urban citizenry are largely literate (1986 National Literacy Test indicated 9.6% illiterate; Carnoy & Samoff, 1990) and there is nearly universal access to primary school. Educational advancement is by examination, and exams are constructed and administered by the government. The educational goals and the political system are both ideologically tied to a socialist system that is derived from Tanzanian collectivist communities, although Arab, British, German, Portuguese, and Asian influence remains as a result of historical political and social events.

All the mothers were native Tanzanians who had at least one child between the ages of 5 and 12 years. More than half the families had relatives who helped care for the children. Child caregivers are common in the countryside of Tanzania, and older siblings and cousins were reported to be responsible for child care for the 33 mothers of Dar es Salaam who worked outside the home. Employed mothers most often worked in shops or business settings. All the children attended the International School of Tanzania (Tanganyika), which serves children of the large expatriate community of Dar es Salaam as well as children of wealthy Tanzanians.

Eighty percent of the Tanzanian mothers were married and 15 were single mothers. The average number of years of education was 14.7, well above average. Mothers' average age was 35.8. The mean number of children in the family was 3.4. The fathers' mean years of formal school was 17.3.

These two samples cannot be equated with respect to socioeconomic status or background because the meaningfulness of demographic characteristics differs across the two groups. However, the families in both samples had selected and had the means to live in affluent communities of their countries. Their children attended schools that were highly regarded and prepared children for higher education (postsecondary level). Fathers and mothers in families from both settings were well educated and fathers held professional and managerial-status jobs. Much of the educational curriculum implemented in the two settings was similar at the time of data collection, although there were some unique aspects to each setting (treatment of history, geography, of seasons, etc., reflected content specific to each country). Instruction occurred in English in both settings. In Tanzania, Swahili was spoken at home, and all mothers were fluent in English as well.

Within the U.S. setting, all families of children in the school district received a letter asking them to volunteer to participate in a study of parental beliefs and children's school achievement. Data regarding school behavior and achievement test scores were also collected from the school district, and these have been reported elsewhere (McGillicuddy-De Lisi, 1992). Questionnaires were mailed to parents who agreed to participate and they were returned by mail.

In Tanzania, mothers were first contacted by telephone. The purpose of the study was explained and if the parent agreed to participate, the child brought the questionnaire home to the mother who returned it with the child to the school.

In both samples, classroom teachers completed a questionnaire that assessed several dimensions of classroom performance and behavior.

## Content of the Questionnaire

The Child Development Questionnaire was constructed to assess the mothers' ideas about the nature of intelligence and the processes that are responsible for cognitive growth in children in general. The questionnaire consisted of 47 items, each of which presented a particular process as responsible for the development of a concept. The processes were taken from a list of definitions compiled on the basis of interviews with 240 American parents (McGillicuddy-De Lisi, 1982b; Sigel & McGillicuddy-De Lisi, 1984). One hundred items representing these processes were distributed to 90 U.S. college undergraduates enrolled in a psychology course, along with definitions of each of seven developmental processes. Students were asked to judge which process each of the items represented. The 47 items comprising the final questionnaire were those items that 99% of the students classified as an instance of the developmental process it represented. The processes were biological, which includes genetics and maturation (6 items); observational learning/imitation (5 items); verbal didactic instruction (8 items);

experimentation by the child (6); active cognitive processing (7); absorption from the environment (8); and reinforcement/punishment (6). An example of items representing each of the seven processes is presented in Table 6.1. There was no opportunity to gather preliminary data from a similar Tanzanian sample of parents and the same questionnaire was used for both American and Tanzanian mothers.

Mothers in each national group were asked to indicate the extent of their agreement or disagreement with each of the 47 statements using a 6-point Likert-type scale (1 = strongly disagree; 6 = strongly agree). A score for belief in each process was obtained by summing over the items that corresponded to each process. Thus, each mother received 7 scores, each representing the mother's degree of agreement that the particular process is responsible for the child's development of

**Table 6.1.** Example of Questionnaire Items Representing Each of Seven Developmental Processes

Biological processes

"Some children are born smarter than others"
"Children with different natures seek out different experiences"

Absorption

"Adults should set up situations in which a child can easily learn"
"Children are motivated to seek experiences that help them to learn"

Didactic instruction

"Verbal instruction is a source of the child's knowledge"
"Children develop an understanding of certain concepts when those
    concepts are explained"

Reinforcement

"The praise that children get from adults is a reason that they learn new
    concepts"
"Children want to acquire knowledge to avoid disapproval from adults"

Cognitive processing

"Children make inferences about the world they see and these form the basis
    of their concepts"
"Children figure ideas out on their own"

Experimentation/discovery

"Children learn through trial and error"
"Children develop concepts by trying out ideas in their play"

Observation

"Children learn by seeing and hearing"
"Copying other people is a way that children learn"

knowledge. Cronbach alpha internal consistency estimates ranged from .35 to .74 for the Tanzanian sample (mean = .69) and from .53 to .75 for the U.S. sample (mean = .74). These estimates suggest that the internal consistency reliability of the questionnaire as a whole was moderate and acceptable.

In addition, each child's teacher was asked to complete the Classroom Behavior Inventory (Schaefer & Edgerton, 1978). The teacher responded to 42 descriptions of child behavior, using a 5-point scale to indicate the degree to which each child in the sample displayed each behavior. The child then received a total score for each of 10 behaviors by summing the teacher ratings over the items that represented each behavior (e.g., intelligent behavior and creative behavior) Cronbach alphas for the Tanzanian sample ranged from .58 to .90 (mean = .78). For the American sample, the range was from .71 to .94 (mean = .85).

## Mothers' Ideas about Intellectual Development

The mothers in the American sample and the mothers in the Tanzanian sample were similar to one another in the educational choices and educational aspirations they held for their children and in their ability to act on those choices relative to other mothers in their societies who were not so advantaged. They chose to send their children to schools that prepare them for postsecondary education and they indicated to researchers that they held high educational goals for their children. We assume that cultural bases of mothers' beliefs occur similarly in both samples in the sense that the process connecting cultural knowledge and personal knowledge operates similarly in these two groups. In spite of similar goals and educational aspirations for their children, we expected that the specific content of mothers' beliefs about the development of their children would differ in ways that reflect and are inseparable from the history and current culture in which those beliefs function today. As a result of these assumptions, the presentation of data relative to mother's beliefs is divided into two parts. First, the content of beliefs within each culture is explored separately for the Tanzanian and for the American mothers in order to examine which processes were seen as more and less responsible for the child's intellectual development within each sample. Second, the beliefs in each of the seven developmental processes are compared between mothers from the two countries. After the content of beliefs has been explored both within and between such beliefs and teacher evaluations of their children's school performance is examined in a separate section.

## Examination of Beliefs of Mothers from Two Cultures

### Mothers from Tanzania

The Tanzanian mothers indicated the strongest beliefs in three very different development processes: (1) biological processes, (2) absorption, and (3) didactic instruction. The mean (and *SD*) level of agreement of Tanzanian mothers with each of the seven developmental processes that were included in the questionnaire is presented in the left portion of Table 6.2. Given that the highest rating was 6, the Tanzanian mothers gave a high level of endorsement to these three processes as responsible for children's knowledge acquisition (average ratings higher than 4.6 for these three processes; see Table 6.2).

The Tanzanian mothers were somewhat less convinced that developmental processes of reinforcement and cognitive processing are responsible for children's intellectual development. These developmental processes were endorsed the least. Processes of learning through experimentation/discovery and through observation received a middle level of endorsement from Tanzanian mothers (see Table 6.2).

The Tanzanian mothers' view of children's knowledge and information acquisition is consistent in many ways with prior reports of views of the nature of children and of parental roles in the rearing and teaching of children in Tanzanian and some East African groups that are similar to those of Tanzania. For example, the Tanzanian mothers reported that direct instruction was important for knowledge acquisition. This is consistent with Harkness and Super's (1991) report that "many East African mothers believe that deliberate instruction is important to the infant's proper development, and that without such training the child would be delayed, or even permanently impaired" (pp. 227–228). Although Harkness and Super were referring to the

**Table 6.2.** Mean (and *SD*) Ratings of Developmental Processes Responsible for Children's Knowledge Acquisition

| Developmental process | Tanzania | United States |
|---|---|---|
| Biological factors | 4.67 (.64) | 5.40 (.51)[*] |
| Absorption | 4.66 (.61) | 4.63 (.42) |
| Direct instruction | 4.61 (.58) | 4.32 (.48)[*] |
| Observation | 4.51 (.62) | 4.89 (.51)[*] |
| Experimentation | 4.35 (.59) | 4.92 (.48)[*] |
| Cognitive organization | 3.92 (.64) | 4.67 (.48)[*] |
| Reinforcement | 3.84 (.82) | 3.73 (.69) |

[*]$p < .05$.

young child's motor development, the finding in the present study that urban Tanzanian mothers believed that direct instruction is important in children's cognitive development suggests that beliefs in didactic teaching methods apply to the acquisition of concepts in the older child's life as well.

The belief in direct instruction as the basis for cognitive development is, however, in conflict with Whiting and Edwards's (1988) report that Kenyan mothers only occasionally explicitly instruct their children, preferring to allow them to learn through observation and imitation, although the Kenyan mothers did view such training as necessary for the development of obedient and responsible behaviors, which were considered an aspect of intelligent behavior. As the definition of intelligence shifts, from home and family life to success through waged work and schooling, for example, perhaps the mothers' beliefs about the source of that intelligent behavior also shifts.

The mothers' view of the importance of absorption though exposure may seem to contradict the reported belief in direct instruction, but this may reflect a differentiation of processes responsible for knowledge in different domains, which was not addressed in the present study. For example, Harkness and Super (1991) reported that the Kenyan mothers who believed training was important for motor development did not see direct instruction as necessary for language acquisition. Children were expected to learn language through everyday experiences with peers and older siblings, acquiring knowledge in some areas through the course of everyday living. In other words, children are expected to develop language through absorption from exposure. There is no particular encouragement or experience that seems necessary.

The lower level of belief in reinforcement as a process responsible for the development of knowledge is consistent with the view that knowledge acquisition is a natural outgrowth of everyday experiences and does not require specific feedback from parents. Furthermore, Whiting and Edwards (1988) reported that many Kenyan mothers believed that praise and approval may lead to negative outcomes, such as a proud child. Although punishment is often used in the training and discipline of children, desired behavior is not often reinforced through praise and rewards. This pattern is consistent with the low level of belief in reinforcements as a source of learning in Tanzanian children.

It was somewhat surprising that observational learning processes were not rated higher than the other processes by mothers in Dar es Salaam. A major difference between items comprising the observation and absorption scales was that absorption items included some purposefulness or structure to environmental events. For example, one can learn about time through observation because it has a structure of its own: The sun comes up, sets, and when it rises again it is a new day. Similarly, language has a structure of its own. The mothers' advocacy of absorption over observation may reflect the view that structure inherent in experiences in the environment is an important component that shapes the child's knowledge acquisition.

The strong belief in biological processes with a concomitant component of individual differences suggests that although individuality may not be a goal of childrearing, mothers observe and accept differences between children. For example, Super and Harkness (1986) note that Kipsigis language socialization is directed toward goals of obedience and responsibility and not toward the goal of verbally expressive individuality. However, these same peoples make judgments about their children's personalities at 5 to 6 years of age. They also increase the complexity of assigned chores in accordance wit the age of the children, suggesting a maturational or stage-like model of development. Thus the mothers see differences among their children, although these are not apparent until the child is somewhat older. Biological factors and individual differences may be salient aspects of the parent's beliefs about the nature of the child in cultures that are characterized as more collectivist than individualistic, although childrearing goals are not centered on fostering the development of individuality.

To briefly summarize the beliefs of Tanzanian mothers, children's development is viewed as a result of biological factors, in conjunction with absorption of knowledge inherent in the structure of the environment, and direct instruction from adults. This presents a view of the child as a recipient of knowledge, although the degree of internalization of information depends on the child's capability to take in that information, which is under biological control. Thus, both internal and external factors are involved in cognitive development. The child's activity or processing, as expressed through experimentation, imitation, and cognitive reorganization, is not thought to be as salient as the processes of imparting knowledge and absorbing knowledge from outside the child. Finally, approval, praise, punishment, and other forms of feedback regarding performance have some role in children's development of knowledge (e.g., 3.84 on a 6-point scale), but these processes are seen as the least important in children's cognitive development.

## Mothers from the United States

Like the Tanzanian mothers, the American mothers most strongly endorsed biological processes as a source of developmental change in children's knowledge (see the right side of Table 6.2). The mean was 5.4 on a 6-point scale, indicating very strong beliefs in biological factors. As Table 6.2 indicates, American mothers strongly believed that children also learn through experimentation and through observation.

American mothers indicated that the child's own cognitive processing and absorption of knowledge from the environment were sources of the development of knowledge, although these constructs were not quite as strongly endorsed as biological, experimentation, or observational learning. Mothers from the U.S. sample gave their lowest endorsement to didactic instruction and to reinforcement as processes responsible for the child's cognitive growth (see Table 6.2).

It was expected that American mothers would evidence beliefs in biological bases for intellectual development. In part, this expectation was based on the emphasis on stage theories and maturational readiness that has characterized the popular literature directed at parents. In fact, Young's (1990) analysis of expert communication to parents through popular publications revealed that biological components of development comprise the area that is most often and clearly communicated to American parents through magazine articles. In the 30 years of popular press reviewed, children were presented as different from one another, and these differences were attributed to "differing physiological and psychological systems and not maternal style" (p. 24).

The expectation that American mothers would express beliefs in biological processes was also based on the assumption that American middle-class families have a positive view of individuality. Hogan and Elmer (1978) proposed that competitive individualism is one of three ideological beliefs that define American life. Developmental researchers posit that American mothers "tune into" individual differences among children in the family, emphasizing and nurturing their development (Rowe & Plomin, 1981). American parents have been found to put emphasis on the concept of stage as a way to gauge their own children's behavior in relation to other children in the same age range, further supporting notions of biological determinism and maturational models of development (Harkness, Super & Keefer, 1992). Such beliefs reflect not only the internalization of ideas presented somewhat formally through the media but also less formally articulated ideas that underlie what Americans value for their children.

The endorsement of children's own experimentation and observational learning as developmental processes was also consistent with views of children and the nature of intellectual growth that are visible in both the recent historical past and current representation of children in the United States. For example, Dr. Spock (1946) influenced parents' ideas when he wrote about the exploration of children as a natural event that leads to discovery of the world, including knowledge about specific objects as well as consequences of actions. Young (1990) reports that *Parents* magazine presented Piaget's theory to the American culture through descriptions of children's experiments as a source of the child's "coherent picture of the world" (p. 24). Beliefs in the child's own activity as a source of knowledge has also been found to be the strongest factor expressed in interviews of middle-class American mothers and fathers (McGillicuddy-De Lisi, 1982a). The relevance of observational learning for children's knowledge acquisition is demonstrated in acceptance of imitation as a mode of learning in parenting and self-help books for parents (e.g., Jensen & Kingston, 1986). Such media presentations both reflect and contribute to views of the active nature of the child and of developmental processes.

The American mothers' lesser belief in constructs of didactic instruction and reinforcement as processes responsible for children's knowledge development is consistent with the historical shift away from the mechanistic models of learning that characterized American psychology in the earlier part of the century (Young, 1990). Thus, these mothers see children first as individuals, with genetic endowment and maturational readiness framing the progress and quality of their children's knowledge acquisition. Children then develop cognitively through a result of their experiences in the world, largely through active experimentation and observation of other people and events. Feedback from the environment in the form of praise, approval, encouragement, and didactic instruction from adults have some role in knowledge acquisition, but these are less important in comparison with the child's own activity.

## Some Comparisons of Beliefs across Cultures

The examination of mothers' beliefs in each of the seven processes revealed that biological factors were the most strongly endorsed factors, and reinforcements were least strongly endorsed by both the American and Tanzanian mothers. There was, however, a noticeable difference in the relative importance attributed to the remaining five processes. Inspection of the mean ratings in Table 6.2 reveals that, after the most strongly endorsed factor of biological processes, absorption was rated most highly by Tanzanian mothers, followed by direct instruction, observation, experimentation, and cognitive processing. The American mothers' ratings followed a different pattern of high to low mean ratings: experimentation, observation, cognitive processing, absorption, and direct instruction.

It seems that the Tanzanian mothers view development in terms of a movement of knowledge from the external environment into the child in a somewhat automatic, natural, or passive (on the part of the child) manner. This conclusion is based on the relatively higher ratings assigned to absorption, direct instruction, and observation than to experimentation and cognitive processes. The American mothers, on the other hand, appear to explain development more in terms of the child's active processing, rating experimentation, observation, and cognitive processes more highly than they rate absorption and direct instruction.

In addition to investigating relative preference for one process over another as an explanation of knowledge acquisition, we wanted to examine whether or not one group of mothers felt more strongly about a particular process as a source of knowledge in children's development. A statistical analysis of the mean differences assigned to each processes was therefore conducted to examine whether the Tanzanian and American mothers differed from one another in the absolute value of the ratings assigned to each process. The analysis revealed that mothers from the two countries differed from one another in their levels of endorsement of biological processes, experimentation, observational learning, cognitive processing, and direct instruction. Mothers from Tanzania and from the United States did not differ from one another in their beliefs concerning reinforcement and absorption as developmental processes. (These findings are based on a multivariate analysis of variance that revealed that Tanzanian and the American mothers differed significantly from one another in their ratings, $F[1,142] = 18.01, p < .01$, and on follow-up univariate analyses of variance revealing significant differences for each process except reinforcement and absorption, $p$'s $< .05$.)

The differences indicate that although both Tanzanian and American mothers viewed biological processes as very important in child's development (having received the highest mean rating in both groups), American mothers indicated greater belief than Tanzanian mothers in biological factors as responsible for the development of knowledge. This was also true for the processes of experimentation, observational learning, and cognitive processing. The Tanzanian mothers believed more strongly in direct instruction as a source of developmental change than American mothers did.

These comparisons are informative and suggest that Tanzanian mothers believe the child is a recipient of knowledge more than American mothers, who view the child as more active in the acquisition of knowledge, processing information, experimenting, and mentally organizing experiences. These contrasts are consistent with Schaefer and Edgerton's (1985) dichotomy of parenting styles. More "traditional" parents were characterized as believing that the child learns in a passive manner and knowledge is instilled. More "modern" parents believed that children are active learners and knowledge is creative rather than static.

Thus, both the examination of the relative endorsement of each type of developmental process and the comparison of mean ratings suggest that biological determinism is an important aspect of the content of beliefs about children's cognitive development among mothers from both samples. However, the Tanzanian mothers endorsed developmental processes that are consistent with a view of children as receivers of knowledge from both the social environment—through didactic instruction—and the physical environment—through absorption of information contained in structured events and objects. American mothers endorsed different developmental processes in conjunction with biological factors. Processes of discovery/experimentation, observation, and cognitive reorganization suggest that the child is mentally active, transforming and abstracting concepts out of experiences, creating rather than receiving knowledge.

## Relationship of Mothers' Beliefs to Ratings of Children's School Behavior

The Tanzanian and American mothers comprising these samples have very different backgrounds, both in terms of their personal lives and the larger sociocultural history. What they have in common is that they hold advantaged positions within their societies and have high educational goals for their children. In spite of the likelihood that the meaning of their educational aspirations of their children differs, there should be a link between the mothers' beliefs about sources of children's knowledge and children's performance in school.

There is some evidence to suggest that beliefs are associated with children's cognitive development. For example, middle-class and working-class American parents' beliefs about child development processes have been linked to children's cognitive development through the teaching strategies that are presumed to stem from those beliefs (McGillicuddy-De Lisi, 1982b) and through more subtle mechanisms that are not as directly open to observation (e.g., cumulative effects over time; McGillicuddy-De Lisi, 1985). Okagaki and Sternberg (1993) have found that achievement test scores, ability scores, and classroom performance scores of children in six immigrant and ethnic groups in the United States were negatively related to parental beliefs in promoting social conformity. Schaefer and Edgerton (1985) report higher ability scores for children of parents who believe that children are active and creative rather than passive learners.

It is not clear, however, whether such relationships will be observed in cultures that have come to define knowledge and intelligence in terms of performance in formal school settings only recently in their social history. Investigations of the relationship between Tanzanian mothers' beliefs and teachers' ratings of their children's school performance were therefore very exploratory.

The behaviors that form the subscales labeled "intelligent behavior" and "creativity" of the Classroom Behavior Inventory were examined in relation to mothers' beliefs in order to investigate whether mothers' beliefs were associated with behaviors in children observed by an independent rater who was familiar with the child's school performance. Tanzanian children were rated as most intelligent by their teachers when their mothers believed children learn through observation ($r = .20$,) $p$'s $< .05$, and were rated as less intelligent when mothers endorsed reinforcement as a source of knowledge acquisition ($r = -.37$). Children rated as more creative had mothers who believed children develop knowledge through their own experimentation (.23) and cognitive organization (.31).

The pattern was similar for American mothers in the sense that belief in cognitive organization was related to teacher ratings for intelligent behavior (.23) and observational learning was related to creativity ratings (.23). In addition, American mothers' belief in biological processes was negatively related to teacher ratings for intelligence (−.23) and creativity (−.33).

With respect to teacher views of cognitive attributes evidenced in intelligent and creative behaviors, children in both samples were rated higher by teachers when mothers espoused beliefs in the child as an active learner (observing, engaged in cognitive processing, and experimenting).

These correlations between maternal beliefs and teacher ratings of children's classroom behaviors were very modest, although statistically significant. It is interesting to note that ratings of children's intelligent and creative behaviors by teachers were associated with processes that suggest the child is an active learner, and that beliefs in these processes have been viewed both as more "modern" and as correlated with school achievement in several settings (see Schaefer & Edgerton, 1985). This association may reflect a correspondence between the ways that teachers in a formal school setting view intelligence and creativity and the ways that mothers see the development of knowledge. Thus, the association may reflect aspects of schooling and how these relate to mothers' beliefs about development. If the child's intelligence and creativity were assessed by a different person in a different setting, the associations might be different. Or when mothers' beliefs about developmental processes are congruent with observers' (in this case, teachers') definitions of intelligent school behavior, the relationship may hold. Multiple definitions of school success and exploration of how different patterns of relations between parental beliefs and children's behaviors might reveal a variety of patterns with attention to the alternative meanings of school success for parent, teacher, and child.

## Conclusions

Three ways that culture and beliefs about children are related to one another have been presented. Tanzanian and American mothers indicated the degree to which they thought that seven possible processes were responsible for the development of children's knowledge. It is important to look beyond the finding that there were differences in these beliefs and examine *how* the beliefs differ. The possible connection of those beliefs to the culture in which these women live and the historical antecedents that created ways of life and views of children that provide the content of the women's lives with children reveal the nature of beliefs as knowledge and the functions they serve for parents that are more salient than mere cultural variability.

Some beliefs strongly endorsed by both the Tanzanian and the American mothers are most easily understood as internalizations from the social world. These are the beliefs connected to culture in the manner that was depicted in Figure 6.1. These beliefs were not a result of reflection and acceptance or conclusion but were absorbed by the individual and are a part of the cultural and personal belief system that is so long-standing and ingrained that the individual is unaware of its existence or any alternative possibility. The mother is startled when asked to explain such a belief any further than stating the obvious truth of it. For example, why does an East African mother believe that children acquire knowledge through absorption? No one has told her that children will learn language through play with other children and that it is a natural event that occurs just by being alive. But she has seen this every day since she was a girl. That is how it has always been. Mothers do not teach their children to talk and yet children speak. When Harkness and Super (1991) press the mother as to why mothers talk to their children, she had no answer except the surprised response, "We love them."

The American mothers studied also appropriated beliefs directly from the culture. American mothers believe that children are active little experimenters because it is in every magazine, the other mothers shared this knowledge, and the supermarkets sell little gadgets to keep the child safe from their own explorations and so on. They have adopted this notion ready-made, just as their Tanzanian counterparts have adopted the notion of absorption.

But some beliefs seem to be connected to cultural origins in a different way, through the shaping of experiences that lead mothers to their beliefs. These beliefs may be a result of conscious reflection on one's experience as a child, as an adult assuming the parent role and as a parent growing in the parenting role. In a sense, the culture canalizes many beliefs. Within the pastoral societies of Tanzania, women and children have eaten and slept together, while men were separate, sleeping in their own huts, or in the hut of a cowife. The mothers worked the fields and older children cared for younger ones, bringing them to the mothers for nursing as necessary. With additional births, older children were trained in more household and farming tasks, and the older children became children of the community rather than being reared only by their mother. This way of life led to experiences and a view of the child as trainable, capable, at an early age. By the time the child is 2 or 3 years old, the child must be taught how to be intelligent (i.e., responsible for tasks necessary for survival), for there is likely to be a new infant and the older child's services are needed in fields, in child care, and in some household tasks (see Harkness & Super, 1992b). Beliefs in direct instruction as a source of the child's knowledge can be seen to have grown out of these experiences as the mothers trained the child to do these tasks, to be intelligent.

The American mothers' beliefs in the child's own cognitive processing as a source of knowledge can similarly be seen to originate in experiences as a parent in the urban industrialized United States. Unlike the pastoral community in which many hands, even little ones, ease the burden of work, the children of America have not had significant responsibilities for many generations. The job of childhood is to play, and the outcome is cognitive development (Rubin, Fein, & Vandenberg, 1983). The child is stimulated to use imagination, to explore, and to express himself or herself through play. As the American parent provides such opportunities for play, it is a natural outgrowth of these parental experiences to conclude that the playful, imaginative explorations are a source of the child's development, rather than direct instruction, because there is little training or didactic instruction occurring.

Finally, the third perspective is apparent throughout much of discussion of the content of beliefs evidenced by the Tanzanian and by the

American mothers in relation to observed customs and changes in the culture. It is difficult to explore the knowledge that is culture and the knowledge that is personal belief to demonstrate this perspective in depth with the data available from the questionnaire format. If one views each of these knowledges as construed by the individuals, then cultural knowledge that is transformed by the individual's action of ascribing meaning to the cultural customs provides content for personal beliefs. Personal beliefs become reality through their application in the culture.

The clearest indication of the confluence of cultural and personal beliefs is available in the historical linkages and transformations in both cultural and personal beliefs when transformations correspond or co-occur. For example, in Tanzania there has been a shift in the value of farming, and many mothers look to waged work in the future of their children. As a cultural shift has occurred in the past thirty years in this belief that the future lies in schooling and waged earning, corresponding shifts have occurred in the value of large families, in the assignment of household versus school responsibilities to the child as a way to fulfill familial obligations, in the manner in which each individual is expected to desire to provide their services to the nation as a whole, to the control that parents have over their children's lives, and so on. These changes reflect adaptations of the personal beliefs and as these personal beliefs are altered, so must be the knowledge of the culture.

It is not possible, necessary, or desirable to try to separate these components of culture from components of beliefs. The individual and the culture can be best understood by examining the relation between them.

## Acknowledgments

Some data presented in this chapter were collected in partial fulfillment of requirements for an Honors thesis submitted by the second author. We are indebted to discussions with Richard De Lisi and Irving Sigel regarding the relation between beliefs and culture.

## References

Blount, B. G. (1982). Culture and the language of socialization: Parental speech. In D. A. Wagner & H. W. Stevenson (Eds.), *Cultural perspectives on child development* (pp. 54–76). San Francisco: Freeman.

Bornstein, M. H., Tal, J., & Tamis-LeMonda, C. S. (1991). Parenting in cross-cultural perspective: The United States, France, and Japan. In M. H.

Bornstein (Ed.), *Cultural approaches to parenting* (pp. 69–90). Hillsdale, NJ: Erlbaum.

Carnoy, M., & Samoff, J. (1990). *Education and social transition in the third world.* Princeton, NJ: Princeton University Press.

Fox, L. K. (1967). Introduction. In L. K. Fox (Ed.), *East African childhood* (pp. i–vi). Nairobi: Oxford University Press.

Goodnow, J. J. (1988). Parents' ideas, actions, and feelings: Models and methods from developmental and social psychology. *Child Development, 59,* 286–320.

Harkness, S., & Super, C. M. (1991). East Africa. In J. M. Hawes & N. R. Hiner (Eds.), *Children in historical and comparative perspective* (pp. 217–239). New York: Greenwood.

Harkness, S., & Super, C. M. (1992a). Parental ethnotheories in action. In I. E. Sigel, A. V. McGillicuddy-De Lisi, & J. J. Goodnow (Eds.), *Parental belief systems: The psychological consequences for children* (2nd ed., pp. 373–391). Hillsdale, NJ: Erlbaum.

Harkness, S., & Super, C. M. (1992b). Shared child care in East Africa: Sociocultural origins and developmental consequences. In M. E. Lamb, K. J. Sternberg, C.-P. Hwang, & A. G. Broberg (Eds.), *Child care in context: Cross-cultural perspectives* (pp. 441–462). Hillsdale, NJ: Erlbaum.

Harkness, S., & Super, C. M. (1992c). The cultural foundations of fathers' roles: Evidence from Kenya and the U.S. In B. S. Hewlett (Ed.), *The father–child relationship: Anthropological perspectives* (pp. 191–212). New York: Aldine.

Harkness, S., Super, C. M., & Keefer, C. H. (1992). Learning to be an American parent: How cultural models gain directive force. In R. G. D'Andrade & C. Strauss (Eds.), *Human motives and cultural models* (pp. 163–178). Cambridge: Cambridge University Press.

Hogan, R., & Elmer, N. (1978). The biases in contemporary social psychology. *Social Research, 45,* 478–534.

Jensen, L. C., & Kingston, M. (1986). *Parenting.* New York: CBS College Publishing.

Kelly, G. A. (1955). *The psychology of personal constructs* (2 vols.). New York: Norton.

Lamb, M. E., & Sternberg, K. J. (1992). Sociocultural perspectives on parental care. In M. E. Lamb, K. J. Sternberg, C.-P. Hwang, & A. G. Broberg (Eds.), *Child care in context: Cross-cultural perspectives* (pp. 1–26). Hillsdale, NJ: Erlbaum.

LeVine, R. A. (1980). Anthropology and child development. In C. M. Super & S. Harkness (Eds.), *Anthropological perspectives on child development* (pp. 71–86) (New Directions for Child Development No. 8). San Francisco: Jossey-Bass.

LeVine, R. (1988). Human parental care: Universal goals, cultural strategies, individual behavior. In R. A. LeVine, P. M. Miller, & M. M. West (Eds.), *Parental behavior in diverse societies* (pp.3–35) (New Directions for Child Development No. 40). San Francisco: Jossey-Bass.

LeVine, R. A., & LeVine, S. E. (1988). Parental strategies among the Gusii of Kenya. In R. A. LeVine, P. Miller, & M. M. West (Eds.), *Parental behavior in diverse societies* (pp. 27–35) (New Directions for Child Development No. 40). San Francisco: Jossey-Bass.

Lightfoot, C., & Valsiner, J. (1992). Parental belief systems under the influence: Social guidance of the construction of personal cultures. In I. E. Sigel, A. V. McGillicuddy-De Lisi, & J. J. Goodnow (Eds.), *Parental belief systems: The psychological consequences for children* (2nd ed., pp. 393–414). Hillsdale, NJ: Erlbaum.

Marcia, J. E. (1980). Identity in adolescence. In J. Adelson (Ed.), *Handbook of adolescent psychology* (pp. 159–187). New York: Wiley.

McGillicuddy-De Lisi, A. V. (1982a). Parental beliefs about developmental processes. *Human Development, 25,* 192–200.

McGillicuddy-De Lisi, A. V. (1982b). The relationship between parents' beliefs about development and family constellation, socioeconomic status, and parents' teaching strategies. In L. Laosa & I. E. Sigel (Eds.), *Families as learning environments for children* (pp. 261–299). New York: Plenum Press.

McGillicuddy-De Lisi, A. V. (1985). The relationship between parental beliefs and children's cognitive level. In I. E. Sigel (Ed.), *Parental belief systems: The psychological consequences for children* (pp. 7–24). Hillsdale, NJ: Erlbaum.

McGillicuddy-De Lisi, A. V. (1992). Parents' beliefs and children's personal–social development. In I. E. Sigel, A. V. McGillicuddy-De Lisi, & J. J. Goodnow (Eds.), *Parental belief systems: The psychological consequences for children* (2nd ed., pp. 115–142). Hillsdale, NJ: Erlbaum.

McGillicuddy-De Lisi, A. V., & Sigel, I. E. (1995). Parental beliefs. In M. H. Bornstein (Ed.), *Handbook of parenting: Vol. 3. Social conditions of parenting* (pp. 333–358). Hillsdale, NJ: Erlbaum.

McGillicuddy-De Lisi, A. V., & Subramanian, S. (1994). Tanzanian and American mothers' beliefs about parents' and teachers' roles in children's knowledge acquisition. *International Journal of Behavioral Development, 17,* 209–239.

Morelli, C. A., & Tronick, E. Z. (1991). Parenting and child development in the Efe foragers and Lese farmers of Zaire. In M. H. Bornstein (Ed.), *Cultural approaches to parenting* (pp. 91–114). Hillsdale, NJ: Erlbaum.

Okagaki, L., & Sternberg, R. R. J. (1993). Parental beliefs and children's school performance. *Child Development, 64,* 36–56.

Pomerleau, A., Malcuit, G., & Sabatier, C. (1991). Child-rearing practices and parental beliefs in three cultural groups of Montréal: Québécois, Vietnamese, Haitian. In M. H. Bornstein (Ed.), *Cultural approaches to parenting* (pp. 45–68). Hillsdale, NJ: Erlbaum.

Rowe, D. C., & Plomin, R. (1981). The importance of nonshared ($E_1$) environmental influences on behavioral development. *Developmental Psychology, 17,* 517–531.

Rubin, K. H., Fein, G. G., & Vandenberg, B. (1983). Play. In E. M. Hetherington (Ed.), *Handbook of child psychology* (4th ed.): *Vol IV. Socialization, personality and social development* (pp. 693–774). New York: Wiley.

Schaefer, E. S., & Edgerton, M. (1978). *Child Behavior Inventory.* Unpublished manuscript. University of North Carolina at Chapel Hill.

Schaefer, E. S., & Edgerton, M. (1985). Parent and child correlates of parental modernity. In I. E. Sigel (Ed.), *Parental belief systems: The psychological consequences for children* (pp. 287–318). Hillsdale, NJ: Erlbaum.

Sigel, I. E., & McGillicuddy-De Lisi, A. V. (1984). Parents as teachers of their children: A distancing behavior model. In A. D. Pellegrini & T. D. Yawkey (Eds.), *The development of oral and written language in social contexts* (pp. 71–92). Norwood, NJ: Ablex.

Spock, B. M. (1946). *The common sense book of baby and child care.* New York: Duell, Sloan & Pearce.

Super, C. M., & Harkness, S. (1986). The developmental niche: A conceptualization at the interface of child and culture. *International Journal of Behavioral Development, 9,* 545–969.

Whiting, B. B. (1980). Culture and social behavior: A model for the development of social behavior. *Ethos, 8,* 95–116.

Whiting, B. B., & Edwards, C. P. (1988). *Children of different worlds: The formation of social behavior.* Cambridge, MA: Harvard University Press.

Young, K. T. (1990). American conceptions of infant development from 1955 to 1984: What the experts are telling parents. *Child Development, 61,* 17–28.

CHAPTER 7

# Japanese Mothers' Ideas about Infants and Temperament

David W. Shwalb
Barbara J. Shwalb
Junichi Shoji

Mothers' perceptions of infants and temperament are to a large extent cultural constructions. As they describe and evaluate their babies' temperament, mothers reveal societal beliefs about personality, individuality, and emotionality. In this chapter, we take an emic approach to examine one aspect of the Japanese system of parental ethnotheories. The data to be discussed concern (1) maternal perceptions of Japanese infant temperament and (2) the use of temperament categories to describe hehavioral style across the Japanese life-span. We investigated native-based categories of temperament and personality, using non-Western measures, and relying at all stages of our research on the interpretations and ideas of Japanese mothers.

In the course of the long history of Japanese childhood, ideas about childrearing and the nature of children appear to have become firmly established as one aspect of Japanese thought. So the words used currently by mothers to describe temperament and personality are a product of the legacy of Japanese history and culture. We think that historical continuity, and the widely held and highly valued role expectations of mothers, may foster homogeneity among Japanese mothers in their values, beliefs and expectations. Further, the strongly ingrained thinking and applied childrearing practices of mothers reflect a parental ethnotheory that is highly resistant to societal changes. We discuss and evaluate these ideas here and offer research findings that support our generalizations.

## Constancy in Japanese Ideas about Infants

Can one really generalize about Japanese mothers' ideas, as the chapter title suggests? We think so. What the Japanese think is not always generalizable (Dale, 1986), yet adults' ideas about infancy and childhood appear to be consistent in Japan across several historical eras. The following three examples suggest such historical continuity.

Kojima (1989) cites the work of an early-18th-century physician, Kazuki (1703/1976), who wrote a systematic manual about child care and education. In the manual, Kazuki writes that if a mother is responsive to the smiling and vocalizations of her baby, it facilitates positive mother–infant interaction and the infant's social and language development. Almost 300 years later, identical advice is still given. The Japan Health and Welfare Ministry (1990) manual for professional infant caregivers at day nurseries says, "Respond gently to a child's smiling or crying, to facilitate the development of communication" (p. 27), and "when feeding hold the child with a relaxed feeling, smiling and talking gently" (p. 28). In addition, the *Mother and Child Health Handbook* (Boshi Aiikukai, 1992), a book given to all expectant mothers by the Health and Welfare Ministry, advises, "Until your baby is about two months old, hold him/her if he/she cries in spite of being dry and not hungry. . . . When your baby cries, talk to him/her" (p. 54). These multigenerational directions indicate a tradition and the importance of responsiveness, gentleness, and communication in the context of a close mother–infant relationship.

A second example concerns the long held Japanese beliefs that babies are pure and spiritually independent. Purity is untainted goodness. In this sense, infants were regarded as superior to adults (Hara & Wagatsuma, 1974) and were described by words reflecting their innate goodness. These beliefs and practices continue. Kosawa, Shand, Takahashi, and Fujimaki (1985) found that nearly their entire sample of Tokyo mothers described their infants as good babies. Infant spiritual independence is an idea rooted in old Japan. As long ago as 900 A.D. children less than 7 years old were thought to "belong to the gods" (Hara & Wagatsuma, 1974, p. 119) rather than to mortals. Mortals tried to keep the gods happy by anticipating and indulging their desires. Though the initial religiously based belief has diminished, the pampering itself has not. Lanham (1966) and many others have observed that modern Japanese mothers cater to babies' every whim. This second example suggests a positive view of infants as independent beings who are to be treated with great importance.

A third example of continuity in adults' ideas concerns childbirth practices. The sociologist Embree (1939) wrote that "childbirth being so secret, a woman never cries out, for if she did, the neighbors would know what she was doing, and she would be ashamed" (pp. 178–179). This quote recalls our own Tokyo childbirth experience five decades after Embree's observations. At a sophisticated modern hospital, nurses derided the second author for crying out during labor, with such comments as "You're a baby!" and "Stop whining like a little girl!" This example indicates the value placed on the cultural norm of a taboo against crying out, as well as sensitivity toward secrecy at childbirth. Here again, an ethnotheory transcends historical eras.

## Infant Temperament and Culture

Japanese socioemotional development has been the subject of cross-cultural research for over four decades (Shwalb & Shwalb, in press), and this database provides a background for the interpretation of current investigations of Japanese infant temperament. Bornstein's (1989) review includes a fine discussion of two comparative investigations of Japanese and American infants. One was Caudill and Weinstein's (1969) report, and the other was Shand and Kosawa's (1985) replication of the Caudill study. Both studies found differences in infant motoric activity. Caudill and Weinstein (1969) reported that there was more motoric activity among American babies than among Japanese babies at 1 year, 3 months, and attributed this primarily to cultural differences in maternal behavior. The Tokyo mothers observed were physically closer and more soothing toward their babies, which led Caudill and Weinstein to write that Japanese mothers "produced" less active infants. Washington, D.C., mothers, on the other hand, stimulated their babies more and elicited higher infant activity levels, according to Caudill and Weinstein. Fifteen years later, Shand and Kosawa (1985) found that Japanese babies were more active than American babies. They stressed biogenetic factors in interpreting their data but added that cultural beliefs were an important influence on the development of infant temperament. Our view is that these opposing findings reflect the different samples (late 1950s vs. late 1970s) and measurement techniques (naked-eye observations vs. intrasecond film analyses) used by the two research teams. We also believe that influence and socialization between mothers and infants is mutual, and that cultural and biological influences on temperament are both universal. Bornstein (1989) adds that together these two studies are useful because they helped suggest an infant temperament dimension (i.e., activity level) of cross-cultural utility.

Such highlighting of salient behaviors can contribute more to an understanding of culture and temperament than would cross-cultural group comparisons. Less useful cultural temperament research is the genre that simply replicates Western-based maternal report measures in non-Western cultures. This type of study (e.g., Hsu, Soong, Stigler, Hong, & Liang, 1981) reports "lower" or "higher" group means on infant temperament scales, most often the Revised Infant Temperament Questionnaire (RITQ; Carey & McDevitt, 1978). The group mean comparisons of infant temperament ratings from different nations do not reflect group differences in actual temperament, or even in maternal perceptions, because the measurement instruments may not be cross-culturally valid. Shoji and Maekawa's (1981) ongoing research has shown the inadequacy of directly translating Western measures and temperament categories, as they adapted the RITQ for Japanese mothers. For instance, based on their clinical observations they eliminated several RITQ items as irrelevant to Japanese mothers and infants.

## Categories of Temperament

We suggest that the categories Western psychologists use to analyze temperament reflect their own ethnotheories; that is, temperament concepts *are* a type of ethnotheory. The data we collected were intended to elicit the cultural "meaning" of temperament rather than to make cross-cultural comparisons. In taking a single-culture approach, self-report data are valuable as a way of eliciting how mothers in one culture categorize developmental phenomena. As White and LeVine (1986) note, the single-culture approach appears at first to contradict the goal of a universal understanding of development. Therefore, we must first study everyday expressions used in different cultures to describe psychological phenomena and then make cultural comparisons between such expressions. The temperament dimensions we found among Japanese mothers suggest both possible cultural similarities and differences.

We asked Japanese mothers themselves to generate dimensions of early infant temperament, rather than simply replicating the RITQ or another Western instrument. By contrast, most other studies on the structure of temperament have taken as their reference point Thomas and Chess's (1977) nine aspects of temperament (Rhythmicity, Activity,

Approach–Withdrawal, Adaptability, Intensity, Threshold, Mood, Distractibility, and Persistence) as measured on the RITQ. To assess dimensionality, researchers have factor-analyzed RITQ or similar data (Hagekull, 1991; Sanson, Prior, Garino, Oberklaid, & Sewell, 1987; Shoji, Soeda, & Yokoi, 1992) and have derived some consistent dimensions across measurement instruments. Rothbart and Mauro (1990) listed the following factors as reported across various measurement instruments: (1) reactions to novelty, (2) general proneness to distress, (3) positive affect, (4) activity level, (5) rhythmicity, and (6) attention span/persistence. While described as the dimensions of infants' temperament, these factors are actually dimensions of maternal perceptions, which reflect ethnotheories in the Western cultures where the questionnaires were created.

## Maternal Perceptions

Maternal perception measures have been criticized in the West as confounded by socioeconomic status, prenatal maternal anxiety, experiences during childbirth, and maternal personality variables (Bates, 1987). But we cannot assume that these particular confounds are universal. It would do better to assume them as part of the cognitive structure for mothers' judgments. We assume, as do Thomas and Chess (1977), Bates and Bayles (1984), Goodnow and Collins (1990), and Rothbart and Mauro (1990), that parents' ideas have a great influence on children's socioemotional development. Indeed recent studies validate their importance. For instance, LeVine, Miller, Richman, & LeVine (Chapter 10, this volume) found cross-cultural differences in parental conceptions of infant development and showed how parental models influence mother–infant communication.

## Previous Japanese Temperament Research

Cross-cultural American/Japanese developmental research related to temperament began with Caudill's previously mentioned study. Caudill's extensive 1962–1964 interviews of the mothers were unfortunately never analyzed, so it is difficult to determine the relationship between the thinking and the behavior of the mothers in his sample. But we think that the ethnotheories of his American and Japanese subjects may have influenced their maternal styles, so that maternal perceptions (and not only maternal behavior) influenced the temperament of the infants observed.

Over the past generation, studies of Japanese socioemotional development have become far more specialized and technical than in Caudill's time (Shwalb & Shwalb, in press). Since about 1980, several Japanese researchers made sophisticated observations of mother and infant behavior (Miyake, Chen, & Campos, 1985; Sengoku, 1983; Shand & Kosawa, 1985) and devised maternal rating scales for infant temperament (Murai, Nihei, Nasu, & Yonemoto, 1982; Shoji & Maekawa, 1981; Soeda, Shoji, Yokoi, & Maekawa, 1991; Sugawara, Aoki, Kitamura, & Shima, 1988).

## Maternal Perception Study

Following the lead of Japanese researchers, we created a maternal report instrument grounded in Japanese mothers' thinking and experiences. Our research elicited Japanese native-based temperament concepts, rather than relying on Western-based categories. The instructions of our first questionnaire defined temperament generally as behavioral style, and thereafter mothers delineated the content and contexts in which temperament appears.

Although Japanese may emphasize collectivism over individuality and dependency over independence (White & Levine, 1986), they have everyday expressions for individuality (*kosei*), temperament (*kishitsu*), and personality (*seikaku*). For example, the *Mother and Child Health Handbook* (Boshi Aiikukai, 1992) emphasizes individual differences with the warning, "There is quite a difference among babies during the infancy period. Do not compare your baby with other babies" (p. 54), and the Health and Welfare Ministry states that the development of an individual personality is the primary goal of infant care. Thus we assume that the respondents were aware of both individual differences and the importance of infant temperament.

### Data Collection

We first asked a sample of middle-class mothers of 50 newborns, 50 3-month olds, and 50 6-month olds to list items they thought reflected their infants' temperament, as follows: "We wish to know the characteristics of *your* baby's behavioral style. . . . Rather than *what* she/he can do, we are asking *how* she/he normally does things. . . . Please list specific items you think reveal your child's character. . . ." Such instructions indicated a focus on the temperament of a specific baby and not on infants in general. Mothers of newborns were given this form at a Tokyo hospital within a week postpartum, and mothers of 3- and 6-month olds were sent forms by mail. Mothers of 26 newborns, 21

3-month olds, and 26 6-month olds returned the forms and listed a total of 566 items. These items were sorted independently by two bilingual research assistants into items grouped by related content (agreement rate = .86). Next, items with similar wordings, as well as those listed by mothers for only one age group, were eliminated. This resulted in a 52-item form, the Japanese Temperament Questionnaire (JTQ). This form was checked for appropriateness of wording by four pediatricians and two clinical psychologists in Tokyo. The items appeared to describe mainly concrete behaviors, which reflects the same tendency found among Western mothers (Rothbart, 1989), that is, to relate temperament to specific contexts and caretaking behaviors rather than to psychological attributes.

Hospital staff attained consent from participants by telephone, and the JTQ was next mailed to 600 middle-class mothers in Tokyo. Over 94% of Japanese families now consider themselves to be middle class (Shwalb, Shwalb, Sukemune, & Tatsumoto, 1992), so it is very difficult to measure social status in Japan. But based on parents' educational history, the hospital's population seemed broadly representative of mothers and babies throughout Japan (Shoji & Maekawa, 1981; Vogel, 1992). Mothers of 146 normal 1-month olds, 165 3-month olds, and 158 6-month olds returned completed forms by mail. On the form, mothers rated the frequency of the 52 items, listed in Table 7.1, on a 5-point scale (1 = never does this; 5 = always does this).

Other demographic information showed that families had an average of two children, and in 431 cases (93%) the mother was the primary daytime caregiver. Mothers' mean age was 29.4 years, and 81 (17%) were currently employed. These data are similar to national demographics of middle-class Japanese mothers and babies (Nippon Aiiku Kenkyujo, 1994; Shwalb, Imaizumi, & Nakazawa, 1987).

**Table 7.1.** Japanese Temperament Questionnaire Items

| | |
|---|---|
| 1 | SMILES OR LAUGHS WHEN with played with or CARESSED. |
| 2 | MOVES head or LIMBS ACTIVELY. |
| 3 | PLAYS awhile BEFORE going to SLEEP. |
| 4 | STARES AT OWN LIMBS, moving objects, OR colored OBJECTS. |
| 5 | MAKES A COOING VOICE when wanting to play or be held. |
| 6 | Is DISTRACTIBLE BY SOUNDS OR FACES when feeding. |
| 7 | CRIES WHEN THINGS are NOT going one's OWN WAY. |
| 8 | JOYFUL WHEN BATHED, kicking limbs about. |
| 9 | Is HAPPY, relaxed, or looks around WHEN TAKEN FOR WALKS. |
| 10 | SMILES joyfully WHEN GIVEN A BOTTLE or breast. |
| 11 | NURSES OR DRINKS WELL. |

*(cont.)*

**Table 7.1.** *(cont.)*

| | |
|---|---|
| 12 | GRABS FOR THINGS (people, toys, own body). |
| 13 | EASY TO CARE FOR (requires very little attention). |
| 14 | Makes many EXPRESSIONS, AND KICKS about playfully, WHEN ASLEEP. |
| 15 | BENDS BACKWARD or throws head back WHEN EMBRACED. |
| 16 | PLAYS, pushes bottle away, OR POUTS WHEN has had ENOUGH MILK. |
| 17 | Is ANNOYED WHEN FACE IS washed or TOUCHED. |
| 18 | Makes HAPPY VOICINGS or smiles back, WHEN smiled at or CALLED by name. |
| 19 | CRINGES or draws legs in WHEN DIAPERED. |
| 20 | LIKES PLEASANT SOUNDS. |
| 21 | SOON CRIES WHEN left ALONE. |
| 22 | FALLS ASLEEP while DRINKING MILK relaxed and slowly. |
| 23 | Often has DIFFICULTY BURPING, OR HICCUPS. |
| 24 | CRIES OUT loudly and IMPATIENTLY when thirsty. |
| 25 | DOESN'T move or EXTEND LIMBS MUCH. |
| 26 | FRETS OR CRIES WHEN BATHING. |
| 27 | EXPRESSES ANGER VISCERALLY, not just by crying. |
| 28 | SLEEPS WELL. |
| 29 | LOVES TO HAVE BODY EXERCISED. |
| 30 | FEEDING and SLEEPING TIMES are basically REGULAR. |
| 31 | FRETS OR CRIES loudly WHEN TIRED. |
| 32 | EASY TO BATHE; loves bathing. |
| 33 | UNSETTLED WHEN DIAPERS NEED a CHANGE. |
| 34 | PUTS TOYS INTO MOUTH immediately. |
| 35 | PUZZLED BY UNFAMILIAR FOOD. |
| 36 | SLEEPS WITH ARMS OUTSTRETCHED in "banzai" position. |
| 37 | Soon DEFECATES WHEN FEEDING or just put into clean diapers. |
| 38 | STARTLES AT SUDDEN or LOUD SOUNDS. |
| 39 | FEEDS SERIOUSLY AND QUICKLY. |
| 40 | Is NOT CAUTIOUS TOWARD STRANGERS. |
| 41 | CRIES LOUDLY WHEN has TROUBLE FEEDING (can't get nipple; milk flows poorly). |
| 42 | MOVES HEAD back and forth when LYING SLEEPILY. |
| 43 | BURIES HEAD IN my NECK or chest WHEN EMBRACED. |
| 44 | CRIES WILDLY, kicking limbs about and TURNING RED. |
| 45 | DOESN'T CRY MUCH. |
| 46 | SUCKS THUMB, FINGERS OR TOES. |
| 47 | Is very WARY OF NEW PEOPLE. |
| 48 | KICKS LIMBS ACTIVELY WHEN CHANGED or undressed. |
| 49 | GRASPS MOTHER'S CLOTHING when feeding. |
| 50 | CAN PLAY ALONE. |
| 51 | CRIES LOUDLY or is upset WHEN NOT HELD. |
| 52 | JOYFUL WHEN head or FACE IS caressed or PATTED. |

## Infancy Results

Maternal scale ratings were factor-analyzed, and for comparison purposes the factor structure of temperament items was explored separately for each age group. Common factor analysis was first applied to each subsample, followed by oblique rotation, with the minimum eigen value relaxed to 1.0, as recommended for such analyses by Hair, Anderson, Tatham, and Black (1992). Table 7.2 lists the temperament items (all loadings .40) for factors derived for 1-, 3-, and 6-month olds, respectively. Table 7.2 item wordings are abbreviated to match the capitalized words within Table 7.1 items. To help the reader compare factors and items across age groups, related dimensions are aligned from left to right in the table. Orders of factor extraction are given in parentheses.

### Factor Structure for Three Age Levels

Factor analysis produced a nine-factor solution accounting for 75% of the common variance. Factors at all three age levels were moderately intercorrelated. Factor analysis of the 3-month-olds' data also resulted in an nine-factor solution, which accounted for 78% of the common variance. Here the individual items comprising each factor differed between the age groups, which was expected given that the experiences and contexts of infant development change rapidly during early infancy. Given the moderate sample sizes for the three age groups and the exploratory nature of the research it was impressive that almost all 1-month dimensions were replicated for 3-month-olds.

For the data on 6-month-olds there was a 10-factor solution, accounting for 79% of the common variance. The factors were quite similar to those found for 1- and 3-month olds, although again the spccific items loading on each factor differed between age groups. Given that temperament dimensions build in complexity throughout infancy (Rothbart, 1989), the continuity between 3 and 6 months was again notable.

### Mother-Generated Labels

In all previous studies of maternal perceptions, professionals have provided the labels for temperament dimensions. But to ground our results in the subject population we had mothers generate dimension labels as well. So lists of items loading on each factor were distributed to a different middle-class sample of 16 mothers, who labeled each cluster of items. Various labels were suggested for every factor; the

**Table 7.2.** Temperament Dimensions' Items for Three Age Groups

| 1-month-old dimensions | 3-month-old dimensions | 6-month-old dimensions |
|---|---|---|
| Ease/difficulty of care (1) | Ease/difficulty of care (1) | Ease/difficulty of care (9) |
| 13 Easy to care for | 2 Moves limbs actively | 13 Easy to care for |
| 28 Sleeps well | 3 Plays before sleep | 33 Unsettled when diapers need change |
| 31 Frets or cries when tired | 4 Stares at own limbs or objects | 45 Doesn't cry much |
| | 8 Joyful when bathes | |
| Intensity of emotions (2) | 9 Happy when taken for walks | Intensity of reactions (6) |
| 7 Cries when things not own way | 10 Smiles when given a bottle | 14 Expressions and kicks when asleep |
| 8 Joyful when bathed | 11 Nurses or drinks well | 15 Bends backward when embraced |
| 9 Happy when taken for walks | | 27 Expresses anger viscerally |
| 15 Bends backward when embraced | Intensity of reactions (6) | 42 Moves head lying sleepily |
| 27 Expresses anger viscerally | 24 Cries out impatiently | |
| 44 Cries wildly turning red | 41 Cries loudly when trouble feeding | Sociability (3) |
| 46 Sucks thumb, fingers or toes | 44 Cries wildly turning red | 10 Smiles when given a bottle |
| | 48 Kicks limbs actively when changed | 16 Plays or pouts when enough milk |
| Sociability (3) | | 20 Likes pleasant sounds |
| 1 Smiles or laughs when caressed | Social responsiveness (5) | 43 Buries head in neck when embraced |
| 3 Stares at own limbs or objects | 1 Smiles or laughs when caressed | |
| 10 Smiles when given a bottle | 5 Makes a cooing voice | Motoric activity (8) |
| 18 Happy voicings when called | 12 Grabs for things | 2 Moves limbs actively |
| | 18 Happy voicings when called | 12 Grabs for things |
| Motoric activity (4) | 49 Grasps mother's clothing | 41 Cries loudly when trouble feeding |
| 2 Moves limbs actively | | |
| 3 Plays before sleep | Motoric activity (2) | Willfulness (1) |
| 11 Drinks or nurses well | 13 Easy to care for | 7 Cries when things not own way |
| 14 Expressions and kicks when asleep | 21 Cries when left alone | 21 Cries when left alone |
| 16 Plays or pouts when enough milk | 28 Sleeps well | 24 Cries out impatiently |
| | 30 Feeding and sleeping times regular | 44 Cries wildly turning red |
| Self-assertiveness (5) | 51 Cries loudly when not held | 50 Can play alone |
| 20 Likes pleasant sounds | | 51 Cries loudly when not held |
| 29 Loves to have body exercised | | |
| 39 Feeds seriously and quickly | | *(cont.)* |

**Table 7.2.** *(cont.)*

| 1-month-old dimensions | 3-month-old dimensions | 6-month-old dimensions |
|---|---|---|
| Self-assertiveness (5) *(cont.)* 43 Buries head in neck when embraced 49 Grasps mother's clothing 52 Joyful when face is patted | Willfulness (3) 6 Distractable by sounds or faces 7 Cries when things not own way 27 Expresses anger viscerally 33 Unsettled when diapers need change 38 Startles at sudden loud noises | Stability/ gentleness (10) 1 Smiles or laughs when caressed 22 Falls asleep drinking milk 37 Defecates when feeding |
| Stability/gentleness (6) 22 Falls asleep drinking milk 37 Defecates when feeding 38 Startles at sudden loud noises | Gentleness (7) 14 Expressions or kicks when asleep 31 Frets or cries when tired 45 Doesn't cry much | Reactivity to change (5) 5 Makes a cooing voice 6 Distractable by sounds or faces 10 Smiles when given a bottle 38 Startles at sudden loud noises |
| Cautiousness (7) 6 Distractable by sounds or faces 35 Puzzled by unfamiliar food 40 Is not cautious toward strangers 47 Is wary of new people | Reactivity to change (4) 34 Puts toys into mouth 35 Puzzled by unfamiliar food 40 Is not cautious toward strangers 50 Can play alone | Social activity level (4) 11 Nurses or drinks well 34 Puts toys into mouth 49 Grasps mother's clothing 50 Can play alone |
| Indulgence/ dependency (8) 5 Makes a cooing voice 21 Cries when alone 33 Unsettled when diapers need change 51 Cries loudly when not held | Indulgence/ dependency (9) 22 Falls asleep drinking milk 23 Difficulty burping or hiccups 43 Buries head in neck when embraced | Sensitive to physical stimulation (2) 6 Distractable by sounds or faces 8 Joyful when bathed 17 Annoyed when face is touched 26 Frets or cries when bathed 32 Easy to bathe |
| Responsiveness to physical contact (9) 17 Annoyed when face is touched 26 Frets or cries when bathing 32 Easy to bathe | Sensitivity to physical contact (8) 17 Annoyed when face is touched 26 Frets or cries when bathing 32 Easy to bathe | Rhythmicity (7) 28 Sleeps well 30 Feeding and sleeping times regular 52 Joyful when face is patted |

responses given most often are listed in Table 7.2 and alternative labels for each dimension are presented in Table 7.3.

The labels were generally everyday expressions rather than technical terms. In addition, sometimes two Japanese expressions with the same English translation were generated for infants of different ages.

## Discussion of Infancy Findings

The procedure of having mothers label the temperament dimensions demonstrated the utility of considering mothers' thinking. We did not leave the labeling entirely to mothers, as each author independently labeled the dimensions. But we often preferred the mothers' wordings to our own (which were laden with psychological jargon), as mothers grasped the dimension labels in simpler real-life terms. It thus seems useful to involve parents in the interpretive as well as the data-collection stage of research.

Sometimes Japanese-perceived dimensions of temperament overlapped conceptually with those from the West, but their context and content often differed. It was notable that nearly every JTQ item had a different wording from items on English-language temperament instruments. And even when a JTQ dimension was analogous to an RITQ or other Western-based dimension, the items making up the dimension were quite different from the English-language items.

## Comparisons between JTQ Dimensions and Dimensions Found Elsewhere

### Similarities

Direct comparisons between the JTQ dimension labels and others (e.g., RITQ) will require concurrent data collection, but the following speculative comments are made to clarify the JTQ dimensions for the benefit of readers familiar with dimensions such as the nine Thomas and Chess (1977) New York Longitudinal Studies (NYLS) dimensions. First, 7 of the 13 Table 7.3 dimensions probably are analogous to RITQ dimensions, as follows: (2) "Intensity of emotional reactions" = RITQ "Intensity," (4) "Activity level" = RITQ "Activity," (6) "Stability/gentleness" = RITQ "Mood" (positive), (7) "Cautiousness" = RITQ "Approach–withdrawal," (7B) "Reactivity to change" = RITQ "Adaptability," (9B) "Sensitivity" = RITQ "Threshold," and (10) "Rhythmicity" = RITQ "Rhythmicity."

The JTQ "Ease/difficulty of care" dimension may be conceptually

**Table 7.3.** Infant Temperament Dimension Labels and Alternatives

| | |
|---|---|
| Factor 1 | Ease/difficulty of care (*te no kakaru/kakaranai*)<br>Nervousness (*shinkeishitsu*)<br>Easy baby (*raku na ko*)<br>Easy-going (*ochitsuita*) |
| Factor 2 | Intensity of emotional reactions (*kanjo no hageshisa*)<br>Strong-willed (*ishi ga suyoi*)<br>Impatient (*matte irarenai*) |
| Factor 3 | Sociability (*shakohsei*)<br>Sociability (*shakaiteki otosei*)<br>Good-humored (*kigen ga yoi*)<br>Rich in emotionality (*iocho yutaka*) |
| Factor 4 | Activity level (*katsudosei*)<br>Curiosity (*kohkishin*)<br>Energetic (*genki na ko*)<br>Lively (*sekkyokuteki*) |
| Factor 5 | Self-assertiveness (*jiko shucho*)<br>Frustrated desires (*yokkyu fuman*)<br>The roots of self (*jiwa no mebae*)<br>Independent (*jiritsusei*) |
| Factor 6 | Stability/gentleness (*anteisei/otonashii*)<br>Goes at own pace (*mai peisu*)<br>At ease (*odayakasa*)<br>Quiet (*shizuka*) |
| Factor 7 | Cautiousness (*shincho*)<br>Curiosity (*khkishin*)<br>Withdrawal from new situations (*hajimete ni kaihiteki keiko*) |
| Factor 8 | Indulgence/dependency (*amaembo*)<br>Mama's baby (*mamakko*)<br>Strongly attached (*kan'aisei ga tsuyoi*)<br>Gentle (*yasashii*) |
| Factor 9 | Responsiveness to physical contact (*shintaiteki setsuzoku no hannosei*)<br>Enjoys skin contact (*sukinshippu*)<br>Enjoys bathing (*ofuro ga suki*)<br>Easy-going (*nonki*) |
| Factor 5B | Willfulness (*wagamama*) (only at 3/6 months; related to above Self-assertiveness)<br>Cries easily (*nakiyasusa*)<br>Ill-spiritedness (*kigen no warusa*)<br>Settled/unsettled (*kai/fukai*) |
| Factor 7B | Reactivity to change (*henka o konomu*) (only at 3/6 months; related to above Cautiousness)<br>Strong curiosity (*kohkishin ohsei*)<br>Interest in things (*kyomi ga aru*)<br>Sensitivity (*kankaku*) |

*(cont.)*

**Table 7.3.** *(cont.)*

| | |
|---|---|
| Factor 9B | Sensitivity (*binkansa*) (only at 3/6 months; related to above Responsiveness to physical contact) <br> Nervousness (*shinkeishitsu*) <br> Unsettledness (*jukai*) <br> Negative responsivity to change (*mushikaku shigeki e no hannosei*) |
| Factor 10 | Rhythmicity (*shuki no kisokusei*) (only at 6 months; not related to above labels) <br> Care-free (*nonki*) <br> Emotionally settled (*jocho antei*) <br> Predictable (*kisokusei*) |

related to the Thomas and Chess notion of the "easy baby," and one alternative label for this factor was indeed easy baby (*raku na ko*). This dimension has appeared in several previous factor-analytic studies of maternal perceptions and was termed "manageability" by Sugawara et al. (1988) and Murai et al. (1982) in Japan, Sanson et al. (1987) in Australia, and Hagekull (1991) in Sweden. Of course, Japanese mothers would not use the expression "manageability," which is a technical term. There is some discussion in the literature as to whether easy baby or manageability dimensions are actually a "general" temperament factor, but in the present study ease–difficulty of care was only one of several dimensions. A Japanese, when describing her baby in brief terms to a visitor, may use a general term such as a "good baby" (*ii ko*) or a more specific descriptor such as "gentle child" (*otonashii*). The "ease of care" (*te no kakaranai*) wording is one of the most frequent colloquial expressions to describe a baby or child.

## RITQ Dimensions Not Found

Two RITQ dimensions were not found among the labels for the JTQ factors: persistence and distractibility. A persistence dimension had been found in two factor analyses of Japanese RITQ data (Shoji et al., 1992; Sugawara et al., 1988). But is persistence an important aspect of Japanese temperament? As indicated by the title of Wagatsuma and DeVos's *Heritage of Endurance* (1984), patience and persistence are keys to understanding Japanese motivation. Only follow-up research can explain why persistence was never included in the free responses of our sample. As for distractibility, observations of young children suggest that young Japanese children learn to resist distraction. As one can see at any Japanese preschool playground, numerous small groups share a very crowded play space and focus on their respective organized games.

Among older children, we are always impressed by the ability of Japanese pupils to concentrate in classrooms despite high noise levels. So did we miss these two important dimensions? Or are distractibility and persistence omitted by parents because all Japanese are assumed to have these traits? Again follow-up research is needed.

### Japanese-Style Dimensions

Perhaps most importantly, five JTQ dimensions seem quite different from those observed elsewhere. Of these, three seem to be related to self-expression and two are related to social responsiveness. In sum, all five seem to reflect the nature of the Japanese mother–infant relationship and are interpersonal in their focus.

Factors 3 (Sociability) and 9 (Responsiveness to physical contact) are related in that both indicate a positive and close relationship between infant and mother. Shoji et al. (1992) likewise found many Japanese RITQ items to be related to social responsiveness. The alternative labels for sociability included "good-humored" and "rich in emotionality," and what these terms have in common is that the baby expresses such humor and emotionality through a close and happy relationship with the mother. The responsiveness dimension included items mainly related to bathing, and as psychologists we were tempted to label this dimension "responsiveness to bathing." But the mothers easily discerned the social and physical aspects of bathing, as cobathing is still common in Japan from infancy through childhood. Here, mothers looked at the temperament items as markers of the mother–infant relationship rather than as characteristics of child alone.

Factors 5 (Self-assertiveness), 8 (Indulgence/dependency), and 5B (Willfulness) express another important aspect of the Japanese mother–infant relationship, which is characterized by both intense interdependence and by free expression of the child's desires (Lebra, 1976). In infancy, indulgent and dependent (8) behavior (*amae*) is thought to be healthy and normal (Doi, 1985) because Japanese mothers believe dependency indicates a close bond that fosters emotional security. As stated in the *Mother and Child Health Handbook,* "Never leave your [six month-old] baby crying. . . . Don't worry about spoiling your baby by allowing him/her to fall into the habit of being held" (Boshi Aiikukai, 1992, p. 54). The mothers treated the related concept of willfulness or *wagamama* (5B) somewhat differently, perhaps as a negative expression of self. The alternative labels for willfulness (including "cries easily" and "ill-spirited") make it clear that the Japanese distinguish between acceptable and unacceptable self-expression. Together these five dimensions distinguish Japanese maternal perceptions from the Western categories used to describe temperament in that our subjects considered the mother–infant relationship *style* as one aspect of temperament. This contrasts with the usual Western psychological focus on the characteristics of the isolated individual. It also reflects the cultural origins of Japanese maternal perceptions, because "the Japanese are extremely sensitive to and concerned about social interaction and relationships" (Lebra, 1976, p. 2).

## Adult Analogues of Infant Temperament Dimensions

Do mothers' ideas about infant temperament concepts extend to their thinking about temperament and personality beyond infancy? To consider our temperament dimensions as possible life-span concepts, an additional sample of 14 middle-class women were asked to explain each of the Table 7.3 labels. They used many everyday expressions about personality, temperament, and development. The women were given only the factor labels and asked to write the following about each: (1) a definition, (2) examples of the trait, and (3) whether the term was "good" or "bad." We were also interested in the age levels depicted by respondents in their various examples.

### Results

Respondents mainly described other adults with the labels and seldom referred to children or infants. Does this mean that labels for infant temperament factors are actually projections of adult personality terms or that adult personality terms are extensions of infant temperament dimensions? In some cases (e.g., "indulgence/dependency" [*amaembo*]), the word is used most often in reference to infants or small children, and its adult usage refers to childish behavior. In other cases, (e.g., "cautiousness") there seemed to be very little connection between the examples of adult behavior and examples clearly describing adult experiences (e.g., "one who can do nothing without formulating a plan") and the meaning of the infant trait (e.g., "withdrawal from new situations"). Of course, psychological characteristics change functionally with development (e.g., an intense baby compared with a passionate adult). But there were varying degrees of continuity between life-span meanings and infancy meanings, depending on the temperament dimension. The following summarizes the women's ideas about the labels, referring first to the nine 1-month factor labels, followed by the three labels derived above for 3- and

6-month-olds, and the one label (rhythmicity) derived only for 6-month olds.

### Ease/Difficulty of Care

Referring to older children, some adult respondents stated that the "difficult child" (*te no kakaru ko*) requires extra time and assistance in all caretaking matters. Additionally, some adults were depicted as relying on their parents for things they actually could do alone. Therefore, ease of care is desirable across the life-span.

### Intensity of Emotions

Intensity (*hageshisa*) was typified by adults with "a violent temper" or "great passion." This trait was described as undesirable, although some noted that a healthy person should have at least some passion.

### Sociability

Sociability (*shakohsei*) was often used to describe someone who has varied and positive social relations and works well with superiors and coworkers in a company setting. This trait was typically seen as desirable among adults.

### Activity Level

This trait was illustrated by a person who has difficulty remaining still or who takes part in sporting activities. This characteristic was generally thought to be good.

### Self-Assertion

Self-assertiveness (*jiko shucho*) was related to the individual who stands out within the group and persists in one's views. An example was the person who stands alone in discussions, taking a persistent minority position. Depending on the situation, this trait was both good or bad.

### Stability/Gentleness

Gentleness (*otonashii*), paired conceptually with stability by mothers, was most often viewed as desirable, related to a person who is meek, quiet, or obedient. Examples of gentility included one who is "kind to everybody" or "compassionate." This trait also had an undesirable side, as in the conforming individual who "loves animals *because animals are obedient like him*" or cannot assert his own opinion.

## Cautiousness

An example of cautiousness (*shincho*) was the adult who measures each word and does nothing without making a plan. Other examples included the person who will "do nothing if there is any doubt" or "always comes early when he has an appointment." This dimension was often thought to be related to age, becoming more prevalent with age.

## Indulgence/Dependency

This characteristic (*amaembo*) was mainly related to children, although the term can also be used to describe a willful adolescent or adult. "Spoiled child" is a common English translation for this expression, but the Japanese word *amaembo* is not always a negative characteristic. It connotes reliance, and examples included asking for a hug and help with toileting, eating, or dressing. At the same time, this trait can be undesirable, as in the child who "is a torment to parents and an embarrassment throughout life." In this latter example, *amaembo*-like behavior could be a permanent trait.

## Responsiveness to Physical Contact

Responsiveness (*hannosei*) was often related to *skinship*, a Japanese word that originated as a play on words on the English expression "kinship." Skinship was defined by one respondent as "an exchange of loving feelings by skin contact" between parent and child. One example given of skinship was the way a parent presses his or her cheek against the child's face. This behavior was seen as very desirable and was said by one adult to facilitate communication. Responsiveness was both a physical and a social expression of emotional closeness.

## Willfulness

Willfulness (*wagamama*) was a 3- and 6-month dimension similar to indulgence/dependency and self-assertiveness. One participant compared it to selfishness, and *wagamama* was generally described more negatively than the other two dimensions. Some thought that this style developed early in life, mostly among only children. Parents were said to encourage such self-centeredness by yielding to a child's every demand.

## Reactivity to Change

This 3- and 6-month label was discussed in relation to children and adolescents. A typical example of negative reactivity was the elementary or junior high school pupil who cannot adapt to the change of class-mates that occurs at the beginning of a school year. Negative reactivity was usually viewed as undesirable.

## Sensitivity

Rather than sensitivity to physical contact, respondents related sensi-tivity (*binkansa*) to social sensitivity in adults. For instance, sensitive individuals were said to "grasp things quickly." This was viewed as a valuable social skill because the sensitive, empathic individual can understand others' thinking and feelings easily. So whereas infant sensitivity was physical, sensitivity among adults was psychological.

## Rhythmicity

In relation to this dimension, which emerged only for 6-month-olds, rhythmicity (*shuki no kisokusei*) was illustrated by adults as a person who "lives a predictable lifestyle" (*nichijo seikatsu no kisokuteki koi*). For instance, children who eat and sleep at predictable times are called patterned or deemed to have "predictability" (*kisokusei*). This type of behavior is considered good for one's health, but predictability some-times was viewed negatively, as in the case of the adult who cannot correct a bad habit. The term "rhythmicity" (*shuki no kisokusei*) was one case in which the label was a technical term, which was difficult for respondents to understand. But in general the respondents readily perceived the infant temperament dimensions as life-span phenomena, suggesting that these dimensions reflect general concepts of Japanese personality.

# Final Comments

As evidenced by the 15 years Shoji and his colleagues have taken to adapt the RITQ for Japanese babies (Shoji & Maekawa, 1981; Shoji et al., 1992), it is very difficult to understand temperament even within a single culture. Thus any universal understanding of temperament is indeed a formidable goal, which must begin with single-culture studies. We hope that replications of the above methodology can be made in other cultures, and we are currently studying maternal and caretaker perceptions of Japanese toddlers and preschoolers. This may help determine whether the consistent dimensionalities reported here persist across culture, age, and/or observer. In addition, concurrent testing of parents with instruments developed in more than one culture would make possible cross-cultural comparisons, and longitudinal research will be necessary to understand how parental thinking about temperament develops.

Our results concerning infant temperament pertained mainly to mothers' ideas about temperament rather than to "actual" temperament or biological factors. There is a consensus among theorists that temperament is to some extent biologically determined (Bates, 1987), but maternal perceptions may be more related to context than to actual temperament. We have not yet explicitly studied the physical and cultural environment in which temperament develops (Super & Harkness, 1986a, 1986b). Yet our data does define one aspect of context, that is, maternal cognitions about temperament. Our data show that (1) when mothers generate the items and factor labels relevant to infant temperament, the structure of temperament is largely consistent between 1 and 6 months of age, and (2) caution is required in applying temperament dimensions or questionnaire items across cultures. As noted earlier, it is possible that the long history of parenting in Japan has produced a consensual set of temperament dimensions. The advice Japanese receive about infants is consistent and humanistic, such that the government can tell all mothers in the *Mother and Child Health Handbook* that "the secret to child care is to do everything slowly and comfortably" (Boshi Aiikukai, 1992, p. 54).

Our pilot study sample of adults generated specific instances in which the infant temperament dimensions were readily applied to children, adolescents, and (most often) adults. This small survey focused on another aspect of context by eliciting examples of the settings in which individuals exhibit each aspect of temperament. It would be interesting in follow-up research to see whether adults in other cultures suggest the same situations in which each dimension of temperament is expressed.

Viewing our findings as a whole, one can see temperament and personality as a system by which members of a culture agree on dimensions they can use to compare and understand individuals. If indeed maternal perceptions are one type of parental ethnotheory, it might be inferred from the pilot study examples that parental ethnotheories about infant temperament are related to adult's general understanding of personality. This reminds one of Kelly's (1955) theory, in which each individual "constructs" personality by using the dimensions salient to himself or herself for evaluating and comparing people. One source of such personal constructs could be the characteristics of infant temperament. Conversely, our views of infant temperament may reflect our general personality constructs. Under Kelly's theory, parental ethnotheories would be a subset of personal constructs relating to the parental role, and the values and beliefs of a particular culture could bias that population to focus on certain dimensions of child personality or temperament. If indeed maternal perceptions of babies are part of a larger cognitive framework, our follow-up research should consider parental ethnotheories as one aspect of the cultural construction of adult personality.

## Acknowledgments

Appreciation is extended to Drs. Shigeo Yokoi, Atsuhiro Soeda, Kihei Maekawa, and Hiroshi Kurimoto. This chapter is dedicated to our children: Lori, Connie, Becky, Davy, Debbie, Daisuke, Kensuke, and Yukori.

## References

Bates, J. E. (1987). Temperament in infancy. In J. D. Osofsky (Ed.), *Handbook of infant development* (2nd ed. pp. 1101–1149). New York: Wiley.

Bates, J. E., & Bayles, K. (1984). Objective and subjective components in mothers' perceptions of their children from age 6 months to 3 years. *Merrill-Palmer Quarterly, 30*(2), 111–130.

Bornstein, M. H. (1989). Cross-cultural developmental comparisons: The case of Japanese-American infant and mother activities and interactions. *Developmental Review, 9,* 171–204.

Boshi Aiikukai (1992). *Mother and child health handbook.* Tokyo: Author.

Carey, W. B., & McDevitt, S. C. (1978). Revision of the infant temperament questionnaire. *Pediatrics, 61,* 735–739.

Caudill, W., & Weinstein, H. (1969). Maternal care and infant behavior in Japan and America. *Psychiatry, 32,* 12–43.

Dale, P. N. (1986). *The myth of Japanese uniqueness.* New York: St. Martin's Press.

Doi, T. (1985). *The anatomy of self: The individual versus society.* Tokyo: Kodansha International.

Embree, J. (1939). *Suye mura: A Japanese village.* Chicago: University of Chicago Press.

Goodnow, J. J., & Collins, W. A. (1990). *Development according to parents.* Hillsdale, NJ: Erlbaum.

Hagekull, B. (1991). *The search for meaning in factor analytically derived dimensions.* Symposium paper presented at the biennial meetings of the Society for Research in Child Development, Seattle, WA.

Hair, J. F., Anderson, R. E., Tatham, R. L., & Black, W. C. (1992). *Multivariate data analysis* (3rd ed.). New York: Macmillan.

Hara, H., & Wagatsuma, H. (1974). *Shitsuke* [Child-rearing]. Tokyo: Kobundoh.

Hsu, C., Soong, W., Stigler, J. W., Hong, C. , & Liang, C. (1981). The temperamental characteristics of Chinese babies. *Child Development, 52,* 1337–1340.

Japan Health and Welfare Ministry (1990). *Guidelines for day nursery child care.* Tokyo: Japanese Government Printing Office (in Japanese).

Kazuki, G. (1976). *A handbook of childrearing.* (Reprinted in M. Yamazumi & K. Nakae [Eds.], *Books on child-rearing,* [Vol. 1, pp. 287–366]. Tokyo: Heibon-sha [in Japanese]) (Original work published 1703)

Kelly, G. A. (1955). *The psychology of personal constructs.* New York: Norton.

Kojima, H. (1989). *An inquiry into the history of Japanese child-rearing.* Tokyo: Shinyosha (in Japanese).

Kosawa, Y., Shand, N., Takahashi, M. & Fujisaki, M. (1985). Maternal ratings in the newborn period as a function to determine the behavioral status of infants at 12 and 16 months of age. Paper presented at the meetings of the Society for Research in Child Development, Toronto.

Lanham, B. B. (1966). The psychological orientation of the mother–child relationship in Japan. *Monumenta Nipponica, 21,* 322–332.

Lebra, T. S. (1976). *Japanese patterns of behavior.* Honolulu: University of Hawaii Press.

Miyake, K., Chen, S. J., & Campos, J. J. (1985). Infant temperament, mother's mode of interaction, and attachment. In I. Bretherton & E. Waters (Eds.), *Growing points in attachment theory and research. Monographs of the Society for Research in Child Development, 50* (Serial No. 209, pp. 267–297).

Murai, N., Nihei, Y., Nasu, I., & Yonemoto, Y. (1982). Stability of individual differences in early infancy. *Tohoku Psychologica Folia, 41*(1–4), 95–106.

Nippon Aiiku Kenkyujo (1994). *Nihon Kodomo Dhiryo Nenkan* Statistical yearbook of children. Nagoya: KTC Chuo Shuppan.

Rothbart, M. K. (1989). Temperament and development. In G. Kohnstamm, J. Bates & M. Rothbart (Eds.), *Temperament in childhood* (pp. 187–247). New York: Wiley.

Rothbart, M. K., & Mauro, J. A. (1990). Questionnaire approaches to the study of infant temperament. In J. Colombo & J. Fagen (Eds.), *Individual differences in infancy: Reliability, stability, prediction* (pp. 411–429). Hillsdale, NJ: Erlbaum.

Sanson, A., Prior, M., Garino, E., Oberklaid, F., & Sewell, J. (1987). The structure of infant temperament: Factor analysis of the Revised Infant Temperament Questionnaire. *Infant Behavior and Development, 10,* 97–104.

Sengoku, T. (1983). Mother–child relationships in Japan through behavioral observation. *Journal of Perinatal Medicine, 13* (Suppl.), 501–504 (in Japanese).

Shand, N., & Kosawa, Y. (1985). Japanese and American behavior types at three months: Infants and infant–mother dyads. *Infant Behavior and Development, 8,* 225–240.

Shoji, J., & Maekawa, K. (1981). Infant temperament: Its significance and a method of assessment. *Journal of Pediatric Practice, 44*(8), 1225–1232 (in Japanese).

Shoji, J., Soeda, A., & Yokoi, S. (1992). *A factor analytic study of the Japanese ITQ.* Paper presented at the 67th annual meetings of the Japanese Association of Child Psychiatry and Neurology, Shizuoka (in Japanese).

Shwalb, D. W., Imaizumi, N., & Nakazawa, J. (1987). The modern Japanese father: Roles and problems in a changing society. In M. E. Lamb (Ed.), *The father's role: Cross-cultural perspectives* (pp. 247–269). Hillsdale, NJ: Erlbaum.

Shwalb, D. W., & Shwalb, B. J. (Eds.). (in press). *Japanese childrearing: Two generations of scholarship.* New York: Guilford Press.

Shwalb, D. W., Shwalb, B. J., Sukemune, S., & Tatsumoto, S. (1992). Japanese non-maternal childcare: Past, present and future. In M. Lamb, K. Sternberg, C.-P. Hwang, & A. Broberg (Eds.), *Childcare in context* (pp. 331–353). Hillsdale, NJ: Erlbaum.

Soeda, A., Shoji, J., Yokoi, S., & Maekawa, K. (1991). *Developmental change in temperamental characteristics: A comparison of infants, 5- and 7-year olds.* Paper presented at the 38th annual meetings of the Japanese Society of Child Health, Asahikawa City, Hokkaido (in Japanese).

Sugawara, M., Aoki, M., Kitamura, T., & Shima, S. (1988). The structure of infant temperamental characteristics. *Shohoku Junior College Bulletin, 9*(8), 157–163 (in Japanese).

Super, C. M., & Harkness, S. (1986a). Temperament, development and culture. In R. Plomin & J. Dunn (Eds.), *The study of temperament: Changes, continuities, and challenges* (pp. 131–149). Hillsdale, NJ: Erlbaum.

Super, C., & Harkness, S. (1986b). The developmental niche: A conceptualization at the interface of child and culture. *International Journal of Behavioral Development, 9,* 545–569.

Thomas, A., & Chess, S. (1977). *Temperament and development.* New York: Brunner/Mazel.

Vogel, E. (1992). *Japan's new middle class* (2nd ed.). Berkeley: University of California Press.

Wagatsuma, H., & DeVos, G. (1984). *Heritage of endurance: Family patterns and delinquency patterns in Japan.* Berkeley: University of California Press.

White, M. I., & LeVine, R. A. (1986). What is an *Ii Ko* (good child)? In H. Stevenson, H. Azuma, & K. Hakuta (Eds.), *Child development and education in Japan* (pp. 55–62). New York: Freeman.

# CHAPTER 8

# Scenes from a Marriage
## Equality Ideology in Swedish Family Policy, Maternal Ethnotheories, and Practice

Barbara Welles-Nyström

## Preface

When asked to prepare this chapter on Swedish parental ethnotheories, I immediately thought of the title, "Scenes from a Marriage." This was a film directed and written by Ingmar Bergman in the early 1970s, which captured a critical historical moment, when many Western societies, including Sweden, were undergoing social upheaval, particularly in regard to relations between the sexes. Using Bergman's title is simply a device for me to paraphrase my own "insider–outsider" status. I am an American who lives and conducts child development and feminist research in Sweden; my husband is Swedish and my children are being raised biculturally. While firmly advocating that the personal is political, in my case, the scientific is also the personal.

## Introduction and Theoretical Background

Equality as ideology is the thread that binds together the cultural fabric of Swedish politics, health care, and child status and is a key element of parental ethnotheories (Super & Harkness, 1986; Harkness & Super, 1992) for infant and child health and development. Equality is defined as the state of being equal, particularly in respect to gender, parent–child interaction, and social class. In Sweden, mothers and government (specifically the progressive and liberal Social Democrats who have held political control until the recent election in 1991) collaborate to assure the primary goal of infant survival and protection followed by goals of enculturaltion, those parental goals LeVine (1974) hypothesizes as universal. In particular I will consider equality, its meaning and interpretation, as a dynamic thread in society connecting family policy and legislation, health care programs, and the special status of the child to maternal theories of child development. I will argue that governmental policy *creates* culture in that certain social programs, particularly those concerned with health care and family policy, amplify and institutionalize public preferences in the population (i.e., first there was support for legislation, then the laws were passed). These policies enable the Swedish child to be reared in ways distinctly new. Equality ideology provides the philosophical "stuff" from which parents construct theories of childrearing and which interface with maternal attitude and behavior.

The purpose of this chapter is to explore the unique situation of the Swedish child and the ideology of equality in respect to psychoanthropological perspectives on child development and cultural milieu. Following two related theories which securely place the child within a culture-specific environment, I will explore the meaning of equality as an instantiation (Harkness & Super, 1992) of Swedish culture and Swedish parental ethnotheory. The first theory concerns aspects of the physical environment, or what Weisner (1984) calls the ecocultural niche. The second theory considers aspects of the child's psychological environment or what Super and Harkness term the developmental niche. The term "niche" implies that this context has not only evolved through time but has also adapted to the constraints imposed by the subsistence base, the climate, and the political economy of the region (Weisner, 1984, pp. 335–336). Domains of the ecocultural niche can be categorized into five clusters: health and mortality, provision of food and shelter, personnel likely to be around children and what they do, specific focus on role of women and mothers in the community, and cultural alternatives available in the community (Weisner, 1984; Whiting & Edwards, 1988). The developmental niche includes the physical and social setting in which the child lives, with culturally regulated customs of child care and childrearing provided by caretakers of certain psychological characteristics. Three components are conceptualized: the physical and social setting in which the child lives, culturally regulated customs of child care and childrearing, and the psychology of the caretakers (Super & Harkness, 1986). Particular attention will be given in this chapter to how maternal attitudes toward equality effect childrearing practices.

In Sweden, I argue, the concept of equality ideology binds together the ecocultural niche and the developmental niche, as mothers, in response to constraints and support in the former, manage and organize the latter in their children's best interest. How Swedish parents do this depends, at least in part, on the ways in which they perceive their own culture, and their attitudes toward culturally accepted values, including equality but also individualism and collectivity.

> Swedish mentality seems to have two opposing tendencies; one towards individualism and the other towards collectivity. The explanation for this is the different meaning that can be given to the concept of individualism. Swedes seem to need social autonomy strongly and seem not to be dependent on other individuals, such as neighbors, relatives, employers, and so on. At the same time, Swedes seem to need collective support for their opinions. Collective solutions are a hallmark of Swedish society and dominate Swedish politics. (Daun, 1991, p. 165).

Swedish parents socialize their children toward individualistic goals, particularly within the family, which are subsequently balanced by needs and demands of the larger social group. The child is perceived as developing "naturally" into a person who incorporates both and one who is guided by the idea of equality.

Ideologically, Sweden has been considered foremost among Western societies on three critical fronts. First, "state feminism's" (Dahlerup, 1993) aspiration was to assure equal opportunities for both genders in the private and public sectors. Basic aspects of this ideology were formalized in the late 1960s when the Swedish government prepared a document, "Status of the Woman in Sweden." In this document, goals for attaining sexual equality were spelled out as the balance between the "rights" of women to participate in the labor market and the "rights" of men to participate in the home—with specific emphasis on housework and child care (Fogarty, Rapaport, & Rapaport, 1971; see appendix for excerpt).

The ideology of equality is also evidenced by Sweden's child and parent-friendly leave policy entitled "Parental Insurance." Briefly, what this insurance provides for the child is reimbursement at 90% of salary for one parent to take care of the infant in the home for a period of up to 1 year. Following this, the parent may choose to remain at home for an additional year at a reduced salary, or reduce the amount of hours involved in the labor market. In either event, the parent will not be penalized and the job must be guaranteed (or one of equivalent status) for the parent when they return to work.

Second, not only is the high status of the child ideologically prominent in the family and society, but the child's human rights are legally protected. These rights have included the right of inheritance regardless of gender (inheritance law, instituted 1845); rights to inherit property from the biological father regardless of marital status (1970), the right to be wanted (liberal abortion law, instituted 1974); a healthy *prenatal* milieu (free prenatal care; paid maternity leave during pregnancy if mother is sick, or if employment is hazardous to health of infant or mother); a healthy *perinatal* milieu (free medical care during the hospitalized management of birth and the early perinatal period) followed by a stable *postnatal* environment with one or both parents caring for the baby during the first year of life (parental leave insurance established 1974, expanded 1980); adequate housing (housing allowance); adequate clothing and food (child-care allowance, instituted 1947); right of parents of young children to a 6-hour workday (instituted 1979) (Carlson, 1990; Bernhardt, 1991; Statistiska Centralbyrån, 1990). Children, by law, are also protected from parental corporal punishment (instituted 1979) (Rädda Barnen, 1991). Thus, ideally, every child is welcome in the society regardless of parent's marital, economic, or ethnic status or the child's gender.

Third, the Swedish socialized health care sector not only links together diverse groups in society, by delivering high-quality medical services for all, but produces culture-specific theories of infant and child health, which are subsequently reproduced within the family when parents act on that information to transform it into parental ethnotheories. The Swedish socialized health care sector supersedes every other source of information to parents about infant and child development, beginning with the conception of the child. Virtually every pregnant woman in Sweden attends the free midwife-run prenatal clinics locally available throughout the country, and her baby's health, growth, and development are charted and followed after delivery through the first 6 years of life by the pediatric nurses who staff the national well-baby clinics. Thus, in Sweden, equality ideology contends not only that both genders are to be equally involved in society, in public and private spheres, which extends to include children, but that every citizen's right (child and adult) is to have assistance in maintaining and improving health through the socialized health care sector. Transformation of equality ideology into reality is a consistent maternal childrearing theme. However, that transformation is problematic as shown by certain ethnographic examples that contrast the "reality" of experienced equality ideology with the ideology itself.

The data for this chapter come from two different studies. The maternal age study, conducted in 1980–1982, investigated certain pre- and postnatal psychosocial variables for 52 Swedish first-time mothers ranging in age from 20 to 40 years (Welles, 1982). Included were attitudinal data about childrearing goals and division of labor and child care in the home and maternal ethnotheories of gender-based behaviors in both parents and children framed by ethnographic observations of community and family life (Welles-Nyström, 1988; LeVine, Miller, & West, 1988; Richman et al., 1988; Welles-Nyström, 1991). The second study, postponed motherhood in Sweden and the United States, conducted in 1987–1990 investigated psychosocial variables for a small comparative sample of late-timing mothers during pregnancy and the early postpartum period. Attitudinal data about gender and behavior were collected and mothers were interviewed about childrearing goals (Welles-Nyström, 1995).

I will limit my discussion of parental ethnotheories to *maternal* ethnotheories, because Swedish women, as research and personal informants, have helped me to better understand culture-specific paradigms of child health and development. My data have been collected primarily in research interviews with new mothers, but I have also relied on information collected in a more "natural" way by living in Sweden, so that certain antecdotal and ethnographic evidence is interwoven through the text. It should be noted that the focus on equality as a key element and ideology in Swedish culture does not deny that other issues are also important, nor does focusing on security and independence exclude the significance of other values. My point is to illustrate how, within an "equality" paradigm, the cultural and political framework of the society interacts and supports a certain type of familial experience for the child that is uniquely Swedish.

## The Ecocultural and Developmental Niche of the Swedish Child

Sweden is a small country in northern Europe about the size of California, with a population of about 8 million (a bit less than that of Los Angeles). The general level of education is high enough so that all citizens are literate, and more newspapers per person are sold (and supposedly read) than in any other country in the world. Most health statistics are superior to those of the United States, with the most noteworthy statistic the low infant mortality rate (see Table 8.1). "Science" is highly respected, and scientists or experts often inform governmental policy, particularly those connected with the child. Sweden also ranks high among urbanized, industrial societies in female labor force participation, male domestic responsibility, and legislative support for sexual equality and the protection of children (Liljeström, 1978). In fact, Sweden's progressive family policies have been termed part of "state feminism" (Dahlerup, 1993) in that feminist goals of gender equality have been directly incorporated into political dogma and realized through family policy supporting women and children. Cradle-to-grave security, although paid for by high taxes, has been nurturant first to its children and directly and indirectly supportive of their mothers. In order to provide *all* children with quality basic necessitites of life, many social programs were developed to support single women with children. (Approximately 12% of children live in single-parent families, predominantly with the mother, while 18% live in mixed families in which the custodial parent lives with a new spouse. About 70% of children live in nuclear families with both parents [Statistiska Centralbyrån, 1991].)

At the larger, ecocultural level, Sweden then exhibits a different ideology of equality from other Western societies, from which individuals construct gender-appropriate roles and behaviors during the life course, including those for taking care of children. Parenting, particularly the ideal message about what mothering is, can be conceptualized as "cultural script" (Willard, 1988). The cultural script is a "rather specific set of ideas about how events should take place so that members of that culture can be guided through major life events and changes." This script works well when "clear cultural expectations are supported by social structures that make it possible for people to carry out their roles in accord with the cultures expectations" (Willard, 1988, p. 226). In Sweden, the cultural script for parenting differs from other Western cultures on several important variables. Swedish fathers, for instance, are expected to be as capable and interested in active caretaking of

**Table 8.1.** Comparative Demographic Statistics

|  | United States | Sweden |
| --- | --- | --- |
| Population[a] | 226,545,805 | 8,360,178 |
| Life expectancy |  |  |
| Men[a] | 71.3 years | 74.16 years |
| Women[a] | 78.3 years | 80.15 years |
| Crude birth rate[a] | 15.9 | 13.6 |
| Infant mortality rate[a] | 9.9 | 6.0 |
| Marriage rate[a] | 9.7 | 5.2 |
| Divorce rate[a] | 4.8 | 2.26 |
| First birth rate[b] | 24.7 | 19.3 |

*Note.* Sources: [a]United Nations (1991); [b]United Nations (1988). Crude birth, marriage, and divorce rates are computed per 1,000 midyear population. Infant mortality rates are per 1,000 live births and first birth rates are the sum of the age-specific fertility rates per woman. First birth rates and cohort-specific first birth rates are computed for total live births in each birth order and age group per 1,000 total female population in specific age group.

offspring, including infants, as are the mothers. This "soft" (*mjuk*) side of manhood has affectionately been called the velveteen daddy phenomenon.

Swedish maternal scripts are also culture-specific. Swedish women generally postpone motherhood until their mid to late 20s, as the vast majority of women are employed, and adult identity for both genders finds its primary definition in relation to employment. Approximately 90% of women ages 25 to 44 participate in the labor force, although 47% of those are part-time workers (Statistiska Centralbyrån, 1990). Even for those women with children under the age of 7, at least 80% are employed, although most do not reenter the labor market until after the child's first, and preferably after the second birthday and then do so in a part-time capacity (Hoem & Hoem, 1988).

Childbirth usually precedes formalized marriage, if marriage occurs at all. For women, the median age for first birth is 26.1 years and first marriage is 27 years, while for men the median age of first marriage is approximately 29.6 years. The age when men first become fathers is not statistically documented (Statistiska Centralbyrån, 1990, 1991). First children are usually born in a nuclear family situation, although they are equally as likely to be born to a married mother as an unmarried one (Hoem & Hoem, 1988). The vast majority of unmarried mothers cohabit with the child's father in a *sambo* (cohabiting) relationship. Expecting a child is not much of an incentive for getting married, and it only marginally affects the decision whether to legalize cohabitation (Hoem, 1985; Popenoe, 1987). Rates of marital instability in Sweden are similar to those of most other Western societies. About half of all marriages (even those without children or without children living at home) end in divorce, with the statistics for cohabitors even higher. According to a recent study conducted by the census bureau, "The most stable families with children are those with married parents, rather than families where parents cohabit" (Statistiska Centralbyrån, 1990, p. 88).

Prior to the moment of conception, the Swedish child is "supposed" to be wanted, desired, and planned, which are values consistent with those projected by midwives at the governmental maternity clinics. To continue a pregnancy (25% of all pregnancies, including those of adolescents, are terminated, [Statistiska Centralbyrån, 1986]) indicates that ideally a women considers herself psychologically and economically capable of taking care of a new baby. Pregnancy is monitored by midwives at local maternity clinics for literally all women in Sweden and is free of charge. The major goal is protective: to assure the best possible uterine environment for the growing fetus. Expectant mothers are informed about health risks to the infant of certain maternal behaviors, such as smoking and drinking, and the positive effects of good diet and exercise, and a great deal of literature concerning the pre- and postnatal period is distributed (e.g., regarding breastfeeding). The fetus's growth is recorded at regular intervals and exercise and natural childbirth classes are organized for new mothers and their mates.

Pregnancy is not considered a "special" time because it is viewed as a normal, developmental part of life. Women are expected to continue to carry on their usual daily routines, which include going to work, and most take a paid leave of absence only when they go to the hospital to deliver. Childbirth is also managed by midwives, who ideally support women's wishes in choice of attendants (usually the father of the baby), labor position, pharmaceutical intervention, and length of stay in hospital. Postnatally, after the mother and child return home after birth, the baby is registered at the national well-baby clinic, where the infant is routinely weighed and measured through age 6. Since 1968, all 4-year-old children undergo a full physical examination, where physical problems can be detected and remedial measures taken. The clinics also sponsor parenting classes for new families.

The health care sector, because it reaches all new babies and their families from conception through the start of school, is a unifying element in Swedish society. Its goal of protecting the infant and ensuring that his or her physical environment as managed by the parents is a secure and well-informed one is thereby an equalizing cultural factor in that *all* infants are included in such care. Ideas about good infant care which mothers report "coincide" with the standardized health care information supplied by the well-baby clinics. For instance, in the mid-1980s when I asked mothers what they could do to protect the health of their infant, women mentioned good nutrition, including breastfeeding, inoculations, adequate sleep, fresh air, and a harmonious environment (Welles-Nyström, 1988). These answers were remarkable because they were so consistently scientific and informed, as if the answers came directly from the well-baby clinic. To test this idea, I recently gave some nursing students the original data to reanalyze. They spontaneously commented on how the answers the mothers provided sounded exactly like information from the well-baby clinics. This antecdotal evidence suggests that health information provided to mothers "reaches" them at some level, and that it also informs maternal theories of infant health.

Swedish children are made to feel welcome in society and much effort is made to assure a secure (*trygg*) physical environment, equal in basic standard to any other child's. Government-funded day care is well organized and generally available. Most Swedish children do not receive formalized child care until after the first year of life, and many not until around the age of 3. Objectives of the day-care system, which was regulated by the Social Services Act in 1982 (Swedish Institute, 1987), are consistent with the general norms of society. They can be summarized by the following key principles: democracy, solidarity, *equality*, security, participation, and responsibility. These key words apply as well to Swedish ideals of adult behavior including the ideal of cooperation (Qvarfort, McCrae, & Kolenda, 1988; Daun, 1991), which is subsumed in the ideal of participation and responsibility.

Enculturation of the Swedish child during the first year of life takes place almost exclusively in the home. The unequivocal belief is that the newborn and young child must be made to feel welcomed, safe, and secure, and that the best place for this to take place is in the home. The Swedish home is still the location in which traditional values such as neatness, orderliness, cleanliness, and comfort are reproduced. Many folk sayings prevail in which the virtues and importance of the home are sung (e.g., "to be away is good; to be home, the best;" and "*hem-kär*" (to be in love with the home). The home symbolizes the strong attachment Swedes have to the family (Popenoe, 1987), whether it be the place of year-round residence or the summer cottages most aspire to own.

Within the home, mothers, or fathers if they are the parent responsible for the daily care of the infant, create safe environments. Halldén (1991) suggests that good parents take time with their children, and this time should be spent within the home environment. Time is recognized as a valuable commodity in Sweden, where the goal for adult behavior is rational use of that commodity. "The home is a place of intimacy, a haven of fewer demands and greater permissiveness, while the outside world stands for all that is foreign and alien" (Halldén, 1991, pp. 338–339). In the privacy of the home, one can more likely "be oneself," or take off the public mask. It is a "free zone for individuality" (Halldén, 1991).

Consistent with the belief that "home is best," legislation provides the economic means with which the infant can, after birth and for at least the first year of life, remain in the home and be taken care of by one parent. Swedish mothers are the primary parent who remain, or rather *return*, to the home after the child is born, and being given the right to "*vara hemma*" (to be at home) is highly valued, not only for the "break" it entails from the work force but because of the opportunity provided to really get to know the new baby and to develop a close relationship.

Gender roles affiliated with home care, however, compete with child care, and many women report conflict in roles and values. On the one hand, as modern, well-educated women, they "know" that they are supposed to "bond" with the baby. Ideas about bonding derived from the popularizing of early attachment research (e.g., Klaus & Kennell,

1972; and in Sweden, DeChateau, 1976, 1979). On the other hand, to be a good traditional Swedish housewife (which in some respects they view themselves as they are "at home" and not "at work"), their house is supposed to be clean and orderly. The tension between these two roles and the work they entail is a distinct element of the passage to motherhood. First-time mothers often mention their interpretation of role responsibility conflicts, and many say that one of the most important things they learned while taking care of their child in the first year was to accept the dust under the bed (Welles, 1982). In contemporary Sweden, the emotional development of the child is the priority when mothers decide to give their time and attention to the baby instead of to cleaning and cooking. However, these household tasks continue to weigh heavily on many women, and complaints about how difficult it is to get "everything done at home," even when they are at home all day, are common.

## Equality as Policy and Maternal Goal

How mothers interpret equality ideology has ramifications for understanding Swedish maternal ethnotheories. It is the framework within which other goals can or cannot be realized. Swedish women are cognizant of the legal aspects of equality legislation particularly in respect to women's rights at the workplace, because so many are gainfully employed outside the home. However, in the home, private decisions between parents about child-care responsibilities and housework are not always negotiated in respect to women's or men's rights. Swedish policymakers continue to legislate for men's increased involvement in child care, but no large-scale radicalization of parental responsibility has occurred. Women continue to be the primary parent. Men, as fathers, assist them.

In respect to equality, what are some hallmarks of political ideology? One area in which there is constant debate and interest is the issue of sexual equality (*jämnställdhet*), which in Sweden has implications and direct consequences for both genders. One inherent idea of *jämnställdhet* derives from the "Status of Women in Sweden," mentioned previously. A section of this document is worth investigating in more detail because it sets the stage for the equality paradigm for gender role and responsibility. The original document stated: "If women are to attain a position in society outside the home which corresponds to their proportional membership of the citizen body, it follows that men must *assume a greater share or responsibility* [emphasis added] for the upbringing of the children and the care of the home" ("Status of Women in

Sweden" quoted in Fogarty et al., 1971, pp. 107–108). That is, women will be "raised" to the level of men in the labor market only when men "help out" more at home (with children and housework).

There is a flaw in the argument that ties in with ideological discrepancies manifest in the reality of current parental behaviors. If the goal in Sweden was that women's position and status in the public sphere should *theoretically* correspond proportionately to their number, then women should represent 50% of all levels of positions in society. And would not the converse argument have been the same for men in the home? Because all children are born to parents who equally represent both sexes (whether or not they are married), should not men have been expected to participate equally in their care rather than only to "assume a greater share of responsibility"?

In fact, the interface between ideology and reality on this point is interesting. Although Swedish women have not reached equal representation in society at large (e.g. women are still not proportionately represented in government, nor do they receive equal wages), men have taken a greater share of parental responsibility, at least with infants and the young child. Studies of fathers have shown that men's use of parental leave has increased slightly from 20.4% in 1978 to 24.5% in 1987 (Sundström, 1991). Particularly active are fathers of newborns, the majority of whom make use of the 10 postpartum "new daddy days" to help out at home (Bernhardt, 1991). And there is evidence that, at least among the younger men in society, fatherhood scripts have been rewritten to mean "real" involvement in child care (Ohlander, 1993). However, whether or not men as fathers strive to realize equality ideology by taking a proportional share of parental responsibility seems unclear. To date, the general pattern continues whereby fathers "assist" the mothers of their children in caring for them, rather than any role reversal which would put men, at least 50% of the time, into the role of parent with real responsibility (Hwang, 1987; Lamb, Frodi, Hwang, Frodi, & Stinberg, 1981; Sandqvist, 1987).

What was fascinating about this paternal policy development was that when the maternal leave policy was expanded to include fathers in 1974, contrary to many other such political decisions, the intention of placing infants in the primary care of their fathers was not based on any "hard" scientific evidence that fathers could do the job (i.e., know how to mother). Rather, the decision was based on an equalitarian ideal of parental androgyny; that is, that men and women were interchangeable in respect to the caregiving and caretaking environments they could provide. There was no evidence or research at the time to support this drastic action; the belief system of equality was the motivational force rather than science. The fact remains, then, that although the goal of sexual or gender equality has existed in Sweden for several decades, it has not yet been realized.

Consistently, from observations made in my daily living experiences in Sweden, from empiricial studies I have conducted, and from those by other Swedish social scientists, it seems that both sexes would like to live the myth of social and sexual equality, or at least that is the way they often discuss it. One of the most common statements heard when asking Swedish women how they manage housework is that they "share" it. The sharing may be organized as a turn-taking endeavor, but it can also be shared according to ability. "He does the cleaning, I do the laundry and baking." Few women admit publicly to being dissatisfied with their mate's participation in the home, even though current studies show that not only do men do less housework than women, even when the women are fully employed outside the home, but that men's leisure time at home (e.g., reading newspapers and some recreational activities) has not noticeably decreased while women's has (Statistiska Centralbyrån, 1991). Hence, as mentioned before, although there is some evidence for a kind of role sharing for housework and child care, it is not yet on an equal (50-50) basis. And there is no evidence as yet for incidences of true gender role reversal. Swedish women to date remain primary caregivers both for their children and for their homes.

Studies conducted on the use of time in Swedish families have shown that men spend fewer hours at home when there is a new infant in the family (men are at their job) and that they do considerably less housework than do women. Postnatally, this is rationalized by the fact that because the mother is "home" with the baby anyhow, she might as well dust and clean. Later on, when women return to work, the child is being cared for by an adult other than the parents, and both parents are involved in the labor market, the father's share of housework does not noticeably increase, although the woman's daily input at home does decrease somewhat. (The total amount of housework completed decreases.) While both "work" about the same amount of hours per week, he is paid for his full-time labor, while she receives only partial reimbursement from her employer and nothing for the domestic labor she does (Statistiska Centralbyrån, 1992).

Given the situation, it is surprising how equality is talked about in the family or home situation. One might suppose that women would complain about their husbands not taking a real responsibility for child care, or helping out more, but they do not. Are the statistics wrong? Or is something else at work here? I have no empirical data to support this notion; but I wonder whether women, in loyalty to the ideology of equality, prefer to keep the mask on about the home situation and contend that *their* partner *shares*, thereby *not* directly confronting the specific division of labor inherent in egalitarian partnerships, the cultural script for family life in Sweden.

The Swedish ethnologist Åke Daun may give some clues to the psychological processes behind my observation. He cites Gullstad's (1989) work in Norway to explain how "members of Swedish culture stress sameness, underestimate communicative difference in social encounters, and strive to 'fit in with' friends, neighbors and relatives. Consequently, many Swedes never express in company where they stand on a controversial issue, especially if they do not have any idea about what the others will say about the same thing" (Daun, 1991, p. 167). As Swedes avoid face-to-face conflict whenever possible, they are perhaps doing so even when interviewed about gender norms. Equality ideology is pervasive in Sweden, but to expose the weaknesses, or reality, in the system is not an accepted way to act.

In respect to maternal attitudes toward gender, there are also discrepancies between ideology and reality. There is a two-step accommodation process whereby a kind of professed loyalty to the ideology of equality is first expressed, followed by an statement of normative values, which are of a nonequal nature. The following examples are illustrative.

## Sex of Child

In the interview situation, and even among friends and acquaintances, it is normative for pregnant women to report not having a sexual preference for their unborn child; rather, the primary "wish was for a healthy child" (Welles, 1982). However, when pressed and asked what they desire if they were given a choice, almost all women made a statement preferring one sex over the other. In both studies I conducted in Sweden, the majority of women wanted girls as first children. Gender is important. There are even folk theories about "reading" a woman's pregnancy: a wide stomach is a girl, a stomach protruding out front is a boy.

## Infant Personality

Mothers of 10-month-old infants stated that infants did not exhibit different personalities or behaviors dependent on sex. Little gender difference is attributed to the infant. However, developmentally it was believed that there was a clear differentiation at around age 3, when mothers said that they either observed other children or anticipated for their own child that boys would play with cars and/or be more active while girls would play more with dolls and/or be more passive or calmer.

*Childrearing*

When mothers were asked whether boys or girls were easier to raise, the majority said as young children they were equally demanding. However, predicting the future, they believed that boys were easier to raise as teenagers because girls caused so much worry, they could get pregnant, and because girls matured earlier than boys, they acted older than their age and indulged in a lot of risk behavior. Many mothers said that they hoped their own daughters would not be the way they had been as teenagers.

*Good Mother versus Good Father Role*

When interviewing mothers about their views about what a good mother was, the vast majority of women reported that caring for the infant's health in the first year of life was most important (e.g., providing warm clothes and good food). This caretaking behavior applied as well to ideals of good fatherhood. Of course, breastfeeding was seen as being gender specific, as was taking care of the child's emotional needs. Mothers comforted their children, and fathers played with them. Further, fathers were seen as playing differently with their children than the mothers did; and they were less likely to change dirty diapers.

*Social Status*

The legal status of the child is not negatively affected by whether or not the child's parents are legally married, but social status is less clear-cut. Although parental decisions about legalizing cohabitation are seen as privately managed, the choice of surname for the child often reflects older traditions whereby the father's surname is given to the offspring even when parents are not legally married. A surprising number of these children bear their father's last name rather than their mother's, which is "rightfully" theirs at birth. Why it continues to be important for parents to name paternity rather than maternity in choice of their baby's surname is not understood.

*The Cultural Roots of Equality Ideology: The "Jante Law"*

Equality ideology also contains aspects that constrain the emotional and psychological development of the child. The underside of the equality paradigm in Sweden includes a psychologically important folk theory called the *Jante Law*. Briefly, this rural Nordic philosophy, formalized by Axel Sandemose (1933/1977), was a collection of "10 commandments" for instilling in children self-inhibition and conformity. These commandments can be summarized briefly as follows:

1. You shall not believe that you are anything.
2. You shall not believe that you can do anything.
3. You shall not believe that you know anything.

I contend that these "commandments" are vestiges of traditional childrearing attitudes (Liliequist, 1991) that have prevailed as a dominant parental theme (even for my own Swedish contemporaries), resulting in the stereotypical characteristics of Swedish personality such as humility, lack of confidence, and shyness. However, today, these same age-mates who are parents, in addition to this traditional psychology, now espouse other, more individual-centered beliefs, such as those presented by non-Scandinavian psychologists Benjamin Spock or Penelope Leach. Consequently, I believe the Jante Law remains an important element in the ideology of equality because it explains how the child is humiliated out of desiring to be extra or special in any way (surely a rather typical goal for well-educated American parents, who espouse parental goals such as "be the best that you can be"). Humility, which was once used to support a hierarchical social order, can now be used to support egalitarian cooperation within the group. The result is that the child is "equalized" or reduced to the level of the group, in that he or she is "no better than anyone else." Parental goals inherent in the Jante Law are humbleness and self-depreciation, which can explain how parents then balance goals of equality with conformity and independence with uniformity.

Although many Swedish parents today would disagree explicitly with these "commandments" in respect to their own childrearing goals, they nonetheless readily acknowledge the Jante Law's existence as a prevailing "modus operandi" of Swedish lay psychology. Parents themselves have informed me of the Jante Law, and it is commonly referred to in the popular psychological literature as well as in the press. Because of the prevalence of group care and the importance of establishing group identity rather than a unique individual identity for the older child who is enrolled in day care, I would suggest that this "law" is alive and well in such institutions of day care, but that it also exists within the home and is in fact reproduced by parents.

For instance, what I have observed in my studies of Swedish mothers is that they will seldom openly admit to being proud of their child but will couch that pride in a self-effacing or critical remark or attitude, making the listener believe that even the mother herself does not think her child "special or unusual." For example, complaints such as the following are common: "She is so much work because she goes anywhere she wants and I have to watch her all the time" (translation: The baby is only 8 months old but she is motorically precocious. I am such a good parent that I let her decide what she wants to do, even if she does walk all over the house and it means extra work for me to watch her so that she does not hurt herself). However, unlike the evil eye of many Mediteranian cultures, Swedish mothers are not really afraid that someone will harm their child when they mask parental pride but rather want to assure others that their child is just like, or "equal to," other children, and they are only mothers like others.

## The Child as Natural

Children in Sweden are admired and respected for their naturalness, directness, and unconventionalilty. In direct opposition to norms of Swedish adult demeanor (rational and controlled, nonpassionate) children's spontaneity and affect are highly valued. One common parental theory about children's nature is that it is "Aristotleian." What there is to develop in the child was there from the beginning. It remains to be seen at what pace and in what order those potentials will come to light" (Halldén, 1991, p. 341). In this view there is a reliance on nature, and development of the child is natural and not anything one needs to worry about. Children are perceived as having unique, individual temperaments, and mothers of young children often lament, although with a somewhat "negative" pride, that their child has a mind of its own and is very demanding. In other words, if the child demands a lot of the mother and the mother responds appropriately, then by definition, the woman is a good mother. Also, it is considered bad mothering to "boast" about your child, so pride is couched in a rather negative manner so that to an outsider, it "sounds like" a complaint.

Theories of discipline build on the ideology of equality and respect. The child is an equal member of society and therefore should not be physically punished. Discipline is accomplished verbally through reasoning or distraction, or if that fails, through shaming. Furthermore, physical punishment is not only to be avoided, it is legally prohibited. The child is encouraged to internalize norms of behavior by watching and learning from others. If the environment is ordered and secure, the child will naturally learn what is right and wrong. Parents do not necessarily believe that their role is an instructive one (Halldén, 1991); rather norms are acquired through a process of "social osmosis." That is, if the environment is properly ordered and logical, the child will "naturally" pick up the behavioral and attitudinal norms of the society, without the parents deliberately instructing the child.

It is believed that the naturalness of the child is well matched with exposure to nature. Mothers also consider it good childrearing to allow children free reign with nature. As there are no poisonous snakes or real dangers in the outdoor environment, short of getting lost in the woods (which occasionally happens with 2- or 3-year-old children who then spend the night there alone), even crawling infants are encouraged to explore nature. In the summer months or weeks, and depending on where in Sweden one lives, babies and young children spend days at a time completely naked, running around on the grass or beach. For the non-toilet-trained child, this is the perfect opportunity to learn about body functions in a natural way, and parents indulge children's desire to be without clothing. Small children almost never wear bathing suits unless they swim in a public swimming pool, and then, most often at age 4 or 5, they begin to wear bikini bottoms in "gender-appropriate" color and styles when they themselves decide it is time to "cover up."

This perception of childhood as being a "natural," back-to-nature kind of life stage extends the boundaries of the real outdoors to include even indoor living. One of the most common health problems with infants is diaper rash. This rash is considered to occur most often in the winter months, when the children are warmly dressed, the houses are dry due to the use of centralized heating and good insulation, and there is a lack of sunlight to kill bacteria. The best remedy is to let the child go naked, at least from the waist down, and that is what Swedish parents sometimes do. In the best situation, if a child is not ambulatory, he or she will sit on a rubberized, cotton-backed sheet to avoid unnecessary soiling of the carpets or floors. But it is not at all unusual that the child moves from this space, which results in the obvious. Swedish parents are very nonchalant about body wastes of young children (as they are "natural" and developmentally normal) and take it all in stride.

## Concluding Remarks

Equality ideology, however conceptualized in Sweden, is the thread that binds together the social fabric of culture in which the child in raised. Social policy has been termed "state feminism" in that programs have been directly supportive of women and their children. The health care sector has equalized people living in Sweden, providing adequate and free care for all, and the status of the child is high. Sweden has therefore been considered an important "case study" for examining parameters of motherhood, fatherhood, cohabitation, health, and security.

State feminism has given individuals support for their own ideas about equality, and has even supported the *potential* for truly equal sharing of public and private spheres of life regardless of gender. But has the welfare state really disturbed male dominance and the underlying gender construction of work, trade unions, and political organizations? Several social scientists think not (Holter, 1984; Hirdman, 1987; Acker, 1990). Men exert economic, political, sexual, and educational control over women and children as evidenced, among other documents, in annual governmental labor reports monitoring gender inequality in respect to wages and upper-level positions. And although machismo and swaggering displays of maleness are not generally accepted in Sweden, where indigenous concepts of dignity and restraint typify male behavior, men do retain and protect their privileged status in society.

Sweden has been an important example of a modern society that explicitly legislates equality and where subsequent policies relating to the family, particularly for women and children, have been truly visionary. However, there remains considerable distance before equality ideology is realized in the home and the workplace. The question that then arises, "Will Sweden continue to strive for actualization of true equality? Will Swedish society continue to provide the means for realizing the vision of equality in respect to parenting and other adult careers?"

The answer is ambiguous at best. Currently what is happening in Sweden is that the very fabric of Swedish culture is starting to tear, perhaps due to the weakness in the thread of equality ideology. Because the Swedish crown has been devalued and the economic condition of the country is unbalanced, and political policy fluctuates, the social welfare state seems to be on the verge of collapse. At present, women and particularly their children are at even more risk for not attaining the good Swedish life as one social program after another is canceled. Policies are being reformulated that are detrimental to children, such as cutbacks in day-care facilities and placements, after-school programs, and amount of reimbursement to parents for parental leave insurance and care for sick children (which was 90% and is now 80%) (Statistiska Centralbyrån, 1995). Previously, Social Democratic policy attempted to construct a society in which *all children* were guaranteed a certain living and opportunity standard. Now, some children will decisively be more "equal" than others, as will some categories of parents. These actions have a direct effect on women, especially those who are not married and those who balance employment and mothering. Unemployment (which is at an all-time high of approximately 10%) is highest for women; unemployment compensation has also been decreased.

Thus, the effect on families who no longer have a security net of social welfare programs will be most drastically felt by those families without two parents. Because the ecocultural niche provided by the state will change, parents will have to make accommodations in order to continue to provide the environment they believe necessary for the growth and development of their child. The local interpretation of cutbacks to families is that "parents" will have to either quit their jobs or reduce hours at work to take care of children when day-care programs are cut. My question is: Which parent do they mean? Assigning women the exclusive care of children, because they as a group earn less than do men, directly challenges equality ideology.

Unless there is a serious rededication to equality ideology in Sweden, what may result is a nonequal situation for children not born to legally married and cohabitating parents, both of whom are gainfully employed. It remains to be seen if the ideal of equality is "culturally deep" or if, in fact, it is purely political (i.e., Social Democratic policy). What happens in Sweden *is* of importance in respect to the evolution of equality ideology, whether in gender, health, or age. Whether the child-friendly aspects of Swedish society, which so clearly have been a model for Western social development, will survive remains to be seen. It may be that the "honeymoon" for children's and women's rights is over. I, for one, hope not.

# Acknowledgments

This chapter was prepared in part (1991–1992) while I was a guest researcher at the Departments of Anthropology and Psychology, and Education, University of California, Los Angeles. Special thanks to Professors Thomas Weisner and Carolee Howes for their kind support. Gratitude is also expressed to ICA Partihandel, Bromma, Sweden, for generous support during our family's academic visit in Los Angeles and to the Stockholm College of Health and Caring Sciences for those resources that enabled me to conduct research at UCLA.

This research was partially funded by The Swedish Institute, Humanities and Social Science Research Council of Sweden, and the Stockholm College of Health and Caring Sciences.

I wish to thank several colleagues for their helpful comments. I am particularly grateful to Prof. Robert A. LeVine, Harvard University, who was guest professor at the Swedish Institute of Social Research in Uppsala, 1992–1993, and associate professor of education, Gunilla Halldén, University of Stockholm. Special thanks also to Dr. Kim Lutzén, Stockholm College of Health and Caring Sciences, and to anthropologists Dr. Eva Poluha and Jónina Einarsdottír for their helpful suggestions.

And to the Swedish women and mothers who have inspired me over the years, *Tack så mycket!*

# Appendix. From the "Status of Women in Sweden"

"A decisive and ultimately durable improvement in the status of women cannot be attained by special measures aimed at women alone; it is equally necessary to abolish the conditions which tend to assign certain privileges, obligations, or rights to men. No decisive change in the distribution of functions and status as between the sexes can be achieved if the duties of the male in society are assumed *a priori* to be unaltered. . . . The division of functions as between the sexes must be changed in such a way that both the man and the woman in the family are afforded the same practical opportunities of participating in both active parenthood and gainful employment. If women are to attain a position in society outside the home which corresponds to their proportional membership of the citizen body, it follows that men must assume a greater share or responsibility for the upbringing of the children and the care of the home. A policy which attempts to give women an equal place with men in economic life while at the same time confirming woman's traditional responsibility for the care of home and children has no prospect of fulfilling the first of these aims. This aim can be realized only if the man is also educated and encouraged to take an active part in parenthood and is given the same rights and duties in his parental capacity. This will probably imply that the demands for performance at work on the man's part must be reduced: a continued shortening of working hours will therefore be of great importance. In this context it would be advisable to study how reductions in working hours could be distributed over the working week with a view to making it easier for husbands to do their share of work in the home." (Report of the Swedish Government to the United Nations [1968]. Cited in Fogerty et al., 1971, pp. 107–108.)

# References

Acker, J. (1990). *A contradictory reality: Swedish women and the welfare state in the 1980s.* Paper presented at the Center for Labor Studies (Arbetslivscentrum), Stockholm, Sweden.

Bernhardt, E. (1991). *Working parents in Sweden: An example for Europe* (Stockholm Research Reports in Demography, No. 66). University of Stockholm, Section of Demography, Sweden.

Carlson, A. (1990). *The Swedish experiment in family politics.* New Brunswick, NJ: Transaction.

Dahlerup, D. (1993). From movement protest to state feminism: The women's liberation movement and the unemployment policy in Denmark. *Nora, Nordic Journal of Women's Studies, 1*(1), 4-2.

Daun, A. (1991). Individualism and collectivity among Swedes. *Ethnos, 56*(3–4), 165–172.

DeChateau, P. (1976). The influences of early contact on maternal and infant behavior in primaparae. *Birth and Family Journal, 3,* 149–155.

DeChateau, P. (1979). "Effects of hospital practices on synchrony in development of the infant–pair relationship. *Seminars in Perinatology, 3*(1).

Fogarty, M. P., Rapoport, R., & Rapoport, R. (1971). *Sex, career and family.* Beverly Hills, CA: Sage.

Gullestad, M. (1989). Small facts and large issues: The anthropology of contemporary Scandinavian society. *Annual Review of Anthropology, 18.*

Halldén, G. (1991). The child as project and the child as being: Parent's ideas as frames of reference. *Children & Society, 5*(4).

Harkness, S., & Super, C. (1991). Parental ethnotheories in action. In I. E. Siegel (Ed.), *Parental belief systems: The psychological consequences for children and families* (2nd ed.). Hillsdale, NJ: Erlbaum.

Hirdman, Y. (1987). The Swedish welfare state and the gender system: A theoretical and empirical study. In *The study of power and democracy in Sweden,* (Rep. No. 9). Uppsala University, Uppsala, Sweden.

Hoem, B. (1985). Ett barn är inte nog: Vad har hänt med svenska ett-barnskvinnor födda 1936-60 [One child is not enough; What has happened to Swedish women with one child born 1936-60?] (Stockholm Research Reports in Demography, No. 25). University of Stockholm, Section of Demography, Sweden.

Hoem, B., & Hoem, J. (1988). The Swedish family. Aspects of contemporary developments. *Journal of Family Issues, 9*(3), 397–424.

Holter, H. (1984). Women's research and social theory. In H. Holter (Ed), *Patriarchy in a welfare society.* Oslo: Universitetsförlaget.

Hwang, P. (1987). The changing role of Swedish fathers. In M. Lamb (Ed.), *The father's role. Cross-cultural perspectives.* Hillsdale, NJ: Erlbaum.

Klaus, M. H., & Kennell, J. (1972). Maternal attachment: Importance of the first postpartum days. *New England Journal of Medicine, 286*(9), 460–463.

Lamb, M. E., Frodi, A. M., Hwang, P., Frodi, M., & Steinberg, J. (1981). Attitudes and behavior of traditional parents in Sweden. In R. Emde & R. Harman (Eds.), *Attachment and affiliative system: Neurobiological and psychobiological aspects.* New York: Plenum Press.

LeVine, R. A. (1988). Human parental care: Universal goals, cultural strategies, individual behavior. In R. A. LeVine, P. Miller, & M. M. West (Eds.), *Parental behavior in diverse societies* (New Directions in Child Development, No. 4, pp. 3–11). San Francisco: Jossey-Bass.

LeVine, R. A. (1974). Parental goals: A cross-cultural view. *Teachers College Record, 76*(2), 226–239.

LeVine, R. A., Miller, P. M., & West, M. M. (Eds.). (1988). *Parental behavior in diverse societies* (New Directions in Child Development, No 4). San Francisco: Jossey-Bass.

Liliequist, M. (1991). *Nybyggarbarn* [Children of the Settlers]. Stockholm: Almqvist & Wiksell International.

Liljeström, R. (1978). Sweden. In S. Kamerman & A. Kahn (Eds.), *Family policy in fourteen countries.* New York: Columbia University Press.

Ohlander, A. S. (1993, April 23-24). *Woman–History's main person.* Paper presented at the 1993 Women's History Conference—The Invisible History, sponsored by the Swedish Council for Planning and Coordination of Research, Stockholm, Sweden.

Popenoe, D. (1987). Beyond the nuclear family: A statistical portrait of the changing family in Sweden. *Journal of Marriage and the Family, 49,* 173–183.

Qvarfort, A. M., McCrae, J. M. & Kolenda, P. (1988). Sweden's national policy of equality between men and women. In P. Kolenda (Ed.), *Cultural constructions of "Woman."* Salem, WI: Sheffield.

Richman A. L., LeVine, R. A., New, R. S., Howrigan, G., Welles-Nyström, B., & LeVine, S. (1988). Maternal behavior to infants in five cultures. In R. A. LeVine, P. Miller, & M. M. West (Eds.), *Parental behavior in diverse societies* (pp. 81–98). (New Directions in Child Development, No. 4). San Francisco: Jossey-Bass.

Rädda Barnen. (1991). *Barnets rättigheter* [Children's rights]. Stockholm: Wahlström & Widstrand.

Sandemose, A. (1977). *En flykting korsar sitt spår* [A refugee crosses his tracks]. Uddevalla: Bohusläns AB. (Orignial work published 1933)

Sandqvist, K. (1987). *Fathers and family work in two cultures. Antecendents and concomitants of fathers' participation in child care and household work.* Stockholm, Sweden: Institute of Pedagogy, University of Stockholm.

Statistiska Centralbyrån. (1986). *Kvinno och mans världen* [The world of women and men. Equal opportunity in Sweden]. Stockholm: Statistics Sweden.

Statistiska Centralbyrån. (1990). *The timing of first birth* (Vol. 1). Stockholm: Statistics Sweden.

Statistiska Centralbyrån. (1991). *Familjebildning och familjeupplösning under 1980-talet* [Family formation and the family dissolution in the 1980s]. Stockholm: Statistics Sweden.

Statistiska Centralbyrån. (1992). *I tid och otid–Kvinnors och mäns tidsanvändning 1990/91* [At all times. How women and men use their time 1990/91]. Stockholm: Statistics Sweden.

Statistiska Centralbyrån. (1995). *Barn och deras familjer 1992–1993.* [Children and their families, 1992–1993]. Stockholm: Statistics Sweden.

Super, C., & Harkness, S. (1986). The developmental niche: A conceptualization at the interface of child and culture. *International Journal of Behavior Development, 9,* 1–25.

Sundström, M. (1991). Sweden; supporting work, family and gender equality. I. Kamerman & Kahn (Eds.), *Child care. Parental leave and the under 3's: Policy innovation in Europe.* Westport, CT: Greenwood.

Swedish Institute. (1987). Child care in Sweden. *Fact sheets on Sweden.* Stockholm, Sweden: Nordiska Tryckeri AB.

United Nations. (1988). *Demographic yearbook 1986.* New York: Author.

United Nations. (1991). *Demographic yearbook 1989.* New York: Author.

Weisner, T. (1984). Ecocultural niches of middle childhood: A cross-cultural perspective. In W. A. Collins (Ed.), *Development during middle childhood* (pp. 335–369). Washington, DC: National Academy Press.

Welles, B. (1982). *Maternal age and first birth in Sweden: A life course study in*

*Sweden.* Doctoral dissertation, Harvard Graduate School of Education, Cambridge, MA.

Welles-Nyström, B. (1988). Parenthood and infancy in Sweden. In R. A. LeVine, P. Miller, & M. M. West (Eds.), *Parental behavior in diverse societies* (pp. 75–78) (New Directions in Child Development, No. 4). San Francisco: Jossey Bass.

Welles-Nyström, B. (1991). The mature primipara and her infant in Sweden: A life course study. In J. K. Nugent, B. M. Lester, & T. B. Brazelton (Eds.), *The cultural context of infancy.* Norwood, NJ: Ablex.

Welles-Nyström, B. (1995). Radical timing? Feminist ideology? Postponed motherhood in the United States and Sweden. Manuscript in preparation.

Whiting, B., & Edwards, C. (1988). *Children of different worlds: The formation of social behavior.* Cambridge, MA: Harvard University Press.

Willard, A. (1988). Cultural scripts for mothering. In C. Gilligan, J. V. Ward, & J. M. Taylor (Eds.), *Mapping the moral domain.* Cambridge, MA: Harvard University Press.

## PART THREE

# INTRACULTURAL VARIATION: THE ROLES OF EDUCATION AND "EXPERTS"

# Parents' and Adolescents' Ideas on Children

## Origins and Transmission of Intracultural Diversity

Jesús Palacios
María Carmen Moreno

Much of the extensive body of literature that has emerged around the subject of parents' ideas on the development and upbringing of their children is less than a decade old. In 1985, when we started our research on this topic at the University of Seville, Spain, some relevant papers had already been published in the field, but a solid body of empirical evidence was still lacking. By drawing partly on the small amount of literature existing and partly on our own intuition, we imagined that experience as parents must play a determining role in the formation and transformation of ideas about children. However, as demonstrated later in this chapter, our findings showed that experience as parents played a very modest role, and experience was definitely not the main source of those ideas.

What our data did show was that there were different groups of parents with regard to their ideas about children, their upbringing, and education; the data also revealed that these differences were most closely related to some sociocultural variables. Our question is easily summarized: If the ideas that parents have about the development and upbringing of their children are not mainly formed in the process of becoming parents, when are they formed? This question led us to study a sample of adolescents using an adaptation of an instrument we had used with adults.

The data obtained over these years of research have resulted in considerable empirical evidence.[1] This evidence enables us to make certain speculations, especially related to the transgenerational transmission of ideas about development, upbringing, and education.

Basically, our data have distanced us from what Schwartz (1981) considered a "pristinism" typical of psychologists (a belief that the world should be reconstructed anew by each individual on the basis of the spontaneous processing of his or her own experience), and they have led us to explore new areas that have emerged in the interdisciplinary crossover that has given rise to labels such as cultural psychology and cognitive anthropology. According to Cole (1990), common to the different formulations existing within cultural psychology is a conception of culture as the unique *medium* of human existence. But cultures are not monolithic or homogeneous entities, and any attempt to describe cultural processes and products should be accompanied by an attempt to describe and understand both what is common and what is diverse within a given cultural group. Otherwise, a part would be taken as if it were the whole and some of the most critical aspects of the culture would be ignored (namely, its heterogeneity and the maintenance of its diversity over the generations). Some of the formulations currently available in cultural psychology fail to recognize the existence of intracultural diversity, as if culturalism were the only alternative to individualism.

Therefore, this chapter basically deals with two subjects: first, the intracultural diversity of the ideas of Spanish parents and adolescents and the wider social and cultural framework within which this diversity may be placed in order to understand it better; second, the transmission of intracultural diversity from one generation to another.

## Diversity of Ideas and Intergenerational Differences: A Selective Review of the Literature

### Diversity of Ideas

When studying the ideas that parents have about the development and upbringing of their children, many authors have concentrated on the differences between some parents and others. The most frequently researched variables have been experience as parents, ethnic–cultural origin, and socioeconomic status (SES). Goodnow and Collins (1990, Chapter 4, this volume) present an excellent summary of research and an interesting set of suggestions for research into sources of parents' ideas.

There continue to be conflicting points of view about experience as parents. It is true that some research has found that parents' ideas undergo changes in the process of parenthood (Holden, 1988; Pharis & Manosevitz, 1980), but the majority of the research has shown that this plays a small or weak role (e.g., Goodnow, Knight & Cashmore, 1985; Miller, White, & Delgado, 1980; Ninio, 1988; Palacios, 1990; Palacios & Hidalgo, 1993).

With respect to the other variables, most of the literature has followed the line of the pioneering work done by Ninio (1979) and Hess, Kashigawa, Azuma, Price, and Dickson (1980). The first of these compared answers given by Israeli mothers from two ethnic groups and two socioeconomic categories (high and low) to a series of questions related to the infant development timetable and the activities involved in bringing up and educating children (stop breast feeding, start story telling, etc). As often occurs in this type of study, ethnic group and SES were confounded, as one of the groups had higher SES than the other. The data analysis shows that there was only one factor, which was defined by Ninio (1979) as the tendency to see the infant as more or less precocious. Mothers with high status and from a European origin received higher scores in this factor.

Hess et al. (1980) also dealt with mothers' expectations with respect to children's acquisition of different competencies. The research was conducted in this case in Japan and the United States, and mothers with different socioeconomic levels were interviewed in both countries. This last variable gave rise to some significant differences (with the mothers with a higher status expecting competencies at earlier ages), but the authors highlight the differences related to cultural origin: Japanese mothers expect earlier control in areas such as emotional maturity, self-control, and politeness, while the North Americans expect greater maturity in the area of verbal assertiveness and peer relations.

In the wake of these studies, there has been much more research analyzing the role of cultural differences, normally making use of the ethnic and cultural diversity existing in the countries in which the research is being conducted. This is the case in Australia, for example, where diverse cultural groups have been used to study the developmental timetables and some associated upbringing practices. In their studies, Goodnow, Cashmore, Cotton, and Knight (1984), Rosenthal and Bornholt (1988), and Rosenthal and Gold (1989) compared mothers with Anglo-Australian, Lebanese, Vietnamese, and Greek origins. Although in some of the research the ethnic and socioeconomic variables seem confounded (in Rosenthal & Bornholt, 1988, for example, mothers with Greek origins had at least 5 years less schooling than Anglo-Australian mothers), in others the effect of the different variables was sufficiently controlled. The results of these studies provide solid evidence leading to the assertion that the differences linked to cultural origin have a greater influence on the contents of ideas than do the differences related to socioeconomic variables. Anglo-Australian mothers usually have earlier expectations and give greater importance to independence, while in other groups (e.g., the Greeks), more value is given to interpersonal relations and the feelings of belonging to a family group.

Interesting research has also been conducted in Israel on the role of culture in parents' ideas. Besides the work of Ninio (1979), Frankel and Roer-Bornstein (1982) compared two generations (mothers and grandmothers) of Kurdish and Yemeni women. The data from this research show the existence of cultural differences in ideas about children and their upbringing, but they also demonstrate that these differences are attenuated in the younger generation as a result of exposure to modernizing influences. In fact, whereas in some respects the younger generation of Kurdish and Yemeni mothers are more similar to their own mothers (cultural differences), in other respects they show greater similarities between each other (generational similarities).

On the American continent, Sameroff (Sameroff, 1975; Sameroff & Feil, 1985) carried out a series of studies that introduced the concept of stages in parents' ideas. In most of the previously mentioned research there is the implicit assumption of a continuum, with some parents (those with more precocious expectations) situated at the beginning of the continuum while others (with less optimistic expectations) are placed at its end. Sameroff's vision has more to do with levels or stages than with a mere continuum in which there is only room for the before or the afterwards. In addition, Sameroff's proposals have led to comparative studies between different cultures with a more elaborate design and with a more sophisticated conceptualization of cultural differences than is normally the case in this type of research.

What interests Sameroff are the theories that parents have about development; to a great extent, those theories are defined by the posture that parents take in relation to the role of heredity, education, and interaction between the two. Sameroff and Feil (1985) maintain that the complexity of parents' ideas depends on the extent to which they are cognitively capable of confronting complexity in general. Establishing a parallelism with the levels of logical complexity described by Piaget, Sameroff (1975; Sameroff & Feil, 1985) proposes the existence of four levels of reasoning to do with children and the causes of their development and behavior, with corresponding transitions between the levels. The levels are (1) the symbiotic or nonreflective (does not recognize the existence of development or the antecedents, "I don't know"–type responses), (2) the categorical (considers a determinant of development as the only cause; the child is given a label and his or her behavior is judged depending on this), (3) the compensating (considers that more than one cause affects development; the labels given to the child are not permanent—they are related to his or her age and level of development), and (4) the perspectivistic (the multiple causes that are considered are situated within a wider hypothetical field and the specific situations with a child represent just a fraction of the many possibilities existing).

The transnational and transcultural studies summarized by Sameroff and Feil (1985) show that in all the cultures that were studied, the most elementary concepts of development were found among people with the lowest SES. With a few exceptions, the most developed concepts were found among people with the highest SES. In an interesting piece of research in which cultural differences were not the object of study, Pratt, Hunsberger, Pancer, Roth, and Santolupo (1993) confirmed and extended some of Sameroff's proposals: The level of reasoning about children bears a relation to the level of formal reasoning, as well as to a measure of cognitive complexity, but not to IQ scores or to scores of information processing by the working memory. In addition, gender and the level of authoritarianism demonstrated their relation to the level of reasoning about children: Women showed more complexity in some of the situations, and authoritarianism correlated negatively with the complexity of reasoning about children.

As for cultural differences, the work of Gutierrez and Sameroff (1990; Guitierrez, Sameroff, & Karrer, 1988) should be highlighted. They compare Mexican-American and Anglo-American mothers varying in SES and level of acculturation (Gutierrez et al., 1988), and Anglo-American and Mexican-American middle-class mothers, with the latter varying in the level of acculturation (familiarity with the English language, ethnic identity, and social networks) and biculturalism (extent to which the mothers feel comfortable in the other culture and level of involvement in the other culture) (Gutierrez & Sameroff, 1990). The results showed the influence of both SES and cultural variables: Mothers with lower SES from both ethnic origins presented less complex levels of reasoning; in the case of mothers with high SES, those who were most acculturated and most bicultural showed more complex levels of reasoning than did monocultural mothers. Furthermore, the combined action of the two variables produced synergistic effects, so that the Mexican-American mothers who scored high in acculturation and biculturalism had more complex levels of reasoning than did the

Anglo-American mothers. Otherwise, the level of complexity in reasoning about children was not related to the mothers' IQs.

On the whole, it seems that it is reasonable to state that there are important differences within certain cultural groups that are linked to socioeconomic level. Belonging to a specific cultural group also influences parents' ideas, and in this case it is important to consider not only ethnic origin but also the degree of implantation in the new culture and the extent of the connection with the culture of origin.

Another line of research not yet mentioned, but which is nevertheless closely related to the question of diversity, deals with questions that are closer to the topic of attitudes, values, and ideology. Schaeffer & Edgerton (1985) developed a scale of parental modernity that allows the evaluation of ideas on topics such as the nature-nurture problem, the level of efficacy parents perceive in themselves as childrearers, the extent to which they value obedience or independence, and the relationship between family and school. Some parents are shown to be progressive and democratic, while others appear more traditional and authoritarian, and a third group appears to agree simultaneously with these conflicting ideologies. As Schaeffer and Edgerton (1985) argued, parental modernity in childrearing and education is probably highly related to individual and psychological modernity. This modernity is shaped by parents' educational and occupational level, at least in industrialized countries.

## Intergenerational Differences

Not much research has focused on adolescents' ideas *qua tale* (Moreno, 1991). Most of the empirical studies have emerged within the context of teenage pregnancies and the possible consequences for parenting and the development of the child. Because the rate of adolescent pregnancies is greater in some social sectors than in others, this poses the problem of socially unbalanced samples. However, some studies have managed to avoid this problem and we have chosen to review two. A second line of research has approached the problem of intergenerational agreements and the convergence or divergence between parents and children; our review will be brief on this subject because, as we explain later on, our data do not allow us to make our own analysis of intrafamily convergence.

In Ninio's (1988) study, the sample was made up of parents (both fathers and mothers) and subjects without children consisting of boys and girls age 16 (students in vocational schools or in high schools) and young adults age 25 (university students of both sexes). The subjects were asked about the timetable of cognitive development of infants and the best time for the introduction of cognitive stimulation. The research contains various interesting findings: educational level—and not experience as parents—seems to play a greater part in determining ideas about children; the cultural group to which people belong also seems to have a certain amount of influence, but not as much as the level of studies. The comparison between parents and nonparents demonstrated that ideas about development and upbringing are already present in late adolescence. For girls, ideas seem to stabilize around age 16, whereas boys continue to learn in the following years, until age 25, when ideas can be detected in their final form in both sexes. Boys and girls from high school and with Western origins had more optimistic expectations than did subjects from vocational schools with Asian or North-African origins. As the latter come from larger families, it seems reasonable to state that more optimistic (and also more exact) ideas are in no way linked to greater contact with children.

Sommer et al. (1993) studied cognitive readiness for parenthood (knowledge, attitudes, interactive style) in a sample made up of pregnant adolescents, nonpregnant adolescents, and pregnant adult women. Age, ethnic origin, IQ, and level of schooling were all controlled. The results showed a gradual increase in the sophistication of reasoning about developmental issues up to mature adulthood. But although adult mothers scored higher in cognitive readiness than did the two adolescent groups, many of these differences weakened or disappeared once the effect of the four previously mentioned variables had been controlled (age, race, IQ, and educational level). As the authors state, the differences found are not due to age but to developmental stage.

There have been several pieces of research that have looked at agreement in ideas between parents and adolescents from the same family. The convergences and divergences have been reviewed by Goodnow (1992). Some of these studies have compared parents and adolescents from families from different ethnic groups; in some groups, age seems to be the homogenizing factor (Cashmore & Goodnow, 1985) whereas in others the effect of ethnicity was greatest (Feldman & Quatman, 1988). Rosenthal and Bornholt (1988), who also found interethnic differences, discovered that intergenerational harmony outweighs disagreement. Investigating an ethically and sociodemographically homogeneous sample, Alessandri and Wozniak (1987, 1989) conducted a longitudinal study in which they explored parent-child agreement in beliefs concerning the child and the child's awareness of parental beliefs. They analyzed two groups of subjects (studied, respectively, when they were 10–11 and 15–16 years old, and then 2 years later) whose parents were also studied, which allowed them to assess the level of agreement between the spouses. On the whole, the data showed a high level of intrafamily agreement, although there were differences between some families and others. Intrafamily agreement was greater in adolescents than in preadolescents; in addition, adolescents were more aware of the beliefs of their parents than preadolescents were. All in all, the existence of intergenerational agreements seems to be documented in the literature, although there are differences between families in the level of agreement they share; there are also age-related differences and, in any case, the existence of agreement does not mean that the younger generation limits itself to simply copying the ideas of the parents.

In an attempt to address some of the problems we have been discussing in the preceding paragraphs regarding diversity of ideas and intergenerational differences, a research program was designed that we have been developing together with our colleagues at the University of Seville. Some of the results obtained so far are summarized here.

## Our Research with Adults and Adolescents

### Adult Population's Ideas about Child Development, Upbringing, and Education

In Seville, in 1985, we studied a sample of 278 subjects (139 couples) between 25 and 30 years old. They varied in their educational background (low—education only at primarily level or less; medium—education at secondary level without university studies; high—university), number of children (the main division was between people with just one or more than one child) and place of residence (rural vs. urban). The subjects that formed our sample were ethnically very homogeneous, thus reflecting the general makeup of the Spanish population. Located in the Andalusian region, Seville and its province are interesting for our studies because in this region a city oriented toward industrial, administrative, and service activities coexists with rural villages oriented toward agricultural production. Although in recent years Andalusia has experienced as many political and social changes as the rest of Spain (see Collier, 1986, for an illustration of changes in rural villages in southern Spain), this does not impede the existence among Andalusian people of a great heterogeneity in social status, mentality, and lifestyle.

The subjects were interviewed for the first time in the hospital they attended for the birth of their child. The instrument designed specifically for this research was the Parents' Ideas Questionnaire, consisting of 106 open-ended questions exploring some areas that have been extensively studied in the literature and others that seemed important to us: the amount of information about pregnancy and upbringing, as well as the origin of this information; capacities attributed to the fetus, baby, and child; nature–nurture in personality, intelligence, and language; mother–child relationship during pregnancy; role of the father; practices of upbringing and education; practices of cognitive–linguistic stimulation; behavioral attributions; gender stereotypes; values, aspirations, and expectations; ideas regarding schooling; and, finally, ideas regarding the composition of the family (e.g., whether being an only child is desirable).[2] The data obtained were analyzed using a Multiple Correspondences Analysis (MCA) and a cluster analysis. The main results may be found in Palacios (1988, 1990). The data analyses showed the existence of three classes or groups of parents according to their ideas about children, upbringing, and education.

### Traditional Parents

These were parents with a low level of education (primary education or less) living in rural areas. They believe that the developmental milestones are acquired at an age later than actual age of acquisition; they also have an innatist concept of the origin of their children's psychological features, think that they will not be able to influence the child and his or her development, and manifest attitudes of an authoritarian nature and stereotyped ideas about differences in the socialization of boys and girls.

### Modern Parents

These parents have a high level of education (university) and live in urban environments. Their developmental expectations generally coincide with actual ages of acquisition; they have a concept of the origin of psychological features as arising from the nature–nurture interaction; they see themselves as being able to influence the child and his or her development; their educational attitudes are authoritative, and they do not have stereotyped ideas with respect to differences in socialization between boys and girls.

### Paradoxical Parents

These parents have either a low or medium level of education and reside in both rural and urban areas. Their developmental expectations are very optimistic and sometimes not realistic; nevertheless, paradoxically, the plans of action with the child that they envisage do not take advantage of such precocity. They are strongly environmentalist, but, strangely, they evince a relatively low estimation of their personal ability to influence the child. They reveal this attitude by frequently attributing to other people rather than to themselves the ability to shape the child's development. Their ideas are sometimes stereotyped and at other times opposed to stereotypes.

The use of the labels traditional and modern ties in with their use by other researchers (e.g., Frankel & Roer-Bornstein, 1982; Inkeles & Smith, 1974; Schaeffer & Edgerton, 1985), and in no way does it include an implicit assessment in terms of worse or better. The labels are just meant to indicate greater or lesser proximity to some of the historical tendencies of Western societies: progressive urbanization, prolonged schooling, the existence of the mass media, decreasing emphasis on gender differentiation, democratic attitudes, and so on.

Forty percent of the subjects analyzed turned out to be paradoxical, 32% traditional, and 28% modern. Chi-square analysis showed that the level of schooling was the variable most strongly linked to the class of ideas ($p < 0.001$): A high proportion of parents with low and medium levels of schooling hold, respectively, traditional and paradoxical ideas, whereas the vast majority of parents with a high educational level have modern ideas. The place-of-residence variable gave rise to a distribution that is also significantly different ($p < 0.001$), but this is a variable that is strongly dependent on the previous one, because the parents with a medium and especially a high level of schooling are underrepresented in the rural population. The differences depending on the number of children were also significant ($p < 0.05$), with paradoxical parents being more likely to have more than one child. Finally, gender differences bore no relation to belonging to one class or another.

As stated elsewhere (Palacios, 1991), our data show that the absolute questions that researchers ask about this subject matter (e.g., Do parents' ideas from coherent systems? and Does experience as parents have any influence?) get relative answers: Parents' ideas form coherent systems in some cases (traditional and modern parents) but not in others (paradoxical parents); experience as parents seems to affect some systems of ideas (paradoxical) but not others (traditional and modern). The fundamental explanation has to do with what the determinants of ideas are considered to be: Traditional parents have a lower level of schooling and a greater dependence on a cultural context loaded with traditional values that are overrepresented in rural areas. Modern parents remained in the schooling system longer, and many of them received an academically oriented education. From the mental background created in those circumstances they draw their way of understanding child development and the processes of rearing and education. For the most part, paradoxical parents lack both the deep roots in tradition that one group of parents has had and the years and the type of schooling that the other group has had. In the absence of these elements of coherence, their ideas seem more influenced by their experience with their own children, from which they draw contradictory lessons that are not surprising given the differences between some children and others (e.g., between first children and later ones).

Drawing on data gathered in this first piece of research, various other studies were set in motion. One of them consisted of the longitudinal tracking of approximately half the parents from the original sample. Palacios, Gonzalez, and Moreno (1992) have discussed how the modern, traditional, and paradoxical classes appear again when the parents are studied 2 years after the first data were collected.

In addition, the study conducted by Oliva (1992) has enabled us, among other things, to analyze parents' ideas in a less local context and with an unusually large sample. In a nationwide study, the ideas of mothers and teachers of children of preschool age were compared. In total, 800 mothers (400 with 2-year-old children, and the other 400 with 4–6-year-old children) and 800 teachers of children of this last age group were interviewed with a questionnaire that reexamined some of the contents already explored in the previous study. Most of the questions that discriminated better between one type of parent and another in the previous questionnaire were used. The sample of mothers was heterogeneous with regard to the level of schooling and occupational level, whereas the sample of teachers was made up almost entirely of people who had some type of academic qualification and was heterogeneous with respect to age (which implies differences both in the type of professional training received and in their experience as teachers). The data were analyzed with similar statistical procedures to the ones used in the previous study.

As far as mothers are concerned, the data from this study illustrated patterns of ideas that Oliva (1992) classified as traditional, modern, and insecure. In this case, the third group presented a pattern of ideas in which uncertainty more than contradictions was the norm; thus the use of a different label. Among the teachers, the classes were modern, restrictive traditional, and protective traditional. In the case of both mothers and teachers, the variables related to the level of schooling (mothers) or professional training (teachers) demonstrated that these variables play a very important role. In the case of mothers, for example, virtually all those with a high level of schooling evinced modern ideas. With the mothers, the age or the number of children did not relate to their ideas, whereas in the case of the teachers, the age and professional experience variables were shown to be determinant with regard to ideas about children and education. The group of teachers between ages 30 and 40, with more recent training and an average or low level of experience, was the one with the greatest presence in the modern class; in contrast, three-quarters of the traditional protectors are the oldest teachers in the sample (over 40), those who received their professional training a longer time ago, before the establishment of teacher training studies at a university level. Articles in preparation will give a much more detailed account of this research.

In another study carried out with 59 teachers of preschool children using the same instrument as that used earlier, Lera (1994) labeled the groups she found in the same way as those in the first study: modern, traditional, and paradoxical. The greatest amount of contrast was again found between the modern and traditional groups, both in relation to their ideas (in the case of modern subjects, developmental timetables in which the overriding elements are exactness and precocity, parent–teacher collaboration, priority to not strictly academic contents, etc.) and in relation to the sociodemographic variables that define the components of the groups (modern teachers are under age 30 and traditional ones over 50). Again, future articles will discuss the details of this research in greater depth.

Taken as a whole, the data from all this research illustrate the existence in Spanish society of two very different groups with regard to ideas about children, upbringing, and education. The labels modern ideas and traditional ideas seem to embrace the content of these two contrasting groups and they seem to us to be very close to those described by Schaefer and Edgerton (1985) in the same terms, although the contents included by Schaefer and Edgerton refer, above all, to attitudes and values, whereas ours cover a broader field. In the case of parents, it seems clearly established that the level of schooling is the sociodemographic variable most strongly linked to that polarity, with a clear predominance of people with university studies among those with modern ideas and a prevalence of people with a low level of schooling among those espousing traditional ideas. People with a medium level of schooling seem to be more irregularly distributed, as they either lead to the creation of a third category (paradoxical, insecure, etc.) or they are distributed between the other possibilities, although their presence is normally greater among those who do not have modern ideas. Valuable research on parents' ideas has also been carried out in Spain at the University of La Laguna, where Triana and Rodrigo (1988) used very different instruments and techniques of analyses from the ones used at the University of Seville. They also found that parents with high levels of schooling and living in urban areas have ideas of an environmentalist–constructivist nature, whereas those with low levels of schooling, especially those living in rural areas, hold innatist–medicalist ideas. Finally, as far as teachers are concerned, the generational variable seems to be clearly linked to developmental–educational ideology, although at present it is not possible for us to determine the relative weight of training and accumulated experience, both of which are variables that affect members of each generation in different ways.

A brief overview of the aforementioned seems to demonstrate the existence of a clear heterogeneity of ideas about development, upbringing, and education in the otherwise rather ethnically homogeneous Spanish society. This diversity does not simply consist of placing developmental predictions a little earlier or a little later in a developmental continuum; it implies two qualitatively different versions of child development, upbringing, and education. From the demographic variables considered for the adults who are not members of the teaching profession, the level of schooling emerges, without a doubt, as the most crucial.

## Adolescents' Ideas about Development, Upbringing, and Education

The data from our first piece of research clearly showed that experience as parents plays a fairly secondary role in the shaping of ideas about children and their upbringing. In our case, experience as parents only showed a certain association with the paradoxical class and in line with our interpretation, experience as parents was effectively an association that contributed to paradoxicality. We then asked ourselves about the moment in which ideas are formed and the elements that contribute to shaping them.

Those questions gave rise to a study where Moreno (1991) explored the ideas that adolescent Spaniards have about children, their upbringing, and their education, using a version of the Parents' Ideas Questionnaire (previously used with adults) adapted for use with adolescents. The research studied a wide sample of 872 adolescents from Seville and its province. The data were collected during 1987, at which time mandatory schooling ended at age 14 (at the end of the eighth grade). Having finished the eighth grade, 10% of Spanish schoolchildren left the educational system (access to the labor market was not legal until age 16). Of those remaining in the system, 63% went on to high schools, leading afterwards to university studies; those that did not take the more academic option went to vocational schools, leading to a more immediate incorporation into the labor market. The choice of a more academic or a more vocational path does not generally happen by chance: It is related to academic performance during obligatory schooling in such a way that those who performed better took the more academic option and those who performed worse opted more frequently for the more vocational path (on entry into the vocational schools, 65% of students were over the normal entrance age as a result of having had to repeat at least one school year they had failed). In addition, the dropout rate after the first year at high school was 20%, whereas the percentage of those at vocational school who did not register for the second year was 40%. Moreover, the choice of a more academic or more vocational path also followed a certain social rationale; for example, in many rural areas there were no high schools, just vocational schools; in cities, a similar logic prevailed, with the presence of high schools and vocational schools clearly related to the sociodemographic characteristics of the neighborhood. In 1990, however, a reform in the education system extended the school leaving age to 16 and introduced significant changes to secondary education. All the above percentages related to schooling actually come from a Ministry of Education document on which the reform of the system was based (Ministerio de Educación y Ciencia, 1990).

The first group in our adolescent study was made up of 304 boys and girls in the eighth grade (13–14 years), which assured us of being able to sample virtually the whole population at this age because 100% of the children ages 13 to 14 were in school. The second group consisted of 362 male and female students between 16 and 18 who were in their third year at high school. Finally, 206 16–18-year-old students of both sexes who were in their second year at vocational school made up the third group. Because a fairly substantial proportion of schoolchildren leave after the first year of secondary schooling, especially in the vocational sector, our sample is representative of 16–18-year-old subjects who are in the education system. The distribution of the sample was balanced with respect to gender, place of residence (rural or urban), and parents' level of schooling (low, medium, high), although some cells have lower numbers (e.g. that of subjects who go to vocational schools and whose parents have studied at university) as a reflection of the social realities of the country. The parents' level of studies was taken from the parent with the highest educational level. Finally, none of the subjects had children and they all saw this probably as being a long way off, as the incidence of pregnancies in Spanish adolescents in secondary education is extraordinarily low.

The subjects gave written answers to the 88 open-ended questions from both the Parents' Ideas Questionnaire and a small questionnaire aimed at gathering sociodemographic information. The data were collected in groups, during school hours, and without the presence of teachers, with at least the main researcher (M.C.M.) to give instructions, sort out any problems, and so on. The adolescents were asked the following types of questions: What things do you think a pregnant woman can do that will be of benefit to the fetus? Do you think it is a good idea to pick up children a lot, or do you think it is best to hold them as little as possible? At what age do you think children can walk on their own? Do you think you could influence a child of yours so that he or she would develop characteristics you would like to see in him or her? Why do you think that among normal children some are more intelligent than others? If you saw a son of yours age 4 playing with a doll or a daughter of yours of the same age playing with toys belonging to a boy, what would you do? What would you like your child to be when he or she grows up?

The use of similar coding systems and data analyses to those used in previous studies allowed the identification of three classes of adolescents:

1. Traditional. Those with innatist ideas, belief in the influence of the unsatisfied cravings of the pregnant mother on the physical characteristics of the fetus, perception of a limited parental capacity to influence the child's development and future, reference to relatives and friends as hypothetical sources for consulting to resolve doubts about development and upbringing, defense of restrictive educational practices (e.g., hold the baby in one's arms as little as possible so as not to spoil it), a secondary role for the father in the child's upbringing, sexually stereotyped expectations and aspirations, exclusive reference to physical aspects when asked about the characteristics that they would like to see in their children, and so forth. Thirty-seven percent of the adolescents studied fit into this group.

2. Modern. Those who defend the nature–nurture interaction, emphasize the repercussion on the fetus of the mother's emotional states, attribute to the parents the capacity for influencing the development and future of the child, refer to sources of specialized information (professionals, printed material) for resolving hypothetical doubts, defend stimulating educational practices (e.g., holding the baby in one's arms to stimulate emotional links), support an active role of the father in the upbringing and education of the child and no gender stereotyping about expectations and aspirations, reference to fundamentally psychological attributes when asked about the characteristics they would consider desirable in their children, and so on. Thirty-eight percent of the adolescents studied came within this group.

3. Uncommitted. The defining characteristic of this group is that they lack clear information and opinions about questions related to child development, upbringing, and education. In fact, from the 88 response modalities that define this class, only about 20 contained specific responses, the most usual type of response being, "I don't

know." On the few occasions when these subjects gave specific responses, they most frequently voiced strongly traditional ideas (insensitivity to the psychological components of the interactions, virtually no importance given to the father, defense of unstimulating and clearly punitive educational practices). Twenty-five percent of the adolescents sampled were classified into this group.

This time a log-linear analysis was applied to the data using the ILOG program (Bakeman & Robinson, 1994).[3] Although the details of this analysis will be given elsewhere, it can be said that the effects of our subjects' level of schooling and their gender turned out to be strong. Adding the simple effect of schooling to a schooling by gender by residence by parents' education factorial model accounted for 47% of the goodness-of-fit chi-square. Adding the simple effect of gender accounted for an additional 22%, and their interaction accounted for an additional 4%. Schooling and gender and the interaction between the two reached a significance value of 0.01. In contrast, residence and parents' education had a relatively trivial effect. In summary, schooling and gender were significant in their own right and more powerful than residence and parents' education.

As a result of these statistics, it seemed logical to study schooling in more detail, looking at its effect on boys and girls separately. In the significance test, an alpha level of 0.02 was maintained. Figure 9.1 presents a graphic illustration of the differences as a function of school level and gender for each of the classes of ideas. In 13 to 14 year old boys and girls (eighth grade), traditional ideas are clearly predominant, whereas modern ideas are clearly prevalent in 16 to 18 year old boys and girls attending high school. Boys and girls of this age at vocational school are not significantly more represented in one group of ideas than in another, with the exception of the low presence of girls in the uncommitted group. As far as differences according to gender are concerned, the conclusions are also fairly clear: Girls have clearer ideas than do boys as far as development, upbringing, and education of children are concerned. The percentage of uncommitted boys is always significantly higher than the percentage of uncommitted girls.

## The Diversity of Ideas and Its Determinants

### Heterogeneity

First of all, our data confirm Sigel's (1985, 1986) proposals for a conceptualization of ideas as systems that integrate subsystems. Both traditional and modern ideas appear as organized sets of ideas within which a high level of coherence exists, so that what one thinks, for example, with respect to the nature–nurture issue, is related to beliefs in one's own ability to influence the chid and his or her development. The ideas about stimulation and discipline also seem to belong to the same family and stereotypes linked to gender and expectations for the child's future are also related.

This vision of ideas about children being integrated in systems becomes clearer the wider the range of contents one tackles. While the exploration of just one content (e.g., developmental timetables) tends to produce results that show a continuum in which some subjects are placed a little before and some a little afterwards, the exploration of many interrelated contents leads more easily to a vision of ideas as ideological systems that integrate and harmonize diverse, but related, contents. As a result, we believe that the vision of the epistemic parent, of whom—as in the Piagetian child—one can only expect variations in timing but not in trajectory, should be substituted by a vision that takes into account different epistemologies and diverse and integrated conceptions. Specific ideas about developmental timetables or practices of upbringing and education that each parent holds should be understood basically as forming part of the wider system to which they belong, and not through reference to their more or less advantaged position with respect to the yardstick constituted by a supposed unitary continuum.

Some have called these systems of ideas or beliefs (Sigel, 1985) cultural models, presupposed and taken-for-granted models widely shared by members of a society, models that specify what is in the world and how it works (Quinn & Holland, 1987, p. 3). As Harkness, Super, and Keefer (1992) pointed out, these models facilitate the flow of daily events and behavior in a larger, meaningful framework. But as we explain in greater detail at the end of this chapter, what characterizes the social groups is the existence in the interior of each one of them, not of a cultural model but of a variety of them (Goodnow, Chapter 13, this volume, uses the terms plurality and multiplicity to express a similar idea). Cultures are characterized more by heterogeneity (Tulviste, 1991; Wertsch, 1991; Wertsch & Tulviste, 1992) or by what Kojima (in press) has called an ethnopsychological pool of ideas, than by a unitary set of ideas. To put it in Wertsch's (1991) terms, within each culture there is a heterogeneity of voices, each with different contents. This polyglossy also exists in the interior of each individual, but, at least with respect to the ideas with which we are concerned here, that multiplicity is gifted with coherence, and that is the coherence manifested in the systems of ideas we have labeled modern and traditional. Although perhaps the coherence we are talking about is not limited to the specific field that interests us here, and perhaps it laps over into other areas (political, religious, etc.; see Sigel, 1985), at least within the field of ideas on children, their development, upbringing, and education, the coherence seems clear. After all, as Quinn and Holland (1987) pointed out, cultural models ensure, if not systematic, at least thematic coherence.

It is true that coherence in ideas is a luxury that not all parents can afford (not to mention the coherence between ideas and behavior). Coherence is not an inherent quality in ideas, and when no organizing principle or element exists, contradictions would tend to be more the exception than the norm, as one would depend on fragments of information collected here and there (Mugny & Carugatti, 1985), which would not lead to anything other than a potpourri of erratic experiences (Bugental & Shenum, 1984). In fact, in our view that is what happens to parents we have labeled paradoxical. The contradictions that are found in their ideas are not lessened by the fact that they all have experience as parents. It may even be the case that experience with children, and especially with more than one, increases the source from which most parents get their ideas. As Ninio and Rinott (1988) pointed out, merely spending time in the vicinity of children is not a sufficient condition for learning about them.

## Social Representations and Schooling

But if ideas do not come from and are not organized on the basis of experience, where do they come from? Many of the ideas we have about children (and, without doubt, about many other things) exist before we do, and they take the form of what Moscovici (1981, 1984) has called social representations. According to Moscovici, contact with reality continually presents us with enigmas and problems in the face of which there are two options: the response of science (the reified universe) and the response of common sense (social representations). Social representations form a set of concepts, statements, and explanations that the person in the street uses to confront daily experiences, so that he or she may understand these experiences and give them meaning. According to Moscovici (1981), in industrialized societies social representations are equivalent to the myths and belief systems of traditional societies; their purpose is to make something unfamiliar, or the unfamiliarity itself, familiar (Moscovici, 1984, p. 24). Therefore, the basic function of social representations is to explain things and events so that they become accessible, comprehensible, and relevant. Social representations form part of our daily communicational landscape: people on the street, in cafes, at their places of work, in hospitals, laboratories,

# ERRATA

*Parents' Cultural Belief Systems:*
*Their Origins, Expressions, and Consequences*
Sara Harkness and Charles M. Super, Editors

The second paragraph of the Acknowledgments in Chapter 1 (pp. 20–21) should read as follows:

Several colleagues in Europe have contributed to the development of this work through their interest and hospitality. We are grateful to Dolph and Rita Kohnstamm, Tom van der Voort, Marinus van IJzendoorn, Pieter and Ineke Kroonenberg, and Dymph van den Boom for acting as our hosts and cultural guides in Holland. We would also like to thank Philip Hwang at the University of Gothenburg and the Association for the Study of Young Children in Sweden, Jesús Palacios at the University of Seville, Andrzej Eliasz of the University of Lodz and the Polish Institute for Psychological Research, and Giovanna Axia at the University of Padua for their invitations to lecture or consult on parental ethnotheories, and their warm hospitality to us and our family during visits to their institutions.

The title for Part Five should be The Consequences of Parents' Cultural Belief Systems for Children's Health and Development.

In the Contents the correct spelling of the fourth author's name in Chapter 15 is Roberto Paludetto. In the list of Contributors Jaan Valsiner and Abraham W. Wolf are Ph.D.'s.

In each pair of bars in Figure 19.1 (p. 454), the left-hand bar represents Cambridge parents and the right-hand bar Bloemenheim parents. For each triad of bars in Figure 19.2 (p. 458), the left-hand bar represents the 4-month-old Cambridge sample, the middle bar the 6-month-old Bloemenheim sample, and the right-hand bar the 10-month-old Cambridge sample.

etc., are always making critical remarks, commenting and concocting spontaneous, nonofficial "philosophies" which have a decisive influence on their relations, their choices, their way of educating their children, making plans, and so on (Moscovici, 1981, p. 183). As Bruner (1986) rightly pointed out, the theories that a person constructs to explain things are seldom original; they are normally taken from the culture in which he or she is brought up, and from there he or she takes its metaphors and day-to-day language.

But whether we talk of cultural models or refer to social representations, the previous discussion about heterogeneity should again be addressed. Data from the different studies we and our colleagues have conducted show the existence of qualitatively different social representations; again and again we come across traditional and modern types of social representations, to refer only to those types imbued with a high level of internal coherence. These representations are not available as in a free market model, to use Goodnow's (1988) fitting metaphor. Not all have the same level of accessibility, as they do not all have the same degree of complexity. Some social representations are simpler, whereas others involve more complex contents and relations. Using Sameroff and Feil's (1985) terminology, it is not the same to move on the level of categorical reasoning as it is to move on that of perspectivistic reasoning; to take different variables situated in different hypothetical contexts into consideration and to relate them simultaneously is cognitively more demanding than to limit oneself to considering just one variable. This is where the role of school and the consequences of schooling come in.

As it is clear from our set of research findings, schooling emerges as the most crucial aspect of those that contribute to shaping ideas about children, their upbringing, and their education. Similar data have been found by many other authors and not just in the area of ideas but also in that of behavior. Because the contents we are discussing do not form part of what school attempts to teach formally, one might ask what school provides that introduces such an important differentiating factor. The specific role played by the school experience in the transformation of the cognitive system has been and still is under debate. Analyses of crosscultural research in child development have brought to question the capacity of the school experience to transform the whole cognitive functioning of schooled individuals. Rogoff (1981) concluded that what school brings about is an ease at handling such cognitive skills as strategic remembering or taxonomic classification. Cole (1992) has contended that the transfer from school to out-of-school activities is greatly restricted. Our data brings us to a more sociologically oriented view of the role played by the school experience. Inkeles and Smith (1974), after analyzing a series of attitudes, values, habits and behaviors of people living in six very different developing countries, concluded that schooling is the most powerful element in modernization, and that the influence of schooling would not be limited to the cognitive area; according to Inkeles and Smith (1974), modernity (the modern personality discussed by Schaeffer & Edgerton, 1985) is a general syndrome that makes modern people share four fundamental characteristics: They are informed citizens taking part in social life, they have a marked sense of personal efficacy, they are highly independent and autonomous with regard to sources of influence of a traditional type, and they have a cognitive openness and flexibility that allows them to face new experiences and ideas (cf. Inkeles & Smith, 1974, p. 290). This view is similar to the one expressed by Bourdieu (1972) when he contends that what school modifies in those attending it is the habitus ("a subjective but not individual system of internalized structures, schemes of perception, conception and action common to all members of the same group or class," p. 81).

As for the social representations of children we find in our society, some are obviously more complex than others: Some belong to the realm of the consensual, whereas others are much closer to the reified world. As Moscovici (1981; Moscovici & Hewstone, 1983) points out, the degree of participation is determined by the level of qualification. The lower the level of schooling, the more probable it is that people will look for information about children and their upbringing in social networks and informal experiences (the commonsense and consensual world), whereas as the level of schooling increases, so does the tendency to read books, consult specialists, and so on (the world of the reified) (see, e.g., Bronfrenbrenner, 1958; Frankel & Roer-Bornstein, 1982; Goodnow, 1988; Ninio, 1979; Palacios, 1988; Sigel, McGillicuddy-DeLisi, & Johnson, 1980).

## Developmental Trajectories

The existence of various levels of complexity makes it necessary to refer to the question of their hierarchy. In accordance with Wertsch (1991), heterogeneity may be considered from three different perspectives: heterogeneity as genetic hierarchy (the forms of representation that emerge later are more powerful and frequently they are also considered to be better), heterogeneity despite genetic hierarchy (there is a genetic gradation in the forms of representation, without this implying that the later ones are more powerful), and nongenetic heterogeneity (there is no ranking either in genetic terms or in terms of power). Because our data on adolescents are not longitudinal, we cannot be sure that many of the boys and girls who were classed as traditional at 13 to 14 years of age will be modern at 16 to 18 years of age, even if they followed the more academic schooling track. Our data suggest the existence of a genetic hierarchy in which the lack of commitment could be considered the less complex level and probably the first to be found in the ontogenetic trajectory, especially among boys, due to differential processes of socialization. Traditional ideology implies a commitment to specific ideas, although in this level only isolated factors are considered (nature, for instance), reciprocal influences (e.g., parents on child and situation on decisions) play a minimum role and rearing criteria are likely to lack flexibility (e.g., with regard to gender roles). Modern ideology, on the other hand, implies considering several factors in reciprocal interaction (e.g., nature and nurture), it is not governed by rigid principles (about discipline or gender roles, for instance), and it seems to imply the handling of more and more exact information. It seems possible then to affirm that modern ideas are more complex and, as a consequence, require more cognitive complexity.

There is nothing in the nature of things that says this complexity is or is not desirable, that it is preferable or better, but we cannot escape the fact that this complexity is there and that not everyone has the possibility of reaching it, because this access demands cognitive resources that are not always available. Clearly, the vast majority of our 13–14-year-old adolescents did not possess this complexity; many of the high school pupils clearly demonstrated that they did it and with it they gained access to a form of reasoning, of taking into consideration diverse elements and their interaction, which is typical of what we have labeled modern. It is interesting that pupils at vocational schools, who are cognitively more complex as a group than the eighth grade schoolchildren (they are 2 or 3 years older, among other things), but who are perhaps without the cognitive resources that high school students have access to, cannot as a group be assigned to any of the ideologies we are considering, whereas eighth graders and high school students can as a group be assigned mainly to the traditional and the modern types, respectively.

The comparison of our data to those obtained by Sameroff and his colleagues is interesting. As frequently occurs in this area of research, the differences in methodology, design, instruments, and so on, hinder a direct comparison. We clearly agree that there are different levels of complexity in the forms of reasoning and that this complexity is related to the socioeconomic level, in our case operationalized through years of schooling. Our data do not include intercultural comparisons as this, with few exceptions, is not a social reality in Spain. Our data do include a piece of developmental (nonlongitudinal) material that partly supports the theses of Sameroff and his colleagues. However, we do not talk of stages of development because our data do not allow us to do so, and also because we do not think that we are dealing with a sequence *à la* Piaget in the sense of a unique trajectory. Our simile would be that of a tree with different branches, some of which would be more likely to develop in earlier periods of development (e.g., lack of commitment), while others would require more complexity (i.e., modern ideas); other trajectories would also be possible (e.g., paradoxical ideas and insecurity).

On the whole, our data also seem to go in a similar direction to those of Ninio (1988), who found well-formed ideas in 16-year-old children. Nothing in our data indicates that these ideas are solidified if solidified means that they are not going to be modified. However, the ideas are already there in adolescents, forming coherent and integrated systems, although the comparison of adolescents and adults with modern ideas from our sample demonstrates that adolescents do not yet present the level of clarity and coherence that is found in adults. The process of formation of ideas about children is probably set in motion at a very early age; one only has to recall the study carried out by Melson, Fogel, and Toda (1986) in which children between 4 and 7 years of age correctly answered questions about babies and baby care.

Other interesting data from our research with adolescents, and in which there is also parallelism with Ninio (1988), refers to differences related to gender. Without doubt, girls have greater clarity in their ideas about development and upbringing than do boys. Looking at it from another perspective, what really stands out is the greater incidence of boys who are uncommitted. Neither do the girl–boy differences in ideas on children emerge in adolescence: they are already there in 5-year-olds (Melson & Fogel, 1988). In all probability, as far as adolescent boys are concerned, we are faced here with what Bourdieu (1972) called learned ignorance (*docta ignorantia*) and which Goodnow (1990) called the socialization of ignorance. According to Mugny and Carugatti (1985), such socialization produces an information anorexia that, in relation to the subjects with whom we are dealing here, clearly has a greater effect on males. Because our data with adults show that as parents men and women do not differ significantly in their ideas about children, males who confront parenthood must have a catch-up process that enables them to get out of this anorexia and organize their ideas using their cognitive resources. Having a cognitive readiness for parenthood (Sommer et al., 1993) does not mean that this capacity is used. As a matter of fact, girls seem to use it before boys.

With the data we have available, we can do no more than speculate about which path the ideas of the adolescents we studied will take. We know from other research (e.g., Roberts, Block, & Block, 1984) and from our own (Moreno & Palacios, 1991) that, in the case of adults, stability predominates over change over the course of time. It is easy to speculate that many of the adolescents in whom we have detected a pattern of traditional ideas are not going to have many opportunities for increasing their cognitive complexity. Remember that at 15 years old, a significant percentage of adolescents to whom we did not have access were already outside the school system. On the other hand, many of the adolescents whose ideas have already appeared at 16 to 18 years as being modern will probably continue to retain these ideas because, as our longitudinal data show, the system of modern ideas is the one that has shown the greatest levels of stability among adults (Moreno & Palacios, 1991). As for the uncommitteds, parenthood will make it necessary for them to convert the unknown into the familiar (Moscovici, 1981, 1984) and transform uncertainty into social reality (Rommetveit, 1974), orienting themselves in the direction set by their cognitive complexity and the social representations that best adjust to this. In a world in which messages are continually arriving via the mass media, the collective social viruses will attempt to find a way to the deepest recesses of the mind of each person (see Lightfoot & Valsiner, 1992, for a study on how popular magazines represent children). To pick up on the metaphor used by these authors, the level of penetration that these messages achieve will depend on the level of elaboration that the ideas system has in each person and, as a result, on the capacity of the ideological antibodies to neutralize the attack.

From all that we know from the research in this and other fields of understanding of social reality, the contents that are acquired greatly depend on both the social position and the context in which the development takes place. For example, Emler, Ohana, and Dickinson (1990) and Jankowski (1992), respectively, show how the understanding of socioeconomic structure depends on the person's own position in that structure and how the development of political attitudes and notions depends on the context of political socialization in which it has grown.

Nor should it be forgotten that social representations are not products that are a historical and independent of surrounding circumstances. The rural and urban adolescents in our sample are exposed to the homogenizing influence of schooling and the mass media more than their parents were. In all probability, the changes introduced in the Spanish education system in recent years will have some impact on the topics we are discussing here, although it is not easy to predict in which direction. Consider, for example that at the time at which the adolescents' data were collected in 1987, 25% of 15–16-year-olds were already outside the educational system and inside there were more boys than girls. At the time of this writing, the percentage of this age group in the education system was 90% and there was an equal balance between the sexes. As in Frankel and Roer-Bornstein's (1982) research, the youngest generation we studied is exposed to cultural influences that can on the whole be classified as being more modern.

## Speculations on Transgenerational Transmission

Because the adults and adolescents in our studies do not come from the same families, we can only speculate on the conditions in which the transmission of ideas through generations takes place. However, we feel that these speculations are relevant because they enable us to be more precise about the way we approach the dynamic of formation and transformation of ideas about children.

First we should emphasize that we are talking about a type of understanding that is clearly different from the understanding of the physical world. We are talking about culture, which has been defined by D'Andrade (1984) as learned systems of meaning, communicated by means of natural language and other symbol systems, having representational, directive, and affective functions, and capable of creating cultural entities and particular senses of reality (p. 116). We are talking of socially shared cognitions (Levine, Resnick, & Higgins, 1993), cognitions that are formed following procedures that are quite different from those that occur in the case of the understanding of physical reality (see, in relation to this, the inversions that Shweder, 1984, proposes to Piaget's basic postulations about how knowledge is acquired).

Moscovici (1990) points out that social representations have a marvelously ethereal quality in the form of their transmission. In spite of the difficulties in pinning down what is ethereal, it seems that a few specific paths of transmission can be highlighted: guided participation, conversations, family life with its many different ingredients, and mass media communication.

The concept of guided participation has been used by Rogoff (1990) to refer to activities in which an adult and a child are often involved, with the former generally organizing and initiating the activities and the latter incorporating his or her actions and representations. Guided participation involves communication that consists of both words and actions and involves the organization of routines and activities of daily life, the handling of the life of the child and his or her peers, and so on; skills, goals, values, and aspirations are conveyed through this participation. Because the child learns by acting, acting upon, and being acted upon, and by acting in prestructured and other-structured scenes and events (Schwartz, 1981), when adolescence arrives, the stock of ideas must be fairly considerable. There will undoubtedly have been many socially guided interaction situations in which the child will have taken part, inside and outside the house, in the street, or at school. Holden and Zambarano (1992) showed that 5-year-old children already share their parents' attitudes with respect to physical punishment. It is also quite likely that, especially in traditional contexts, this socialization will have been different for boys and girls, as the socialization for girls will more probably have been loaded with elements related to children and looking after them (see, e.g., Goodnow, this volume, Chapter 13, on the subject of the distribution of domestic tasks).

One of the most likely ways in which guided participation occurs is through conversations. In most cases these are probably not explicit conversations; however, this certainly does not stop the child's learning the lesson. As Rommetveit (1974) has stated, ellipsis is one of the most important characteristics of human language: What is essential goes without saying because it comes without saying (Bourdieu, 1972, p. 167).

Family life is without doubt another source of influence. In each family there are paradigms, myths, stories, and rituals (Sameroff & Fiesse, 1992) and a series of delivery methods among which Goodnow (1992) includes the following list: explicit statements, vague statements, practices without words, displays of affect, protection from outside, or competing messages. The literature tells us that intergenerational agreement is easier when the father and mother in a family share points of view, criteria, and practices (Block, 1972; Cashmore & Goodnow, 1985). It is not out of place to recall here Alessandri and Wozniak's (1987, 1989) data according to which intrafamily agreement is a fairly frequent reality.

The mass media definitely constitute a powerful transmitter of images, representations, aims, and so forth (see Lightfoot & Valsiner, 1992, both for the examination of how social suggestions to parents have changed over this century and for an interesting analysis of the image of children given by a popular magazine for parents). Although they are not readers of magazines for parents, adolescents are habitual consumers of the mass media and they must certainly receive a fairly important number of social suggestions this way.

Joint actions, conversations, family life, and mass media are not completely independent phenomena. Collective culture is full of coded meanings with a high level of redundance (Valsiner, in press) that encourage circular reinforcement that is at the base of collective beliefs (Bourdieu, 1972). Filtered by the way in which people assimilate this redundance—which mainly depends on years of schooling—this cumulative voice of the community (Goodnow, 1992, p. 313) is converted into what Bourdieu (1972) calls a conductorless orchestration of the habitus (those systems of subjective but not individual meaning that Bourdieu terms the durably installed generative principle of regulated improvisations).

However, we are not suggesting that ideas about children are transmitted in such a way that a perfect reproduction takes place. Even if it were only for the fact that cultural models are normally transmitted fragmentarily and their hidden coherence has to be inferred (Keesing, 1987), a certain margin for individuality would still remain. That is where we would find the manifestation of the novelty-constructive nature of the internalization process that Valsiner mentions in this volume and to which others, such as Harkness et al. (1992), have also referred. As Schwartz (1981) put it, for a culture to develop it is necessary that some degree of creativity survive the prior requirement of stability. It is in this context in which the processes of transformation will occur that Collins (1990, in press) has described as typical of adolescence and that adjust more to what happens than those of absolute continuity or absolute discontinuity.

Finally, the intergenerational transmission we are talking about is not limited to the area with which we are dealing here, nor is it unidirectional. Using a wide sample of subjects from three generations, Glass, Bengston, and Dunham (1986) have shown how intergenerational agreement also appears in such other areas as politics and religion; they have also shown that this transmission occurs in part due to heredity or transmission of social status and in part through the transmission of attitudes. Finally, they have demonstrated that transmission does not occur just from older to younger generations; it also occurs in the other direction, although their data are confined to relations between adults and their parents.

# Conclusions

At the University of Seville we have carried out intracultural studies analyzing ideas about children, their upbringing, and their education in different groups: parents, teachers, and adolescents. In this chapter, we have focused on data from samples of parents and adolescents whose ideas were explored using a similar instrument.

Our data show first the existence of a clear heterogeneity, with three different systems of ideas being detected in parents: traditional, modern, and paradoxical. The level of schooling is the variable that is most strongly associated with this differentiation. In the case of adolescents, we studied a wide sample of subjects varying in age, gender, and type and length of schooling and detected the existence of three groups: traditional, modern, and uncommitted. On the whole, the research data obtained with adolescents appear to be entirely compatible with and related to the data obtained with adults, with a transgenerational perspective being added that undoubtedly enriches the findings from the research with adults.

The data with adolescents have also produced an interesting difference linked to gender, as in all the groups considered there was always a higher percentage of uncommitted boys than girls. This point is of interest because it enables us to refer to a different rhythm of acquisition in boys and girls, although, as far as we know from our studies with adults, once they become parents these differences disappear (at least as far as ideas are concerned).

Although the data reviewed in this chapter are not longitudinal, they have enabled us to speculate on the origin and development of ideas and the problem of their transmission from one generation to another. The concept of social representations has enabled us to reflect on both phenomena. This concept has allowed us to go beyond the strictly individual level and reflect on mechanisms of formation and transmission of ideas that are located in the sphere of socially caused, socially shared, and socially transmitted phenomena of understanding.

Finally, the analysis of intracultural differences has brought us into contact with issues related to the social diversity existing within any cultural group. We would like to close this chapter with some reflections on social diversity and its place in research into areas similar to the one we have been dealing with here.

## Coda: Cultural Psychology, the Exotic and the Everyday

When ideas about children are approached from a sociogenetic perspective such as the one we present here, such concepts as culture, cultural models, shared mental frameworks, and transmission of knowledge, become important issues. Therefore, it seems natural to move toward a discipline situated at the interface of anthropology, psychology, and linguistics (Shweder & Sullivan, 1993) to look for a wider framework in which to situate the data on the genesis and diversity of social representations. Cultural psychology is this interdisciplinary subfield. Cultural psychology and cognitive anthropology are not unitary disciplines. As Cole (1990) has analyzed it, within cultural psychology there are different traditions and viewpoints. The following reflections on some of the limitations of cultural psychology and cognitive anthropology do not apply to all versions but only to those represented by the referenced authors (see Quinn & Holland, 1987; Schwartz, White, & Lutz, 1992; Shweder & LeVine, 1984; Stigler, Shweder, & Herdt, 1990).

According to Shweder and Sullivan (1993) the objectives of cultural psychology are to spell out the implicit meanings that shape psychological processes, to examine the distribution of these meanings across cultural groups and to identify the manner of their social acquisition. According to these authors, cultural psychology emerges to a certain extent in the opposite direction of cognitive psychology, which has been in ascendance in recent years. Cognitive psychology has searched for basic universal psychological processes (unity without diversity) whereas cultural psychology attempts to illustrate the local character (i.e., what is specific for one culture but not for another) of these processes (diversity without unity), giving way to cognitive anthropology. According to Shweder (1984), cognitive anthropologists draw inferences about the minds of persons by studying the ideas and actions of exotic peoples. Some approximations from developmental psychology have gone in the same direction (see, e.g., Ogbu, 1981). And, although as developmental psychologists we have learned much thanks to the work of transcultural comparisons, we feel that it should be possible to make a cultural psychology that takes intracultural differences into consideration and is more sensitive to them.

In fact, a large part of the work that is grouped under the labels of cultural psychology or cognitive anthropology (cf. the aforementioned edited volumes) fits within what Rommetveit (1984) has qualified as a basically monistic outlook (p. 331) in which the fundamental reason for diversity between some people and others lies in the culture they belong to; underneath this, only strictly individual characteristics exist. Thus there is talk of the cultural model of American marriage (Holland & Quinn, 1987), as if there was just one marriage model from the Bering Straits to Cape Horn (or in the United States, if that is what they meant by America), there is talk of the mental model of illness in Ecuador (Holland & Quinn, 1987), as if once in this country the only differences that could be found would be strictly idiosyncratic. As Keesing (1987) rightly pointed out, cognitive anthropology remains . . . curiously innocent of social theory, constructing models that at the very least ignore the status quo, whether they be models of Hinduism that reinforce and perpetuate the position of Brahmin priests or the models of illness among the Ecuadorian poor that allow the masses to contend with grim struggles of life and death while the country's oligarchs go to the Mayo

Clinic" (p. 388). It could be argued that cultural psychology or cognitive anthropology are involved in searching for the minimal knowledge shared (Holy & Stuchlik, 1991, p. 18) by all members of a society. But as Holy and Stuchlik (1991) point out, that conception would be rather useless, as it would be difficult to imagine a situation in which an individual would behave simply as an undifferentiated member of a society without any further specification.

Pursuing these differences, researchers interested in cultural psychology frequently search for the exotic. This would, however, be a perfectly legitimate exercise were it not for the fact that interest in far-off differences often means that what is near at hand is ignored. Mugny and Carugatti (1985) and Sternberg, Conway, Ketron, and Bernstein (1981) showed that we do not have to do more than walk out of our front door and ask people about their notion of intelligence for significant differences to emerge between people; differences that, returning to an expression of Bourdieu's used earlier, are subjective but not individual. So differences are not just the territory of Third World specialists (Mugny & Carugatti, 1985) and we do not have to get on a plane to Polynesia or sub-Saharan Africa to find them: We can do it by taking a ride to the end of the bus route. Of course, going to remote places is one of the possibilities that exists and thanks to these expeditions we have learned some of the most interesting things that we know about children and their development. However, this should not mean that we overlook the diverse, heterogeneous, and unequal nature of our own society, in which differences exist that are related not just to rhythm of acquisition but also to profound differences of content on the whole; differences that, given what we are interested in here, affect parents, the process of parenting, children, and their development. Moreover, it is clear that research designs that are limited to comparing illiterate and schooled populations do not go far enough. As our data show unequivocally, we need to know how much and what type of schooling if we really want to gauge the impact of education on variables such as ours. We agree with Lightfoot and Valsiner (1992) when they state that the notion of cultural heterogeneity is not widespread in cultural anthropology or cross-cultural psychology. Years ago, Pelto and Pelto (1975) used a variety of expressions (resistance to heterogeneity, false picture of homogeneity) to refer to the same phenomenon. More recently, Boster (1987) has considered intracultural variation to be a neglected problem in cultural anthropology.

What happens when instead of ignoring intracultural differences we focus on them? To begin with, we discover how often ethnic and sociodemographic variables are confused (Laosa, 1981). We discover how inappropriate it is to make generalizations related to culture, applying the same things people preach about the Navajo to the Hopi (after all, they are native Americans) or, regardless of whether they are of Cuban or Mexican origin, saying that all Hispanic people are the same and bring up their children in a similar way (see Garcia Coll, 1990, for a review sensitive to the differences). There is no need for great abstractions to see how inadequate generalizations based on cultural labels are, and as a simple example we can refer to the fact that educational level bears a close relation to the amount of times Hispanic parents consult doctors about their children (Guendelman & Schwalbe, 1986). It is doubtful that one can talk in general of a homogeneous Hispanic culture in the United States. What is clear is that Hispanics, like Asians or African-Americans, constitute socially heterogeneous groups that, as far as the subject we are dealing with in this chapter is concerned, have all the features of social division within them. To be able to pick up the subtle points (or even the general outline) of these differences and this heterogeneity, it is vital that the methodological approaches should be sufficiently complex and that the appropriate distinctions between groups and subgroups should be made (e.g., Gutierrez & Sameroff, 1990).

The lack of interest in intracultural differences is all the more surprising taking into account the excellent work done in the 1940s and 1950s both on our subject in this chapter and on other work that is not far from the question of social representations (see, e.g., Bronfenbrenner, 1958; Davis & Havinghurst, 1946; Loevinger, 1959; or, in a different area, Hollingshead & Reddlich, 1958). The interest in intracultural differences seemed to wither away after those decades, and Cole and Scribner's (1974) recommendation that the most useful type of intergroup comparisons would most probably be those made within a culture seemed to fall on deaf ears. Pelto and Pelto (1975) were not much more successful with their emphasis on the need to study intracultural diversity.

Cultural psychology and cognitive anthropology have often ignored intracultural differences,[4] and, as is usual when this happens, they have confined themselves to mystifying such differences as when cultural diversity is presented as frame switching (Shweder, 1984). There can be nothing more socially ingenuous than considering that the ethnopsychological pool of ideas (Kojima, in press) present in any culture can be accessed as in a free market model (Goodnow, 1988), taking this today and that tomorrow from it without any more restrictions than the variables of personality that each person imposes. The idea of frame switching involves cognitive resources and implies mental flexibility; rather than following the criteria of the culture or ethnic group, these are distributed mainly following the criteria of the social group. Cultural capital (Bourdieu & Passeron, 1970) is unequally shared between different groups, and this inequality is also present within each of these groups.

According to Shweder (1984), there have been two main traditions in cognitive anthropology: the enlightenment and the romantic traditions. Among those belonging to the first are authors such as Socrates and Spinoza, Voltaire and Diderot, the early Wittgenstein and Levy-Strauss, Chomsky and Piaget (to shorten Shweder's list), who considered the human being as fundamentally rational and scientific and their mental processes as universal. The romantic tradition (the Sophists and Leibnitz, Goethe and Schiller, the later Wittgenstein and Levy-Bruhl, Whorf and Feyerabend) has defended the nonrationality of ideas and the arbitrary nature of culture. This is probably a good classification, among other reasons because it illustrates the absence in cognitive anthropology of a sociological and sociogenetic tradition to which Democritus and Epicurus, Balzac and Dickens, Marx and Weber, Bernstein and Bourdieu, Vygotsky and Wallon belong. Only by ignoring this tradition is it possible for a discipline situated at the interface of anthropology, psychology, and linguistics to embark on a journey around the world in search of diversity without unity. No doubt, traveling around the world is a worthwhile endeavor for social sciences. But it can be even more worthwhile if one recognizes that diversity linked to (not always very romantic) social differences is an integral part of any complex society and transcends the limits of nationalities and ethnic groups.

## Acknowledgments

This chapter was written while the first author (J.P.) was spending a sabbatical year as Visiting Professor at the Institute of Child Development, University of Minnesota, where professional and material support were of great help to him. The stay at the Institute of Child Development was made possible thanks to a grant from the Dirección General de Investigación Científica y Técnica, Ministry of Education and Science, Spain.

A number of colleagues and friends have been kind enough to read previous versions of this chapter, and they all came up with useful suggestions; some expressed disagreements ranging from minor to strong with our viewpoints. This chapter, of course, only represents the point of view of its authors.

## Notes

1. A large quantity of the data used in this chapter has come from doctoral theses that have been finished but not yet published. Articles that are presently in preparation will give a more detailed picture of the results obtained and will

give fuller technical explanations. In the context of this chapter, we use the data to back up our argument rather than concentrating on specific points that will appear in other publications.

2. Copies of this questionnaire (as well as copies of other questionnaires mentioned in this chapter) can be obtained from Jesus Palacios, Psicologia Evolutiva y de la Educación, Universidad de Sevilla, 41080 Sevilla, Spain.

3. Roger Bakeman was kind enough to do the log-linear analysis for us. His excuse was that our data would allow him to try out a new program he had just prepared (ILOG), but we are sure that we needed his help more than he needed our data. It has been a privilege and a pleasure to work with Roger. We are very grateful to him.

4. Even when there is an attempt to analyze intracultural diversity, it is interesting to see the theoretical models and the research designs that are used. Thus, in the volume of *American Behavioral Scientist* on intracultural variation edited by Boster (1987), some of the papers (the ones by Romney, Batchelder, and Weller (1987); Weller (1987); and D'Andrade (1987), all in the same 1987 volume) take as a frame the cultural consensus theory (Romney, Weller, & Batchelder, 1986), a model wherein one of the very basic assumptions is the existence in a culture of modal answers or a common truth; intracultural variability, however, often consists of different truths being in existence. In other cases, the research designs adopted to explore diversity consisted of comparisons between university students of different gender (Holland, 1987) or between black and white economically disadvantaged women (Quandt, 1987). It is therefore less than surprising that the amount of intracultural variability found in these studies was frequently less than expected.

# References

Alesandri, S. M., & Wozniak, R. H. (1987). The child's awareness of parental beliefs concerning the child: A developmental study. *Child Development, 58*, 316–323.

Alessandri, S. M., & Wozniak, R. H. (1989). Continuity and change in intrafamilial agreement in beliefs concerning the adolescent: A follow-up study. *Child Development, 60*, 335–339.

Bakeman, R., & Robinson, B. F. (1994). *Understanding log-linear analysis with ILOG: An interactive approach*. Hillsdale, NJ: Lawrence Erlbaum.

Block, J. H. (1972). Generational continuity and discontinuity in the understanding of social rejection. *Journal of Personality and Social Psychology, 22*, 333–345.

Boster, J. S. (1987). Introduction [Special issue]. *American Behavioral Scientist, 31*, 150–162.

Bourdieu, P. (1972). *Esquisse d'une théorie de la pratique, précédé de trois études d'ethnologie kabyle*. Geneve: Librairie Droz [English translation: Outline of a theory of practice. Cambridge, UK: Cambridge University Press, 1977].

Bourdieu, P., & Passeron, J.-C. (1970). *La réproduction dans l'éducation, la societé et la culture.* Paris: Les editions de Minuit [English translation: Reproduction in education, society and culture. London: Sage, 1977].

Bronfenbrenner, U. (1958). Socialization and social class through time and space. In E. E. Maccoby, T. M. Newcomb, and E. L. Hartley (Eds.), *Readings in social psychology* (pp. 406–425). New York: Holt, Rinehart & Winston.

Bruner, J. (1986). *Actual minds, possible worlds.* Cambridge, MA: Harvard University Press.

Bugenthal, D. B., and Shennum, W. A. (1984). Difficult children as elicitors and targets of adult communication patterns: An attributional-behavioral transactional analysis. Monographs of the Society for Research in Child Development, 4 (Serial Number 205).

Cashmore, J. A., & Goodnow, J. J. (1985) Parent–child agreement on attributional beliefs. *International Journal of Behavioral Development, 9,* 191–204.

Cole, M. (1990). Cultural psychology: A once and future discipline? In J. J. Berman (Ed.), Nebraska Symposium on Motivation, 1989. Cross- cultural perspectives (pp. 279–335). Lincoln: University of Nebraska Press.

Cole, M. (1992). Cognitive development and formal schooling: The evidence from cross-cultural research. In L. C. Moll (Ed.), Vygotsky and education. Instructional implications and applications of socio-historical psychology (pp. 89–110). New York: Cambridge University Press.

Cole, M. & Scribner, S. (1974). *Culture and thought. A psychological introduction.* New York: Wiley.

Collier, J. F. (1986). From Mary to modern woman: The material basis of Marianismo and its transformation in a Spanish village. *American Ethnologist, 13,* 110–107.

Collins, W. A. (1990). Parent–child relationships in the transition to adolescence: Continuity and change in interaction, affect, and cognition. In R. Montemayor, G. Adams, and T. Gullotta (Eds.), *From childhood to adolescence: A transitional period?* (pp. 85–106). Beverly Hills, CA: Sage.

Collins, W. A. (in press). Relationships and development: Family adaptation to individual change. In S. Shulman (Ed.), *Relationships and social–emotional development.* New York: Ablex.

D'Andrade, R. G. (1984). Cultural meaning systems. In R. A. Shweder & R. A. LeVine (Eds.), *Culture theory. Essays on mind, self and emotion* (pp. 88–119). New York: Cambridge University Press.

D'Andrade, R. G. (1987). Modal responses and cultural expertise. *American Behavioral Scientist, 31,* 194–202.

Davis, A., & Havighurst, R. J. (1946). Social class and color differences in child-rearing. *American Sociological Review, 2,* 698–710.

Emler, N., Ohana, J., & Dickinson, J. (1990). Children's representations of social relations. In G. Duveen & B. Lloyd (Eds.), *Social representations and the development of knowledge* (pp. 47–69). Cambridge, UK: Cambridge University Press.

Feldman, S. S., & Quatman, T. (1988). Factors influencing age expectations for adolescent autonomy: A study of early adolescents and parents. *Journal of Early Adolescence, 8,* 325–343.

Frankel, D. G., & Roer-Bornstein, D. (1982). Traditional and modern contributions to changing infant-rearing ideologies of two ethnic communities. *Monographs of the Society for Research in Child Development, 47* (Serial Number 196).

Garcia Coll, C. T. (1990). Developmental outcome of minority infants: A process-oriented look into our beginnings. *Child Development, 61,* 270–289.

Glass, J., Bengtson, V. L., & Dunham, C. C. (1986). Attitude similarity in three-generation families: Socialization, status inheritance, or reciprocal influence. *American Sociological Review, 451,* 685–698.

Goodnow, J. J. (1988). Parents' ideas, actions and feelings: Models and methods from developmental and social psychology. *Child Development, 59,* 286–320.

Goodnow, J. J. (1990). Using sociology to extend psychological accounts of cognitive development. *Human Development, 33,* 81–107.

Goodnow, J. J. (1992). Parents' ideas, children's ideas: Correspondence and divergence. In I. E. Sigel, A. V. McGillicuddy-DeLisi, and J. J. Goodnow (Eds.), *Parental belief systems: The psychological consequences for children (2nd ed.)* (pp. 293–317). Hillsdale, NJ: Erlbaum.

Goodnow, J. J., Cashmore, J., Cotton, S., & Knight, R. (1984). Mothers' developmental timetables in two cultural groups. *International Journal of Psychology, 19,* 193–205.

Goodnow, J. J., Knight, R., & Cashmore, J. (1985). Adult social cognition: Implication of parents' ideas for approaches to social development. In M. Perlmutter (Ed.), *Social cognition: Minnesota Symposia on Child Psychology* (vol. 18, pp. 287–324). Hillsdale, NJ: Erlbaum.

Goodnow, J. J., & Collins, W. A. (199). *Development according to parents: The nature, sources and consequences of parents' ideas.* Hillsdale, NJ: Erlbaum.

Guendelman, S., & Schwalbe, J. (1986). Medical care utilization by Hispanic children. How does it differ from black and white parents? *Medical Care, 24,* 925–940.

Gutierrez, J., & Sameroff, A. J. (1990). Determinants of complexity in Mexican-American and Anglo-American mothers' conceptions of child development. *Child Development, 61,* 384–394.

Gutierrez, J., Sameroff, A. J., & Karrer, B. M. (1988). Acculturation and SES effects on Mexican-American parents' concepts of development. *Child Development, 59,* 250–255.

Harkness, S., Super, C. M., & Keefer, C. H. (1992) Learning to be an American parent: How cultural models gain directive force. In R. G. D'Andrade & C. Straus (Eds.), *Human motives and cultural models* (pp. 163–178). New York: Cambridge University Press.

Hess, R. D., Kashigawa, K., Azuma, H., Price, G. G., & Dickson, W. (1980). Maternal expectations for early mastery of development tasks and cognitive and social competence of preschool children in Japan and in the United States. *International Journal of Psychology, 15,* 259–271.

Holden, G. W. (1988). Adults' thinking about a child-rearing problem: Effects of experience, parental status, and gender. *Child Development, 59,* 1623–1632.

Holden, G. W., & Zambarano, R. J. (1992). Passing the rod: Similarities between parents and their young children in orientations toward physical punishment. In I. E. Sigel, A. V. McGillicuddy-DeLisi, & J. J. Goodnow (Eds.), *Parental belief systems: The psychological consequences for children* (2nd ed. pp. 143–172). Hillsdale, NJ: Erlbaum.

Holland, D. (1987). Culture sharing across gender lines. *American Behavioral Scientist, 31,* 234–249.

Holland, D., & Quinn, N. (Eds.) (1987). *Cultural models in language and thought.* New York: Cambridge University Press.

Hollingshead, A. B., & Reddlich, F. C. (1958). *Social class and mental illness. A community study.* New York: Wiley.

Holy, L., & Stuchlik, M. (1981). *The structure of folk models.* London: Academic Press.

Inkeles, A., & Smith, D. H. (1974). *Becoming modern. Individual change in six developing countries.* Cambridge, MA: Harvard University Press.

Jankowski, M. S. (1992). Ethnic identity and political consciousness in different social orders. In H. Haste & J. Torney-Purta (Eds.), *The development of political understanding* (pp. 79–93). New Directions for Child Development No. 56. San Francisco, CA: Jossey-Bass.

Keesing, R. M. (1987). Models, "folk" and "cultural." Paradigms regained? In D. Holland & N. Quinn (Eds.), *Cultural models in language and thought* (pp. 369–393). New York: Cambridge University Press.

Kojima, H. (in press). The construction of child-rearing theories in early modern to modern Japan. In J. Valsiner & M. da C. Lyra (Eds.), *Construction of psychological processes in the course of interpersonal communication.* Norwood, NJ: Ablex.

Laosa, L. M. (1981). Maternal behavior: Socio-cultural diversity in modes of family interaction. In R. W. Henderson (Ed.), *Parent–child interaction: Theory, research and prospects* (pp. 125–167). New York: Academic Press.

Lera, M. J. (1994). *Ideas de profesores y práctica educativa [Teachers' ideas and their educational activities].* Unpublished doctoral dissertation, University of Seville, Spain.

Levine, J. M., Resnick, L. B., & Higgins, E. T. (1993). Social foundations of cognition. *Annual Review of Psychology, 44,* 585–612.

Lightfoot, C., & Valsiner, J. (1992). Parental belief systems under influence: Social guidance of the construction of personal cultures. In I. E. Sigel, A. V. McGillicuddy-DeLisi, & J. J. Goodnow (Eds.), *Parental belief systems: The psychological consequences for children* (2nd ed., pp. 393–414). Hillsdale, NJ: Erlbaum.

Loevinger, J. (1959). Patters of parenthood as theories of learning. *Journal of Abnormal and Social Psychology, 59,* 148–150.

Melson, G. F., & Fogel, A. (1988, March). The development of nurturance in young children. *Young Children,* 57–65.

Melson, G. F., Fogel, A., & Toda, S. (1986). Children's ideas about infants and their care. *Child Development, 59,d 259-285.*

Miller, S. A., White, N., & Delgado, M. (1980). Adults' conceptions of children's cognitive abilities. *Merrill-Palmer Quarterly, 26,* 135-151.

Ministerio de Educación y Ciencia. (1990). *Libro blanco para la reforma del sistema educativo [White paper for the reform of the educational system].* Madrid: Author.

Moreno, M. C. (1991). *Las ideas evolutivo-educativas. Un estudio longitudinal y transgeneracional [Ideas on development, upbringing and education. A longitudinal and transgenerational study].* Unpublished doctoral dissertation, University of Seville, Spain.

Moreno, M. C., & Palacios, J. (1991). *Parents' ideas, child's daily life organization and interaction in a book-reading situation.* Paper presented at the eleventh biennial meetings of the ISSBD, Minneapolis.

Moscovici, S. (1981). On social representations. In J. P. Forgas (Ed.), *Social cognition. Perspectives on everyday understanding* (pp. 181-209). London: Academic Press.

Moscovici, S. (1984). The phenomenon of social representations. In R. M. Farr & S. Moscovici (Eds.), *Social representations* (pp. 3-69). Cambridge, UK: Cambridge University Press.

Moscovici, S., & Hewstone, M. (1983). Social representations and social explanations: From the naive to the amateur scientist. In M. Hewstone (Ed.), *Attribution theory: Social and functional extensions* (pp. 164-185). Cambridge, UK: Cambridge University Press.

Moscovici, S. (1990). Social psychology and developmental psychology: Extending the conversation. In G. Duveen & B. Lloyd (Eds.), *Social representations and the development of knowledge* (pp. 164-185). Cambridge, UK: Cambridge University Press.

Mugny, G., & Carugetti, F. (1985). *L'intelligence au pluriel: Les représentations sociales de l'intelligence et son dévelopment.* Cousset: Editions Delval [English translation: *Social representations of intelligence.* Cambridge, UK: Cambridge University Press].

Ninio, A. (1979). The naive theory of the infant and other maternal attitudes in two subgroups in Israel. *Child Development, 50,* 976-980.

Ninio, A. (1988). The effects of cultural background, sex and parenthood on beliefs about the timetable of cognitive development in infancy. *Merrill-Palmer Quarterly, 34,* 369-388.

Ninio, A., & Rinnot, N. (1988). Fathers' involvement in the care of their infants and their attributions of cognitive competence to infants. *Child Development, 59,* 652-663.

Ogbu, J. U. (1981). Origins of human competence: A cultural–ecological perspective. *Child Development, 52,* 413-429.

Oliva, A. (1992). *Madres y educadores. Diferentes concepciones de la educación infantil [Mothers and teachers: Different conceptions of early childhood education].* Unpublished doctoral dissertation, University of Seville, Spain.

Palacios, J. (1988). *Las ideas de los padres sobre la educación de sus hijos [Parents' ideas on their children's upbringing]*. Seville: Instituto de Desarrollo Regional.

Palacios, J. (1990). Parents' ideas about the development and education of their children. Answers to some questions. *International Journal of Behavioral Development, 13,* 137–155.

Palacios, J. (1991). *Parents' ideas about their children and parent–child interaction.* Invited address given at the eleventh biennial meetings of the ISSBD, Minneapolis, MN.

Palacios, J., González, M. M., & Moreno, M. C. (1992). Stimulating the child in the zone of proximal development: The role of parents' ideas. In I. E. Sigel, A. V. McGillicuddy-DeLisi, and J. J. Goodnow (Eds.), *Parental belief systems: The psychological consequences for children* (2nd ed., pp. 71–94). Hillsdale, NJ: Erlbaum.

Palacios, J. & Hidalgo, M. V. (1993). *Parents' ideas and contextual factors in the transition to parenthood.* Paper presented in a symposium on Contextual factors in parenting (R. S. L. Mills & J. Palacios, co-conveners) at the twelfth biennial meetings of the ISSBD, Recife, Brazil.

Pelto, P. J. & Pelto, G. H. (1975). Intra-cultural diversity: Some theoretical issues. *American Ethnologist, 2,* 1–18.

Pharis, M. E., & Manosevitz, M. (1980). Parental models: A means for evaluating different prenatal contexts. In D. B. Sawin, R. C. Hawkins, L. O. Walker, & J. H. Penticuff (Eds.), *Exceptional infant* (Vol. 4, pp. 215–233). New York: Brunner/Mazel.

Pratt, M. W., Hunsberger, B., Pancer, S. M., Roth, D., & Santolupo, L. (1993). Thinking about parenting: Reasoning about developmental issues across life-span. *Developmental Psychology, 29,* 585–595.

Quandt, S. A. (1987). Intracultural variation in American infant diet. *American Behavioral Scientist, 31,* 250–265.

Quinn, N., & Holland, D. (1987). Culture and cognition. In D. Holland & N. Quinn (Eds.), *Cultural models in language and thought* (pp. 3–40). New York: Cambridge University Press.

Roberts, G., Block, J. H., & Block, J. (1984). Continuity and change in parents' child-rearing practices. *Child Development, 55,* 586–597.

Rogoff, B. (1981). Schooling and the development of cognitive skills. In H. C. Triandis & A. Heron (Eds.), *Handbook of cross-cultural psychology* (Vol. 4, pp. 233-294). Rockleigh, NJ: Allyn & Bacon.

Rogoff, B. (1990). *Apprenticeship in thinking: Cognitive development in social context.* New York: Oxford University Press.

Rommetveit, R. (1974). *On message structure: A framework for the study of language and communication.* London: Wiley.

Rommetveit, R. (1984). The role of language in the creation and transmission of social representations. In R. M. Farr & S. Moscovici (Eds.), *Social representations* (pp. 331–359). Cambridge, UK: Cambridge University Press.

Romney, A. K., Weller, S. C., & Batchelder, W. H. (1986). Culture as consensus: A theory of culture and informant accuracy. *American Anthropologist, 88,* 313-338.

Romney, A. K., Batchelder, W. H., & Weller, S. C. (1987). Recent applications of cultural consensus theory. *American Behavioral Scientist, 31,* 163-177.

Rosenthal, D., & Bornholt, L. (1988). Expectations about development in Greek- and Anglo-Australian families. *Journal of Cross-Cultural Psychology, 19,* 19-34.

Rosenthal, D., & Gold, R. (1989). A comparison of Vietnamese-Australian and Anglo-Australian mothers' beliefs about intellectual development. *International Journal of Psychology, 24,* 179-193.

Sameroff, A. J. (1975). Early influences on development: Fact or fancy? *Merrill-Palmer Quarterly, 21,* 267-294.

Sameroff, A. J. & Feil, L. A. (1985). Parental concepts of development. In I. E. Sigel, A. V. McGillicuddy-DeLisi, & J.J. Goodnow (Eds.), *Parental belief systems: The psychological consequences for children* (2nd ed., pp. 347-369). Hillsdale, NJ: Erlbaum.

Schaefer, E. S., & Edgerton, M. (1985). Parent and child correlates of parental modernity. In I. E. Sigel (Ed.), *Parental belief systems. The psychological consequences for children* (pp. 287-315). Hillsdale, NJ: Erlbaum.

Schwartz, T. (1981). The acquisition of culture. *Ethos, 9,* 4-17.

Shweder, R. A. (1984). Anthropology's romantic rebellion against the enlightenment, or there's more to thinking than reason and evidence. In R. A. Shweder & R. A. LeVine (Eds.), *Culture theory: Essays on mind, self and emotion* (pp. 27-66). New York: Cambridge University Press.

Shweder, R. A., & Sullivan, M. A. (1993). Cultural psychology: Who needs it? *Annual Review of Psychology, 44,* 497-523.

Sigel, I. E. (1985). A conceptual analysis of beliefs. In I. E. Sigel (Ed.), *Parental belief systems: The psychological consequences for children* (pp. 345-371). Hillsdale, NJ: Erlbaum.

Sigel, I. E. (1986). Reflections on the belief-behavior connection: Lessons learned from a research program on parental belief systems and teaching strategies. In R. D. Ashmore & D. M. Brodzinsky (Eds.), *Thinking about the family: Views of parents and children* (pp. 35-65). Hillsdale, NJ: Erlbaum.

Sigel, I. E., McGillicuddy-DeLisi, A V., & Johnson, J. E. (1980). *Parental distancing, beliefs and children's representational competence within the family context* (ETS RR 80-21). Princeton, NJ: Educational Testing Service.

Sommer, K., Whitman, T. L., Borkowski, J. G., Schellenbach, Cl., Maxwell, S., & Keogh, C. (1993). Cognitive readiness and adolescent parenting. *Developmental Psychology, 29,* 389-398.

Sternberg, R. L., Conway, B. E., Ketron, J. L., & Bernstein, M. (1981). People's conceptions of intelligence. *Journal of Personality and Social Psychology, 41,* 37-55.

Stigler, J. W., Shweder, R. A., & Herdt, G. (Eds.). (1990). *Cultural psychology: Essays on comparative human development.* Cambridge, UK: Cambridge University Press.

Triana, B., & Rodrigo, M. J. (1988). *Parental knowledge and parental beliefs.* Paper presented at the Third European Conference on Developmental Psychology, Budapest, Hungary.

Tulviste, P. (1991). *Cultural-historical development of verbal thinking: A psychological study.* Commack, NY: Nova Science.

Valsiner, J. (in press). Culture and human development: A co-constructivist perspective. In P. van Geert & L. Mos (Eds.), *Annals of Theoretical Psychology* (Vol. X). New York: Plenum Press.

Weller, S. C. (1987). Shared knowledge, intracultural variation, and knowledge aggregation. *American Behavioral Scientist, 31,* 178–193.

Wertsch, J. V. (1991). *Voices of the mind. A sociocultural approach to mediated action.* Cambridge, MA: Harvard University Press.

Wertsch, J. V., & Tulviste, P. (1992). Lev S. Vygotsky and contemporary developmental psychology. *Developmental Psychology, 28,* 548–557.

# Education and Mother–Infant Interaction
## A Mexican Case Study

Robert A. LeVine
Patrice M. Miller
Amy L. Richman
Sarah LeVine

From decades of research on mother–infant interaction we have learned much about its psychological consequences but relatively little about the cultural and socioeconomic conditions under which it occurs. In this chapter we examine data from a study in urban Mexico to identify some of the factors that influence maternal beliefs about communicating with infants and the effects of such beliefs on maternal behavior and child development. Our goals are "to enhance predictability of belief to action" (Sigel, 1985, p. 346) in the study of parental behavior and more generally to demonstrate the role that educational processes play in shaping mother–infant interaction.

Parents' assumptions about infant care and child development are generated in large part by cultural models that set the prevailing standards of "common sense" in their local communities. The actual behavior of parents, however, is influenced by a variety of factors, including their personal histories of participation in such social institutions as schools. In a rapidly changing society like that of urban Mexico, with a large population of recent migrants from the countryside, traditional cultural models may constitute the common background for parents who are otherwise differentiated by personal histories of social participation. The reproductive and parental practices of a particular local population at a specific historical moment can be seen as the outcome of an interaction between *parameters of tradition* (i.e., agrarian goals and norms for infant care and child development), and *parameters of transition* (i.e., urban residence, employment, income levels, declining birth and death rates, and rising school enrollment ratios). The transition parameters reflect the extent to which institutions organized at a national or regional level have redirected the social participation of individuals and (potentially) their priorities as parents. From this perspective, the school attendance of women seems to be an important link between the macrosocial processes of institutional change and the domestic practices of individual parents. But whether and how schooling during childhood and early adolescence influences the ideas and practices of women as mothers years later requires direct investigation.

Populations in the midst of major social transformation, however difficult to characterize culturally, offer some advantages for investigation of parental behavior over populations at early and advanced stages of such historical processes as demographic transition or school expansion. When the rates of child mortality and fertility have recently dropped and are continuing their decline and the average level of women's schooling rises with each 5-year birth cohort, the magnified variations at a particular historical moment permit relatively controlled research into their co-occurrence in a way that is not available when rates of birth, death, and schooling are more stable and concentrated at the high or low ends of their dimensions. The urban–industrial societies of Europe and North America, for example, have advanced so far in their expansion of schooling that women with incomplete primary school attainment are rare and found only in the most economically deprived enclaves. On the other hand, in many rural villages of Latin America, Africa, and much of Asia, women who have completed primary school are still too few to study quantitatively at the local level.

Mexican cities in the early 1980s, however, included childbearing women with a wide range of school attainment levels from culturally similar rural backgrounds living under similar economic conditions—the results of migration from villages with limited or no schooling to urban areas with expanded opportunities for girls to attend school. Even within the same family there were older women raised in the countryside who had little schooling and their younger sisters whose urban childhoods gave them the chance for lengthier school attendance. This situation made it possible to study the impact of formal education on maternal behavior at the level of individual differences without confounding the effect of variation in schooling with that of membership in different social strata. Our research was conducted from 1983 to 1985 in two low-income *colonias* (neighborhoods) of Cuernavaca, a city of about 200,000 at that time (in a metropolitan area of some 600,000) and capital of the state of Morelos 50 miles south of Mexico City. One was an old working-class *colonia* near the center of town ("Inner City"), the other—"Squatter Settlement"—was a recently inhabited residential area located farther from the center. We studied mothers of the same rural cultural background with from 1 to 9 years of schooling, living on the same streets under a limited range of socioeconomic conditions, to discover how schooling might have differentiated their reproductive ideas and practices. Our quantitative findings are summarized in an article, "Women's Schooling and Child Care in the Demographic Transition: A Mexican Case Study" (LeVine et al. 1991), our ethnographic findings in a monograph, *Dolor y Alegria: Women and Social Change in Urban Mexico* (LeVine, 1993).

In this chapter we focus on maternal beliefs about the infant's communicative ability that might be affected by schooling and might influence in turn how mothers interact with their infants. We begin by considering whether there are cross-cultural variations in the extent to which infants are represented as capable of vocal communication. Then we turn to the Cuernavaca study and ask four questions at the level of individual differences: (1) Does the school experience of mothers affect their personal models of the infant's communicative ability? (2) Do these personal models affect maternal responsiveness during the first 6 months after birth? (3) Are there differentials in verbal interaction by maternal schooling later in the first year and in the second year of the child's life? (4) Is there evidence that variations related to maternal schooling have a psychological impact on the child that lasts beyond the second year?

In attempting to answer each of these questions we are concerned with *how* the school experience might influence early interaction and subsequent child development in the context of a central Mexican culture. Our central hypothesis is that the number of years a mother spends in school increases her tendency to view her infant as ready for verbal interaction, to engage in verbal interaction with the infant during its first 2 years, and thereby to enhance the child's verbal ability at an older age. Figure 10.1 portrays the pathways involved in terms of the specific variables measured in the Cuernavaca study, presented in detail later in the chapter.

## Cultural Models

Recent studies indicate wide variation in cultural models of infants as possible conversational partners. In some cultures, infants are conceptualized as incapable of both talking and understanding speech, and protoconversation with infants is absent as a convention. This is reported by Ochs (1988) for Samoans and Schieffelin (1990) for the Kaluli of Papua New Guinea; both investigators also claim that infant-directed speech is rare or absent. From the Solomon Islands, however, Watson-Gegeo and Gegeo (1986) report interactive speech routines involving 6-month-olds among the Kwara'ae people. Thus, in the Pacific region alone it is clear that beliefs about infant ability to communicate and the conventional forms of maternal behavior associated with those beliefs vary from one culture to another, apparently due to different cultural traditions rather than formal education or other socioeconomic factors. As we have concluded elsewhere:

> [Proto-conversation] between mother and infant is not a universal script, and mother–infant interaction is further differentiated by a variety of culture-specific norms that exempt babies from verbal interaction altogether, prescribe formulaic routines such as lullabies that are not overtly designed to initiate a communicative exchange, direct the mother to attend to crying and ignore babbling, or specify the variable terms of what Schieffelin and Ochs (1986) called "communicative accomodation" to the infant's capacities. (Richman, Miller, & LeVine, 1992, p. 614)

The conclusion that there is cultural variation in ideas and practices concerning infant abilities to participate in verbal interaction is

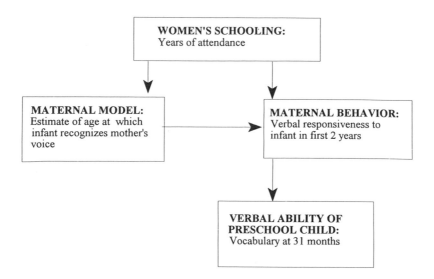

**FIGURE 10.1.** Hypothesized pathways from schooling though maternal belief and behavior to child's verbal ability.

consistent with Konner's (1977) comparison of reciprocal vocalization among the Kalahari San with Guatemalan villagers and working-class and middle-class Bostonians and Field and Widmayer's (1981) comparison of ethnic groups in Miami. Observations by our own research group provide quantitative evidence indicating the rarity of infant-directed speech among the Gusii of western Kenya (LeVine et al., 1994). Older Gusii women, who had not attended school, considered it foolish to talk to children less than 2 years old, as they thought them incapable of understanding speech.

This body of evidence as a whole, though hardly comprehensive, strongly suggests that cultures vary not only in the degree to which their dominant models represent infants as capable of understanding vocal communication but also in the associated practice of speaking to infants by mothers. Women who grow up without attending school are nonetheless *educated* in these dominant cultural models, which they acquire as their own personal models in the course of their participation in family interaction, child care and other social activities during childhood and adolescence (see Rogoff, 1990; Lave & Wenger, 1990).

In the Cuernavaca study, for reasons that are worth considering, we did not investigate directly the cultural models for infant care and development prevailing in the rural villages of Morelos and Guerrero, from which our sample mothers or their parents had come. The pace of social change over the four decades prior to our research had obscured their traditional beliefs and norms. The mothers were 25 years old on average in 1983, which means they were born around 1958 and grew up in the 1960s and early 1970s, when Mexican child mortality was declining but fertility was extremely high. In 1970, for example, infant mortality for Mexico as a whole was variously estimated at between 66 and 83 deaths in the first year for every thousand live births, down from at least 124 in 1940, and the total fertility rate was 6.7 live births per woman (LeVine et al., 1991). Thus, our mothers entered their childbearing years when the demographic situation of *their* mothers had been altered by improved child survival rates permitting large sibship groups to grow up together. In the early part of this period, breast feeding for at least a year was universal, but by 1975, 44.5% of Mexican mothers breast-fed less than 6 months or not at all (LeVine, 1993). This decline in breast feeding, beginning in the 1960s, meant (prior to widespread contraception) an abbreviation of the birth interval and a contraction of the period of care in which a mother had only one young child to attend to. Both of these trends (i.e., the increase in effective sibship size due to improved infant survival and the reduced period of exclusive care by the mother due to briefer breast feeding) led to a domestic situation with more children, closer in age, than there had been in the 1950s. Furthermore, these trends appeared first and were strongest in the rapidly growing cities, where modern health services and other new influences were more available, so that the family's move to the city often coincided with a major change in infant care. Thus, the mothers in our Cuernavaca sample themselves had been children of a transitional period in which traditional concepts and norms were rapidly changing.

It is nonetheless possible to reconstruct some aspects of infant care before Mexico's demographic transition (i.e., when child mortality and fertility were both high). Babies were breast-fed intensively for at least a year, sleeping with the mother during that time, and were weaned when the mother found she was pregnant. Mothers too poor to afford cow's milk weaned later, around 18 months. One older informant said, "If you didn't wean a child by the time he learned to talk, he'd become *muy chillon* (whiny)" (LeVine, 1993, p. 146). Mothers were explicitly concerned about infant disease, and folk medicine was practiced by women in the home as well as specialists from outside. After the infant's health, its docility was the most cherished goal; the ideal infant is described as one who makes few demands for interaction but sleeps or lies quietly in bed. The baby was nonetheless held a good deal in the daytime by elder siblings and women of the older generation in the family as well as by the mother; physical care and such expressions of positive affect as hugging and kissing did not usually involve contingent, conversation-like interaction. Toddlers were expected to be somewhat troublesome and to have tantrums, but mothers were also expected to punish physically, with light spankings (*nalgadas*) on the hands and buttocks during the first year, with a switch by the time a child was 2 or 3, and with a belt by the age of 4. Boys were considered to be less compliant and more troublesome than girls, who were expected to work closely with the mother. Communication between parents and children tended to be formal, not only with the father, who was often a distant figure, but also with the mother, who depended on a measure of formal distance to maintain her authority in the household. Many of these patterns changed when families moved to the city and became involved in its institutions, including schools.

## School Effects I: Maternal Models

Our study in Cuernavaca concerned the impact of maternal schooling and included two forms of data collection. The first was a survey of mothers with young children in two low-income *colonias*. This survey covered 333 mothers ranging in age from 15 to 37, each of whom had attended school at least 1 and no more than 9 years and was currently rearing a child under 48 months of age. The average mother was 25 years old, had been to school for 6 years, and had 3 children. The second form of data collection was home observation of a subsample of mother–infant dyads. The home observations were conducted on 72 mother–infant dyads when the infants were 5 and 10, or 10 and 15, months of age. (See LeVine et al., 1991; Richman et al., 1992, for a fuller account of the settings, samples, and procedures.)

To test the hypothesis that a mother's school experience influences her personal model of the readiness of infants for vocal communication (see Figure 10.1), we examined the survey data. The mothers were asked for their estimate of the age, in months, at which infants can recognize the mother's voice. We assumed that mothers who view their children as ready to communicate during infancy would give an earlier estimate of that age. Table 10.1 shows that when the mothers are divided into three levels of schooling, those with more schooling gave significantly earlier age estimates. The correlation of schooling as a continuous variable with the age estimate is also significant ($r = -.26$, $p < .001$).

It is possible, of course, that maternal schooling is associated with other variables, such as socioeconomic status, which may also have strong effects on maternal beliefs about children's abilities. In order to explore this possibility, we compared three regression models (see Table 10.2). The first model examined only socioeconomic and other associated background variables: the neighborhood in which the mother lived, the husband's level of school attainment, and the number of consumer durables (e.g., major appliances) in the home. These variables, together, accounted for roughly 4% of the variance in the age estimates of the mothers, suggesting that they are not very important in accounting for the mothers' estimates of the infants' communicative abilities. The second model added in the number of children borne by the mother, which may represent the effect of the amount of childrearing experience on the mother's estimation of infant communicative ability. This variable contributed significantly to the estimate of the

**Table 10.1.** Mother's Estimate of Age at Which Infant Recognizes Mother's Voice, by Level of Maternal Schooling ($N = 333$)

| Maternal schooling | Mean estimate (months) ± SD |
|---|---|
| 1–5 years ($n = 82$) | 5.3 ± 3.8 |
| 6 years ($n = 108$) | 4.0 ± 3.1 |
| 7–9 years ($n = 143$) | 3.1 ± 2.8 |

Note. $F(2,330) = 12.8$, $p < .001$.

**Table 10.2.** Regression: Mother's Estimate of Age at Which Infant Recognizes Mother's Voice, Predicted by Number of Children and Maternal Schooling ($N = 333$)

| Variable | df | Parameter estimate | T | p | $R^2$ |
|---|---|---|---|---|---|
| Intercept | 1 | 6.40 | 6.10 | .0001 | |
| *Colonia* | 1 | .74 | 1.85 | .065 | |
| Husband's schooling | 1 | −.04 | −.71 | − | |
| Consumer durables | 1 | .02 | .20 | − | .037[*] |
| Number of children | 1 | −.29 | −2.22 | .027 | .039[*] |
| Maternal schooling | 1 | −.40 | −4.56 | .0001 | .10[***] |

[*]$F_{(3,306)} = 3.94, p < .01$; [**]$F_{(4,305)} = 3.09, p < .02$; [***]$F_{(5,304)} = 6.79, p < .0001$.

dependent variable, suggesting that mothers with more children—those with more experience in infant care—gave lower age estimates; however, it added little to the variance accounted for. Adding maternal schooling, in the third model, contributed significantly to both the estimate of the dependent variable and the variance accounted for. Overall, this analysis suggests that mothers with more schooling gave significantly lower estimates of infants' communicative abilities, even when socioeconomic and experience factors were controlled for. It is important to note that the variance accounted for, while significant, is still relatively small (10%).

## School Effects II: Maternal Behavior

Does a mother's personal model of infant communicative ability affect her behavior toward the infant? Because the mean estimates of the age at which infants recognize their mother's voice ranged from 3.1 for the mothers with the most schooling to 5.3 for the mothers with the least schooling, the behavior observations at 5 months are most relevant to find out whether this particular belief has an impact on maternal behavior. There is observational information on 29 mother–infant dyads at that age. We calculated the conditional probability that any of five maternal behaviors (look, talk, hold, physical, and feed) would follow (in the next interval) the infant's nondistress vocalization as an indicator of the tendency to treat the infant at 5 months as a communicative partner. These conditional probabilities are shown in Table 10.3 for each of three levels of maternal schooling. The mothers with incomplete primary school (1–5 years) responded to a significantly smaller proportion of infant vocalizations than those who had attended school longer. Using schooling as a continuous variable, its correlation with the maternal behavior variable is .36, which is not significant in this small sample. As Table 10.4 shows, however, the correlation between the maternal estimate of infant communicative abilities and observed responsiveness to vocalization *is* statistically significant at −.39 ($p < .05$); that is, mothers who gave a younger age for infant recognition of the mother's face responded to a larger proportion of infant vocalizations at 5 months. Because maternal schooling is related to both the belief variable (age estimate of recognizing mother's voice) and the behavior variable (responsiveness to infant vocal activity), the question is raised as to whether the apparent belief–behavior relationship does not simply reflect their co-variation with schooling. This question was addressed with a regression analysis, shown in Table 10.5, which indicates that even when maternal schooling is controlled for, the mothers' belief with respect to infants' communicative abilities significantly increases maternal responsiveness. Thus, the belief variable shown to be correlated with maternal schooling in the survey sample is an important *independent* predictor of maternal responsiveness in the smaller 5-month observation sample. The model that includes both schooling and maternal beliefs about infant abilities accounts for almost a third of the variance in observed responsiveness. This is consistent with the model of Figure 10.1, in which the impact of maternal schooling on responsiveness is mediated by maternal belief as well as operating "directly" (i.e., through other, unspecified, variables).

These findings (from Tables 10.2 and 10.5) taken together, suggest that schooling influences mothers to believe that infants are ready for communication at an earlier age, and that having acquired such beliefs, mothers are more likely to be responsive to their own infants when they are babbling.

If the relationship between maternal and infant behavior that was shown above existed only at 5 months of age, it might have little developmental significance. Analyses of the observational data for the

**Table 10.3.** Mother's Responsiveness to Infant Vocalization in Home Observations at 5 Months of Age, by Level of Maternal Schooling ($N = 29$)

| Maternal schooling | Mean proportion of infant vocalizations to which mother responded |
|---|---|
| 1–5 years ($n = 8$) | .44 |
| 6 years ($n = 10$) | .68 |
| 7–9 years ($n = 11$) | .65 |

*Note.* $F(2,26) = 3.5$, $p < .05$.

**Table 10.4.** Correlations of Maternal Schooling, Mother's Estimate of Age at Which Infant Recognizes Mother's Voice and Maternal Responsiveness to Infant Babbles in the 5-Month Sample (*N* = 29)

| | Schooling | Estimate | Responsiveness |
|---|---|---|---|
| Schooling | — | −.24 | .36 |
| Estimate | — | — | −.39* |
| Responsiveness | — | — | — |

*$p < .05$.

larger sample of 72 mother–infant dyads, displayed in Table 10.6, show the relationship of maternal schooling to responsiveness variables to be significant at 10 and 15 months, when children are moving into the most critical period for language acquisition. Notice that maternal responsiveness to infant vocalizations and looking is positively correlated with maternal schooling, whereas noncontingent maternal holding is negatively related to schooling, particularly as the infant gets older.

Mother–infant interactions in which mothers respond contingently to infant vocalizations resemble interactions that take place in schools. The apprenticeship in verbal communication between an adult expert and a child novice that takes place in schools provides a pedagogical model that could be acquired by mothers and applied in the domestic setting of infant care, especially as women with more formal education become convinced that even young infants are capable of communication. This effect may be particularly forceful for women from agrarian communities in which traditional apprenticeship tends to involve gradual participation in productive activities with a minimum of verbal instruction from adults. For them, the verbally based interactions of the school classroom represent a novel learning relationship. The longer they attend school, the more fully are they socialized into this

**Table 10.5.** Regression: Maternal Responsiveness to Infant Vocalization at 5 Months, as Predicted by Maternal Schooling and Mother's Estimate of Age at Which Infant Recognizes Mother's Voice (*N* = 29)

| Variable | *df* | Parameter estimate | *T* | *p* | $R^2$ |
|---|---|---|---|---|---|
| Intercept | 1 | .504 | 3.89 | .0001 | — |
| Maternal schooling | 1 | −.028 | −1.61 | n.s. | .14* |
| Mother's estimate | 1 | .028 | 2.62 | .01** | .32** |

*$F(1,27) = 4.35, p < .05$; **$F(2,26) = 6.07, p < .01$.

**Table 10.6.** Correlations between Maternal Schooling and Maternal Responsiveness to Infants, Cuernavaca

|  | Infant age (months) | | |
|---|---|---|---|
|  | 5 | 10 | 15 |
|  | (*n* = 29) | (*n* = 72) | (*n* = 44) |
| Proportion of infant vocalizations followed by maternal speech | .37[*] | .28[*] | .28 |
| Proportion of infant looks followed by maternal speech | .11 | .28[*] | .36[*] |
| Proportion of infant looks followed by maternal looks | .04 | .22 | .35[*] |
| Proportion of infant motor acts followed by maternal speech | .40[*] | .24[*] | .38[**] |
| Proportion of infant vocalizations followed by no maternal response[a] | −.36[*] | −.14 | −.07 |
| Frequency of mother holding infant | −.01 | −.16 | −.33[*] |

[a]This is the reciprocal of maternal responsiveness.

[*]$p < .05$; [**]$p < .01$

new pedagogical model and the more likely they are to think it appropriate in the situation of infant care.

This explanation of the data may not be the only plausible one, but it is certainly worthy of further investigation. We have found a connection between belief and behavior in that the mother's estimate of an early age for infant recognition of maternal voice is linked to her responsiveness to vocalizations at 5 months. We suggest that this is the start of a different pathway for language socialization among infants of more educated mothers, one based on contingent responsiveness that becomes elaborated as the child becomes more capable of speech. This process as we have studied it among the mothers of Cuernavaca, Mexico, is embedded in a broader context of school-associated change, in which mothers who attended school longer bear fewer children and more frequently seek medical care during pregnancy. These relationships are statistically significant even when associated socioeconomic factors are controlled for (LeVine et al., 1991, Tables 6 and 11). Other findings from the same sample show that mothers with more schooling express a greater desire for further education, a greater exposure to the media, more egalitarian family attitudes, higher occupational aspirations for their children, and lower expectations of material returns from them. The breadth of these differentials in belief, expectation, and practice within two low-income *colonias* suggests that schooling has influenced (directly or indirectly) not only the discretionary behavior patterns of these women but also their social identities, parental investment strategies, and conceptions of personal development and interpersonal relations (LeVine et al., 1991, p. 485).

To summarize, models of infant communicative ability vary across cultures, as confirmed by ethnographic reports that in some, but not all, societies infants are believed incapable of communication and are not engaged in conversation. That schooling affects maternal beliefs concerning infant communicative ability has been confirmed by our survey in urban Mexico, showing that women who attended school longer give younger estimates of the age at which infants recognize the maternal voice. This belief is part of a larger set of changing family attitudes influenced by schooling. The question whether maternal beliefs acquired in school influence mother–infant communication has been partially answered by the results of our home observations at 5 months, in which women who gave younger estimates responded to a larger proportion of infant vocalizations. Observations at 10 and 15 months on the larger sample show consistent relationships between the mother's schooling and her verbal responsiveness to the infant. The next question is whether these apparent effects of schooling on maternal belief and behavior have an impact on the child's development.

## School Effects III: The Child's Verbal Ability

We conducted a follow-up assessment when the infants were 31–32 months of age, attempting to find the original 72 mother–infant pairs that had been observed earlier. A total of 31 families could be located. Three instruments were administered to the child: The Stanford–Binet intelligence test, the four-boxes task (Vandell, 1979), and the Quiroz measure of language development, constructed in Mexico for use with children ages 24 to 36 months (see Table 10.7). In this chapter we present only the results from the Stanford–Binet and the Quiroz.

The Stanford–Binet was administered in Spanish by a trained Mexican administrator who recorded the number of items the child passed for 2, 2½, and 3 years of age. An overall score was also obtained. An examination of the means for these four scores showed an increasing mean number of items passed, up until the 2½-year age point. The 3-year items showed a drop in mean number of items passed. Because the sample children were roughly 2½ years of age, and the scores obtained at age 2½ seemed to reflect their optimal performance, it is those scores that will be presented here. These scores showed very high correlations with the total Stanford–Binet scores ($r = .85$).

**Table 10.7.** Quiroz Measure of Language Development

| | |
|---|---|
| Item 1: | Child has to point to parts of his/her body that are named |
| Item 2: | Child has to identify common objects, such as a cup |
| Item 3: | Child has to follow simple commands (e.g., sit down) |
| Item 4: | Child's has to construct a negative sentence (show child cup, ask if it is a ball) |
| Item 5: | Child has to identify a new object among a collection of related objects |
| Item 6: | Child has to identify the function of common objects |
| Item 7: | Picture vocabulary from the Stanford–Binet |

Correlational analyses of the Quiroz indicated that all the items except item 4 (constructing a negative sentence) were highly intercorrelated. Given the high degree of intercorrelation, it made sense to construct a Combined language measure. Items 1, 2, 3, and 6 were included in this Combined language measure. Item 5 was omitted because it was scored on a different scale from the other items (a 0–1 scale instead of a scale showing degrees of competence). Item 7, the picture vocabulary from the Stanford–Binet was omitted in order to avoid unnecessary overlap with the scores from the Stanford–Binet test.

To investigate the question whether maternal schooling and observed patterns of maternal responsiveness in the first and second years of life have consequences for the child's cognitive and language development during the third year, we first examined the correlations of mother's schooling and verbal responsiveness at 10 and 15 months with the Stanford–Binet scores and with the Combined language measure. These correlations, seen in Table 10.8, show that maternal verbal responsiveness at 15 months is significantly related to both the Combined language score and the Stanford–Binet scores at 31 months. Maternal verbal responsiveness at 10 months shows a nonsignificant trend in the same direction. It is also apparent that the Combined language score, at least, is significantly positively related to the amount of schooling that the mothers had. As Table 10.6 showed that maternal schooling is also somewhat related to responsiveness, we decided to explore the relative contributions of maternal schooling and maternal responsiveness to the 31-month outcome variables using regression analyses.

The results of the regression analyses for the Combined language measure, as predicted by maternal schooling and maternal verbal responsiveness to infant verbal behavior, are shown in Table 10.9. These

**Table 10.8.** Correlations between the Combined Language Measure, the Stanford–Binet Test Scores, Mother's Schooling, and Maternal Verbal Responsiveness to 10- and 15-Month-Old infants

|  | Combined language | Stanford–Binet Score |
|---|---|---|
| Mother's schooling | .51[*] | .17 |
| Maternal verbal responsiveness to 10-month-old infant verbal behavior | .35 | .31 |
| Maternal verbal responsiveness to 15-month-old infant verbal behavior | .53[**] | .48[**] |

[*]$p < .01$;  [**]$p < .05$.

analyses show that maternal schooling is a significant predictor of the Combined language scores in both the equation containing the 10-month-old responsiveness measure and in the equation containing the 15-month-old age point. Mother's verbal responsiveness to infant verbal behavior at 10 months does not significantly predict the child's Combined language score at 31 months, but mother's verbal responsiveness at 15 months does, even when controlling for mother's schooling. These findings for maternal verbal responsiveness to infant verbal behavior are essentially replicated in parallel regression analyses of maternal verbal responsiveness to infant looking and to infant motor behavior (not shown). In addition, the findings for the Stanford–Binet are essentially the same; there is significant predictability from the measures of maternal verbal responsiveness at 15 months to the 31-month Stanford–Binet score (controlling for maternal schooling), but not from the equivalent measure at 10 months.

Findings from the follow-up at 31 months indicate that children whose mothers have been more verbally responsive to them at 15 months perform better on vocabulary tests 16 months later. Although the data as a whole do not demonstrate that the causal sequence illustrated in Figure 10.1 must be operating, they do show that all the linkages predicted by that theoretical model—some of which are temporally prior to others—are present in this urban Mexican sample. A longitudinal data collection program with a larger sample would be needed to provide a stronger basis for inferring that the connections are causal ones. We interpret these data as meaning that the school experience of mothers leads them to construe their infants as ready for conversational interaction in the first months after birth, to engage them in reciprocal vocalization from 5 months of age, and to respond verbally to their vocal, visual, and motor actions at 10 and 15 months.

**Table 10.9.** Regression Analyses: Combined Language Measure as Predicted by Maternal Verbal Responsiveness to Infant Verbal Behavior at 10 and 15 Months

| | df | Parameter estimate | Standard error | T |
|---|---|---|---|---|
| | | Regression 1: Mothers of 10-month-olds | | |
| Intercept | 1 | 1.72 | .46 | 3.72[**] |
| Mother's schooling | 1 | 0.15 | .05 | 3.13[*] |
| Maternal verbal responsiveness | 1 | 0.13 | .25 | 0.50 |
| | Adjusted $R^2$ = .32, $F(2,24)$ = 7.16, $p$ < .004 | | | |
| | | Regression 2: Mothers of 15-month-olds | | |
| Intercept | 1 | 2.45 | .38 | 6.58[**] |
| Mother's schooling | 1 | 0.12 | .04 | 2.86[*] |
| Maternal verbal responsiveness | 1 | 0.67 | .22 | 2.96[*] |
| | Adjusted $R^2$ = .50, $F(2,15)$ = 9.67, $p$ < .002 | | | |

[*]$p$ < .01; [**]$p$ < .001.

This early and consistent engagement in verbal interaction by mothers with more schooling during the first 2 years has detectable effects on the child's vocabulary and intelligence test scores at 31 months, precursors of school readiness. In other words, we believe the evidence suggests that the schooling of girls in urban Mexico influences their beliefs and practices as mothers so as to provide their children with the kind of skill that confers an advantage in school: verbal ability. If we are right, this study of mother–infant interaction in Cuernavaca indicates the kinds of microsocial processes through which the expansion of schooling over several generations can change the beliefs and practices of an entire population. In receiving the children of rural migrants, the school as an institutional environment in the low-income neighborhoods of urban Mexico disseminates new models of verbal communication that reshape not only parental behavior but the life cycle in its adaptive dimensions.

# Acknowledgments

The Cuernavaca field research reported in this chapter was supported by the Population Council (Subordinate Agreement CP 82.47A), the Rockefeller Foundation (Population Sciences Division), the Ford Foundation, and the John D. and Catherine T. MacArthur Foundation. Analyses were supported by the Spencer Foundation.

# References

Field, T. M., & Widmayer, S. M. (1981). Mother–infant interactions among lower SES Black, Cuban, Puerto-Rican and South American immigrants. In T. M. Field, A. M. Sostek, P. Vietze, & P. H. Leiderman (Eds.), *Culture and early interactions*. Hillsdale, NJ: Erlbaum.

Kaye, K. (1982). *The mental and social life of babies*. Chicago: University of Chicago Press.

Konner, M. J. (1977). Infancy among the Kalahari Desert San. In P. H. Leiderman, S. R. Tulkin, & A. Rosenfeld (Eds.), *Culture and infancy: Variations in the human experience*. New York: Academic Press.

Lave, J., & Wenger, M. (1990). *Situated learning*. New York: Cambridge University Press.

LeVine, R., LeVine, S., Richman, A. L. , Tapia Uribe, F. M., Sunderland Correa, C., & Miller, P. M. (1991). Women's schooling and child care in demographic transition: A Mexican case study. *Population and Development Review, 17*, 459–496.

LeVine, R., Dixon, S., LeVine, S., Richman, A., Keefer, C., Leiderman, P. H., & Brazelton, T. B. (1994). *Child care and culture: Lessons from Africa*. New York: Cambridge University Press.

LeVine, S. (1993). *Dolor y Alegria: Women and social change in urban Mexico*. Madison, WI: University of Wisconsin Press.

Ochs, E. (1988). *Culture and language development*. New York: Cambridge University Press.

Richman, A. L., Miller, P. M., & LeVine, R. A. (1992). Cultural and educational variations in maternal responsiveness. *Developmental Psychology, 28*(4), 614–621.

Rogoff, B. (1990). *Apprenticeship in thinking*. New York: Oxford University Press.

Schieffelin, B. B. (1990). *The give and take of everyday life: The language socialization of Kaluli children*. New York: Cambridge University Press.

Sigel, I. E. (1985). A conceptual analysis of beliefs. In I. E. Sigel (Ed.), *Parental belief systems: The psychological consequences for children*. Hillsdale, NJ: Erlbaum.

Vandell, D. L. (1979). Effects of a playgroup experience on mother–son and father–son interaction. *Developmental Psychology, 15*(4), 379–385.

Watson-Gegeo, K. A., & Gegeo, D. W. (1986). Calling out and repeating routines in Kwara'ae children's language socialization. In B. B. Schieffelin & E. Ochs (Eds.), *Language socialization across cultures*. London: Cambridge University Press.

# CHAPTER 11

# The Contrasting Developmental Timetables of Parents and Preschool Teachers in Two Cultural Communities

Carolyn Pope Edwards
Lella Gandini
Donatella Giovaninni

In many nations around the world today, but especially in Europe, East Asia, and North America, preschools and child-care centers increasingly have become a part of the strategy for nurturing, socializing, and teaching young children prior to the start of formal schooling (Olmstead & Weikart, 1989; Tobin, Wu, & Davidson, 1989). More and more, the cultural tasks of making sense of infant and child development and translating values and goals into trusted practices no longer remain in the sole hands of parents and extended family but instead are shared with experts or paid practitioners who design, oversee, and provide early childhood services. Such a new sharing of responsibility raises many questions concerning fundamental changes in socialization processes—questions focused on what Bronfenbrenner (1979) calls the mesosystem, the intersection between two developmental contexts—in this case, home and early childhood education setting. For example, how are young children affected when their upbringing is divided between two groups of people who are relative strangers to one another, groups that may or may not hold similar childrearing beliefs and values? And how are the value conflicts mediated? Is there any evidence that parents and professionals move toward greater agreement in their beliefs, methods, and goals? If so, are parents influenced more by the professional experts or vice versa?

All these questions presuppose that there *are* substantial gaps between the socialization beliefs of parents and professionals, but is this so? Perhaps both groups are more deeply guided than they realize by the childrearing approaches (folk systems) preserved from their own childhood memories as well as embedded in the symbolic and communication systems of the surrounding community (Harkness & Super, Introduction, this volume). Or perhaps both groups are similarly influenced by observation and personal experience with young children, or by "expert advice" available from child development research. This exploratory study seeks to determine the distance in child development beliefs between parents and professionals, using as samples two communities, one in Northeastern United States and one in Central Italy, as a way to consider how, when, and why parental and professional belief systems come to differ.

*Developmental expectations*, or *timetables*, are the component of belief systems we have chosen to study. Adult beliefs about children and childrearing have many dimensions, certainly, but timetables have emerged as one dimension that is both theoretically interesting and empirically accessible (Goodnow & Collins, 1990; Miller, 1988). Timetables relate to the boundaries, or *zones*, for acceptable behavior that adults draw around their internalized norms for child development; they measure what adults consider to be normal in the way of earliness or lateness for particular child competencies to appear. The expectations may serve as internal guidelines for adult behavior; adults who expect early development in an area may be more likely to focus on that area and reward or punish children's performance (Holloway & Reichhart-Erickson, 1989). As Spindler (1987) put it, child development is susceptible to "cultural compression"; high expectations on the part of adults for mature behavior may translate into early and strong demands for mature behavior in that domain.

Mothers' timetables have been compared across a number of cultural communities. Israeli mothers of European background had early expectations for infant cognitive development compared to the expectations of Israeli mothers of African or Asian background (Ninio, 1979). Israeli Yemenite Jews were found to have earlier milestones for infant perceptual, language, social, and emotional development than did Israeli Kurdish Jews (Frankel & Roer-Bornstein, 1982). Italian mothers from a traditional city near Rome were found to have late expectations for infant crawling, self-feeding, and sitting unsupported—skills that they actively discourage—relative to a group of mothers in Boston, Massachusetts (New, 1984).

Robert Hess and an intercultural research team (Hess, Kashiwagi, Azuma, Price, & Dickson, 1980) developed an inventory they called the Developmental Expectations Questionaire (DEQ) to assess adults' expectations for specific child competencies. The instrument, a sorting task, involves 38 items reflective of social and emotional maturity and some early school-related skills. The items were created in joint sessions of Japanese and Americans to sample seven major categories of observable behavior (Emotional maturity, Compliance, Politeness, Independence, School-related skills, Social skills, and Verbal assertiveness) that children in both countries were normally expected to master during the childhood years. Hess et al. (1980) found that Japanese mothers from Tokyo and Sapporo had earlier expectations for emotional control, compliance with adult authority, and courtesy, whereas mothers from San Francisco had earlier expectations for social skills with peers (e.g., showing sympathy, taking initiative, negotiating, standing up for their rights) and verbal communication (seeking information, stating own needs, explaining ideas).

Social skills with peers and verbal assertiveness have consistently been found to be expected early by mothers of certain cultural communities. In a study of U.S. day-care children living in metropolitan Washington, D.C., Holloway and Reichhart-Erickson (1989) found that the mothers of more socially competent children not only expected earlier acquisition of 15 DEQ items than did mothers of less competent children but also selected high-quality child-care programs that emphasized sociability and prosocial values. A study conducted in Sydney, Australia, in which Goodnow, Cashmore, Cotton, and Knight (1984) used 32 items of the DEQ to compare timetables of native-born mothers of preschool children with Lebanese immigrants, showed similar findings. The Lebanese-Australian mothers said they valued early school entry but only a few had sent their children to preschool, in contrast to most of the Anglo-Australian mothers. On the DEQ, the Anglo-Australians had significantly earlier expectations; the areas of strongest difference were for social skills with peers and verbal assertiveness.

The DEQ has also proven useful in comparing maternal beliefs with those of preschool teachers. The instrument was first used this way to compare San Francisco mothers of preschool children with local preschool teachers (Hess, Price, Dickson, & Conroy, 1981). In this case, the mothers were found to press for earlier mastery of most social skills than did the professionals. On the other hand, opposite findings appeared in a study of mothers and female day-care providers in Puebla, Mexico, using seven items from the DEQ concerned with independence, cooperation, and obedience. Mothers' expectations were typically about a year behind those of the day-care providers (Holloway, Gorman, & Fuller, 1988). The same was found in Lima, Peru, where mothers showed later expectations than preschool teachers on nine DEQ items; moreover, in this cultural community, later expectations on the part of both mothers and teachers correlated with higher child competence (Gorman, 1987; Gorman & Holloway, 1987). Thus, it is not clear when and why parents and teachers might have different developmental expectations, what is the source of the differences, and what might be the significance.

# Methods

## Study Communities

This study used the full 38-item DEQ plus four items added by our research team to compare parents and early childhood professionals in two focal communities that have been the subject of our own previous research on parental and teacher expectations, childrearing practices, and early childhood education (Edwards & Gandini, 1989; Edwards, Gandini, & Nimmo, 1992, 1994; Gandini, 1988, 1993; Nimmo, 1992). These two communities were selected as comparable along several dimensions. Both are relatively small, stable, cohesive cities with high-quality early childhood education services for children under 6 and a core group of early childhood teachers/caregivers having a professional identity. (In both cities, multiple and conceptually overlapping terms were commonly used to designate early childhood professionals, e.g., in Amherst, "caregiver," "day-care provider," "educator," and "teacher," and in Pistoia, *operatore, educatore, insegnante*. For simplicity, therefore, and because we felt the work of all these adults involved a combination of educating and caregiving, we chose one term, "teacher," to use in this chapter.) Finally, in both communities, there is some division between the cultures and demands of home and school; teachers are aware that their work involves parents as well as children and try to help children feel at ease in both settings and move confidently back and forth between them.

Amherst, Massachusetts (population about 35,000) is a small city in rural western Massachusetts. Founded in 1755, it is known for its several area universities and colleges, as well as for its historic town-meeting form of governance and citizen participation and long-standing traditions of intellectuality and political liberalism. With regard to early childhood programs, Amherst is well-serviced by U.S. standards, possessing public and private day-care centers, nursery schools, and kindergarten programs, as well as a town-supported resource and referral agency. Amherst citizens place a high value on education, as evidenced in tax support for public schools and use of adult education opportunities; most of the child-care providers in our sample had college-level degrees, and many were taking postgraduate professional courses at the local state university. Multicultural education has been a topic of great concern within the community in general and the educational community in particular, and teachers responded to our research with interest and willing participation.

Pistoia, Italy (population 100,000) is an ancient city near Florence in the region of Toscana. A prosperous provincial capital and agricultural and industrial center, it is known for the manufacture of textiles, leather crafts, train cars, and buses and as a center of nurseries and horticulture. A series of progressive (Communist) local administrators have made child and family services a high priority. Pistoia has a recognized and respected system of municipal child-care centers, fulfilling the demand for infant–toddler (age 3 months–3 years) and preprimary (age 3–6 years) care and education, along with an innovative system of *Area Bambini* ("Children's Places") offering family-centered, part-day, after-school, and infant–toddler programs. These various programs are staffed by relatively well-paid professionals who receive continuous, high-quality, in-service professional training under the auspices of the municipal Department of Education. This in-service training, along with other support systems offered, has led to the evolution of a cohesive community of early childhood teachers with a shared pedagogy and belief in a common educational project. This has been especially true for teachers at the infant–toddler level, many of whom entered the system with postsecondary education and have been notably responsive to a multiyear program of professional development and in-service training, in collaboration with leaders from central administration. They see research as a valuable source of information for their individual and collective professional development and incorporated our research into their own program of work. Citizens of Pistoia have been consistently supportive of their town's early childhood services, as reflected in tax support and strong rallying when needed to resist central government cutbacks.

### Sample

Our sample consisted of 240 adults divided equally between Amherst and Pistoia and the four subgroups: mothers, fathers, infant–toddler caregivers, and preprimary teachers. The parents (mothers and fathers were not from the same families) were recruited from five or more child-care centers in each community, whereas the professionals were recruited through in-service courses or meetings run by the municipal Department of Education (in Pistoia) or the local state university (in Amherst).

## Research Instrument

The subjects were given a written questionnaire version of the 38-item DEQ, in English or Italian, to which four items were added that were of special interest for the U.S.-Italian comparison. These four new items (Table 11.1 items 39-42) included two hypothesized by the research team to be earlier for Pistoia, where parents were observed to stress manners and graciousness to others, and two hypothesized to be earlier for Amherst, where parents were observed to stress personal autonomy in self-care. The items were helping a peer when help is needed, refraining from interrupting mother when she is talking to someone else, sleeping the entire night in one's own bed, and getting completely dressed without help. The original 38 items were grouped into seven summary variables, following Hess et al. (1980): Emotional maturity (mean of 4 items), Compliance (mean of 5 items), Politeness (mean of 2 items), Independence (mean of 8 items), School-related skills (mean of 3 items), Social skills with peers (mean of 6 items), and Verbal assertiveness (mean of 5 items). Subjects were instructed that each item on the questionaire represented a skill that develops in childhood; they were asked to "think about children in general" and check off when they believed that children usually acquire the capacity to do that skill: (1) at age 6 years or above; (2) between ages 4 and 6; or (3) younger than 4 years.

# Findings

Table 11.1 presents the mean scores on the DEQ for the Amherst and Pistoia mothers and fathers, infant–toddler and preprimary teachers, for each of the 42 separate items and the 7 summary scales. Visually inspecting the means, it can be seen that the Pistoia mothers and fathers generally have *later* developmental expectations (lower mean scores) than do the Pistoia teachers on respective items, whereas the Amherst mothers and fathers generally have *earlier* expectations (higher mean scores) than do the teachers in their community. The Pistoia parents also seem to have later expectations relative to the Amherst parents,

**Table 11.1.** The Developmental Expectations of Parents and Teachers from Two Communities: Mean Ratings for 8 Subgroups on Items from Hess Questionnaire of Expected Time Skills Appear

| Developmental Expectations Items, as rated on scale:<br>3 = expected before age 4<br>2 = expected between ages 4–6<br>1 = expected after age 6 | Pistoia Mothers (n = 30) | Pistoia Fathers (n = 30) | Pistoia Teachers Inf–Tod. (n = 30) | Pistoia Teachers Preprim. (n = 30) | Amherst Mothers (n = 30) | Amherst Fathers (n = 30) | Amherst Teachers Inf/Tod. (n = 30) | Amherst Teachers Preprim. (n = 30) |
|---|---|---|---|---|---|---|---|---|
| EMOTIONAL MATURITY (Mean of 4 items) | 1.80 | 2.00 | 2.10 | 1.98 | 2.11 | 2.14 | 1.93 | 1.90 |
| 1. Does not cry easily | 1.86 | 2.13 | 2.37 | 2.14 | 2.00 | 1.90 | 1.83 | 1.87 |
| 2. Can get over anger by him/herself | 1.93 | 2.07 | 2.28 | 1.87 | 2.20 | 2.24 | 1.87 | 1.83 |
| 3. Stands disappointment without crying | 1.37 | 1.80 | 1.55 | 1.69 | 1.93 | 1.87 | 1.73 | 1.63 |
| 4. Does not use baby-talk | 2.07 | 2.00 | 2.28 | 2.23 | 2.33 | 2.53 | 2.30 | 2.30 |
| COMPLIANCE (Mean of 5 items) | 2.00 | 2.25 | 2.36 | 2.07 | 2.34 | 2.26 | 2.18 | 2.20 |
| 5. Comes or answers when called | 2.68 | 2.90 | 2.97 | 2.69 | 2.77 | 2.83 | 2.80 | 2.80 |
| 6. Does not do things forbidden by parents | 1.93 | 2.21 | 2.07 | 1.90 | 2.31 | 2.04 | 1.89 | 2.07 |
| 7. Stops misbehaving when told | 1.97 | 2.20 | 2.50 | 2.00 | 2.34 | 2.30 | 2.30 | 2.16 |
| 8. Does task immediately when told | 2.00 | 2.23 | 2.63 | 2.23 | 2.37 | 2.20 | 2.03 | 2.27 |
| 9. Gives up reading or TV to help mother | 1.50 | 1.70 | 1.58 | 1.48 | 1.87 | 1.90 | 1.83 | 1.70 |
| POLITENESS (Mean of 2 items) | 2.25 | 2.13 | 2.60 | 2.42 | 2.52 | 2.47 | 2.32 | 2.35 |
| 10. Greets family courteously, "Good morning" | 2.33 | 2.23 | 2.83 | 2.60 | 2.37 | 2.40 | 2.21 | 2.37 |
| 11. Uses polite forms, "please," to adults | 2.17 | 2.03 | 2.34 | 2.23 | 2.67 | 2.53 | 2.40 | 2.33 |

*(cont.)*

Table 11.1. (cont.)

| INDEPENDENCE (Mean of 8 items) | 1.62 | 1.62 | 1.76 | 1.65 | 1.72 | 1.74 | 1.63 | 1.62 |
|---|---|---|---|---|---|---|---|---|
| 12. Stays home alone for an hour or so | 1.07 | 1.07 | 1.20 | 1.07 | 1.03 | 1.03 | 1.00 | 1.03 |
| 13. Takes care of own clothes | 1.27 | 1.23 | 1.27 | 1.30 | 1.23 | 1.40 | 1.17 | 1.17 |
| 14. Makes phone calls without help | 1.67 | 1.40 | 1.67 | 1.70 | 1.47 | 1.40 | 1.27 | 1.33 |
| 15. Sits at table and eats without help | 2.70 | 2.67 | 2.93 | 2.70 | 2.77 | 2.83 | 2.70 | 2.67 |
| 16. Does regular household tasks | 1.17 | 1.13 | 1.27 | 1.13 | 1.48 | 1.57 | 1.57 | 1.60 |
| 17. Spends own money carefully | 1.03 | 1.03 | 1.14 | 1.03 | 1.10 | 1.03 | 1.18 | 1.03 |
| 18. Can entertain self alone | 2.70 | 2.73 | 2.90 | 2.73 | 2.90 | 2.87 | 2.73 | 2.70 |
| 19. Plays outside without adult supervision | 1.30 | 1.67 | 1.69 | 1.50 | 1.80 | 1.79 | 1.37 | 1.40 |
| SCHOOL-RELATED SKILLS (Mean of 3 items) | 1.29 | 1.34 | 1.40 | 1.27 | 1.52 | 1.41 | 1.28 | 1.24 |
| 20. Can tell time up to quarter hour | 1.40 | 1.40 | 1.27 | 1.37 | 1.42 | 1.47 | 1.23 | 1.07 |
| 21. Read aloud a 30-page picture book | 1.37 | 1.47 | 1.53 | 1.21 | 1.63 | 1.47 | 1.27 | 1.37 |
| 22. Look up things in picture encyclopedia | 1.10 | 1.17 | 1.40 | 1.23 | 1.50 | 1.30 | 1.33 | 1.30 |
| SOCIAL SKILLS (Mean of 6 items) | 2.04 | 2.25 | 2.50 | 2.16 | 2.43 | 2.46 | 2.25 | 2.21 |
| 23. Waits for his or her turn in games | 2.07 | 2.17 | 2.72 | 2.07 | 2.37 | 2.37 | 2.20 | 2.13 |
| 24. Shares his/her toys with other children | 2.14 | 2.33 | 2.43 | 2.17 | 2.57 | 2.73 | 2.43 | 2.43 |
| 25. Sympathetic to feelings of children | 1.93 | 2.20 | 2.27 | 2.00 | 2.63 | 2.43 | 2.53 | 2.20 |
| 26. Resolves disagreements without fighting | 1.53 | 1.79 | 2.07 | 1.63 | 2.07 | 2.23 | 1.67 | 1.90 |
| 27. Gets own way by persuading friends | 2.17 | 2.40 | 2.53 | 2.50 | 2.33 | 2.23 | 2.07 | 2.00 |

(cont.)

**Table 11.1.** (cont.)

| | | | | | | | | |
|---|---|---|---|---|---|---|---|---|
| 28. Takes initiative in playing with others | 2.45 | 2.60 | 2.93 | 2.60 | 2.63 | 2.73 | 2.57 | 2.60 |
| VERBAL ASSERTIVENESS (Mean of 5 items) | 2.20 | 2.27 | 2.42 | 2.15 | 2.46 | 2.55 | 2.33 | 2.22 |
| 29. Answers a question clearly | 2.17 | 2.17 | 2.66 | 2.40 | 2.47 | 2.60 | 2.23 | 2.37 |
| 30. States own preference when asked | 2.30 | 2.47 | 2.60 | 2.28 | 2.87 | 2.93 | 2.63 | 2.67 |
| 31. Asks for explanation when in doubt | 2.47 | 2.43 | 2.43 | 2.21 | 2.40 | 2.53 | 2.20 | 2.01 |
| 32. Can explain why s/he thinks so | 1.80 | 1.90 | 1.93 | 1.63 | 2.27 | 2.20 | 2.27 | 1.80 |
| 33. Stands up for own rights with others | 2.27 | 2.37 | 2.48 | 2.24 | 2.30 | 2.50 | 2.30 | 2.20 |
| Items Not in Any of Above Clusters | | | | | | | | |
| 34. Uses pointed scissors without supervision | 1.40 | 1.43 | 1.68 | 1.50 | 1.60 | 1.73 | 1.40 | 1.47 |
| 35. Keeps feet off furniture | 2.27 | 2.40 | 2.48 | 2.43 | 2.03 | 1.82 | 1.75 | 2.03 |
| 36. Disagrees w/o biting or throwing | 2.33 | 2.50 | 2.53 | 2.34 | 2.69 | 2.60 | 2.30 | 2.37 |
| 37. Answers the telephone properly | 1.97 | 2.16 | 2.53 | 2.14 | 2.03 | 1.87 | 1.90 | 1.70 |
| 38. Resolves quarrels without adult help | 1.43 | 1.63 | 1.83 | 1.50 | 1.60 | 1.67 | 1.60 | 1.53 |
| Items Added by Present Researchers | | | | | | | | |
| 39. Sleeps entire night own bed without getting up | 2.14 | 2.33 | 2.43 | 2.17 | 2.57 | 2.73 | 2.43 | 2.43 |
| 40. Gets completely dressed without help | 1.86 | 1.67 | 1.97 | 1.66 | 2.33 | 2.10 | 2.07 | 1.87 |
| 41. Helps a peer when help is needed | 1.93 | 2.07 | 2.47 | 2.10 | 2.40 | 2.53 | 2.50 | 2.33 |
| 42. Doesn't interrupt mother when she is talking to someone else | 1.27 | 1.57 | 1.50 | 1.47 | 1.27 | 1.60 | 1.50 | 1.50 |

whereas the results comparing the teachers across the two communities vary by item in an inconsistent way.

How do these findings on mothers relate to those from the two earlier studies using the DEQ (Hess et al., 1980; Goodnow et al., 1984)? The means from all three studies are presented and compared in Edwards (1992). Comparing these means for six groups of mothers, it is evident that the Pistoia mothers actually have quite early expectations for social skills with peers and verbal assertiveness; their mean scores are comparable to the San Francisco and Anglo-Australian samples. But the Amherst sample is simply more extreme and has, in fact, the earliest social and verbal expectations of any group studied to date with the DEQ.

All these scores for mothers can be summarized and integrated into one visual representation by the statistical technique of multidimensional scaling. We used the ALSCAL procedure of the Statistical Package for the Social Sciences (SPSS, 1990) to create a two-dimensional model of how the six mother groups stand in proximity to one another across all their means on the 32 DEQ items they have in common, considered at once. The model starts from a proximities matrix (in our case, a correlation matrix based on the table of means for the six cases (the six mother groups) intracorrelated across variables (the 32 DEQ items). By means of an alternating least-squares algorithm, ALSCAL derives the best *n*-dimensional solution to represent the distances between the cases. In our case, a virtually perfect (stress = .007) solution in two dimensions appears (see Figure 11.1).

The model confirms that a strong first dimension spreads the six groups, with Lebanese-Australian mothers occupying the extreme left end (generally "latest expectations"), Amherst mothers taking the extreme right end (generally "earliest expectations"), and all other groups occupying the center (generally "medium expectations"). The second dimension, explaining much less variance than the first, relates to earliness of expectations for particular domains: Emotional maturity (not crying easily, mastering anger by oneself, standing disappointment without crying) and Independence (staying home alone for an hour, taking care of one's clothes, doing regular household tasks, etc.)—early among the Tokyo/Sapporo mothers and late among Pistoia and Lebanese-Australian mothers.

Returning to the new findings, we wished to compare our eight groups of Amherst and Pistoia parents and teachers to one another. To test whether the differences between the various group means are statistically significant, analyses of variance (*F*-tests) were performed. However, because of the large number of items, and because various items were omitted by different subjects, these tests were performed only for the seven summary scales. A three-step process was used. First, the parents in the two communities were compared with each other to see whether parent gender (mothers/fathers), cultural community (Amherst/Pistoia), or their statistical interaction predicts parental developmental expectations. Second, the teachers in the two communities were compared to see whether teaching level (infant–toddler/preprimary), community (Amherst/Pistoia), or the interaction predicts teachers' developmental expectations. Finally, pooled parents and pooled teachers were compared to each other to see whether adult role (parents/teachers), community (Amherst/Pistoia), or the interaction predicts adult developmental expectations across the whole sample.

Table 11.2 indicates the *F*-test results for the two-way analysis involving parents only. Mothers and fathers are not significantly different for any variable. In contrast, the cultural community differences are prominent. Cultural main effects are statistically significant for all seven

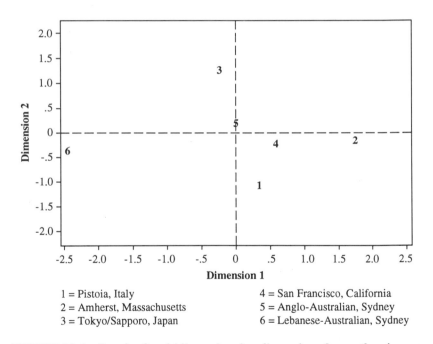

1 = Pistoia, Italy　　　　　　　　　4 = San Francisco, California
2 = Amherst, Massachusetts　　　　　5 = Anglo-Australian, Sydney
3 = Tokyo/Sapporo, Japan　　　　　　6 = Lebanese-Australian, Sydney

**FIGURE 11.1.** Graph of multidimensional scaling values for mothers' mean Developmental Expectations Questionaire (DEQ) scores in six cultural communities. ALSCAL of proximities matrix; stress = .007 in two dimensions. From Hess et al. (1980), Goodnow et al. (1984), and this chapter. Refer to Edwards (1992) for complete table of DEQ means for six groups of mothers.

**Table 11.2.** Pistoia and Amherst Parental Expectations: Results of *F*-Tests Comparing Mothers and Fathers

| | Main effects | | Interactions |
|---|---|---|---|
| DEQ summary scales | Culture | Parent gender | Culture × gender |
| Emotional maturity | 6.85** | | |
| Compliance | 5.19* | | 4.89* |
| Politeness | 9.48** | | |
| Independence | 9.43** | | |
| School-related skills | 4.38* | | |
| Social skills with peers | 20.45*** | | |
| Verbal assertiveness | 16.32*** | | |

*Note.* Only significant *F*-test results (*df* = 1,116) are reported. All tests of significance are two-tailed.
*$p < .05$; **$p < .01$; ***$p < .001$.

summary scales, with most significant differences ($p < .001$) found for Verbal assertiveness and Social skills with peers. The Amherst parents definitely have earlier expectations than do the Pistoia parents. For only one variable, Compliance, is there a significant interaction effect: Pistoia mothers have later expectations for Compliance than do Pistoia fathers, whereas the reverse is true in Amherst. Overall, however, the Amherst parents have earlier expectations.

Table 11.3 indicates the *F*-test results for the two-way analysis involving teachers only. Here the results are also fairly clear-cut. With respect to teaching level, on most variables (Emotional maturity, Independence,

**Table 11.3.** Pistoia and Amherst Teachers' Expectations: Results of *F*-Tests Comparing Infant–Toddler and Preprimary Teachers

| | Main effects | | Interactions |
|---|---|---|---|
| DEQ summary scales | Culture | Teaching level | Culture × level |
| Emotional maturity | | | |
| Compliance | | | 3.98* |
| Politeness | | | |
| Independence | 4.00* | | |
| School-related skills | | | 4.52* |
| Social skills with peers | 6.91** | | |
| Verbal assertiveness | | 5.53* | |

*Note.* Only significant *F*-test results (*df* = 1,116) are reported. All tests of significance are two-tailed.
*$p < .05$; **$p < .01$; ***$p < .001$.

School-related skills, Social skills with peers, and Verbal assertiveness), infant–toddler teachers have *earlier* expectations than do preprimary teachers in both communities, though the effects are significant only for Verbal assertiveness (as a main effect) and Social skills with peers (as an interaction, with the teaching level difference much stronger in Pistoia than in Amherst). On the two other variables (Compliance and Politeness) infant–toddler teachers have earlier expectations in Pistoia but not in Amherst, with the interaction effect reaching significance for Compliance. With respect to community, the situation is the opposite of what it was with parents: Pistoia teachers have *earlier* expectations than do Amherst teachers on all seven variables, with community differences significant for Independence and Social skills with peers.

Finally, Table 11.4 presents the analysis of variance results for the pooled groups of Amherst and Pistoia parents and teachers. Again, the interaction effects (significant for six of the seven variables) are what is most striking: These arise because parents have *earlier* expectations than do teachers in Amherst, but *later* expectations in Pistoia. That is, the two groups of teachers are much more like each other than are the two pooled parent groups; the parent groups occupy the extreme positions—Amherst parents early and Pistoia parents late.

All these DEQ findings can again be integrated by means of a multidimensional scaling (Figure 11.2). Following the same ALSCAL procedure described earlier, a two-dimensional model was created to represent how the eight groups stand in proximity to one another across all their means on all the 42 DEQ items considered at once. A very good two-dimensional solution resulted (stress = .044).

The model shows that a strong first dimension spreads the eight groups, with *Amherst parents* occupying the extreme left end with generally earliest expectations, *teachers from both cultures* (Amherst infant/toddler, Amherst preprimary, Pistoia infant–toddler) taking the middle with generally medium expectations, and *Pistoia parents joined by preprimary teachers* occupying the extreme right end with generally latest expectations. (The second dimension, explaining much less variance, does not seem readily interpretable.) We speculate that Pistoia preprimary teachers are closer to Pistoia parents than to infant–toddler teachers because they have been less influenced by postsecondary education and professional development experiences and hence may more closely reflect the cultural traditions of the local community.

## Summary and Discussion

This study has found that in two communities mothers and fathers were similar to each other in their developmental timetables, even though

**Table 11.4.** Parents' Versus Teachers' Expectations: Results of *F*-Tests Comparing the Adult Roles in Pistoia and Amherst

| | Main effects | | Interactions |
|---|---|---|---|
| DEQ summary scales | Culture | Adult role | Culture × adult role |
| Emotional maturity | | | 9.00[*] |
| Compliance | | | |
| Politeness | | | 12.81[***] |
| Independence | | | 12.51[***] |
| School-related skills | | 3.87[*] | 5.38[*] |
| Social skills with peers | 3.87[*] | | 16.14[***] |
| Verbal assertiveness | 5.97[*] | | 7.08[**] |

*Note.* Only significant *F*-test results (*df* = 1,116) are reported. All tests of significance are two-tailed.

[*]*p* < .05; [**]*p* < .01; [***]*p* < .001.

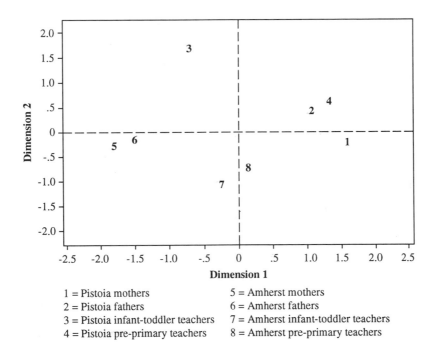

1 = Pistoia mothers      5 = Amherst mothers
2 = Pistoia fathers      6 = Amherst fathers
3 = Pistoia infant-toddler teachers      7 = Amherst infant-toddler teachers
4 = Pistoia pre-primary teachers      8 = Amherst pre-primary teachers

**FIGURE 11.2.** Graph of multidimensional scaling values for group means on DEQ for mothers, fathers, infant–toddler teachers, and preprimary teachers in Amherst and Pistoia. ALSCAL of proximities matrix; stress = .044 in two dimensions.

they were not recruited from the same families; however, the pooled groups of parents differed strongly and consistently according to culture. The Amherst (United States) parents were found to have very early social expectations, the earliest of any group yet studied, whereas the Pistoia (Italy) parents tend toward the middle range of what has been found in past studies of Japanese, U.S., and Australian mothers. The areas in which the Amherst and Pistoia parents were found to differ most sharply concern certain social skills with peers (turn taking, sharing toys, negotiating, offering help) and verbal assertiveness (using words instead of fighting, biting, or crying; being able to state preferences and explanations)—the same areas stressed by Anglo-Australian and U.S. mothers studied previously, though not with such early expectations as the Amherst parents. The behavioral areas in which the Amherst and Pistoia parents differed least were the summary categories having to do with School-related skills and Compliance, as well as for many specific items such as avoiding baby talk, mastering anger independently, greeting people courteously and not interrupting, taking care of one's clothes, eating without assistance, entertaining oneself, and respecting household property, which both groups of parents stressed in similar ways. We did not find areas in which the Pistoia parents had earlier expectations than Amherst parents, a finding that rather surprised us because in our experience, Italian parents expect more maturity than do U.S. parents for many key competencies, such as being able to participate in a social group in a way agreeable to others (demonstrating patience, stamina, and empathy as required), make greetings and good-byes, share desirable resources, and respond to requests so as to make others feel welcome and at ease (Edwards & Gandini, 1989). Perhaps the DEQ instrument—developed by U.S. and Japanese research teams—is not worded to tap into these areas well.

Although cultural background strongly predicted the parents' responses, the same was not true for the teachers. Amherst and Pistoia teachers were nonsignificantly different on most of the summary variables, and for Social skills with peers and Independence, it was the Pistoia teachers who had the earlier expectations. Clearly, expertise— whether arising from coursework and training or from observation and contact with large numbers of children—has influenced the Pistoia and Amherst teachers and made their perspectives different from those of the parents in their communities. A multidimensional scaling revealed that while the parental perspectives were more extreme, the teacher perspectives diverged from the parent groups toward a common middle ground; this was expecially true for Amherst teachers and Pistoia infant–toddler teachers. We therefore conclude that the teachers have expectations that in part reflect their particular cultural traditions and societal ideologies (and which they share with the families with whom they work) but equally reflect a sort of professional culture shared internationally with other practitioners of parallel or equivalent education and training and experience with children. Perhaps this finding is not surprising because there is much overlap in the theoretical and empirical knowledge base of child development and pedagogical practice between the United States and Western Europe, based on common philosophical traditions and much current exchange of scientific and educational ideas and findings. Furthermore, Amherst and Pistoia, as described earlier, are the kinds of educationally oriented and politically progressive communities where educators seek out the most up-to-date knowledge about child development and where administrators tend to support educational innovation and professional development.

The results do raise the natural question of whether children in Pistoia and Amherst differ in actual achievement of developmental milestones or whether it is just the adult belief systems that vary by culture. Furthermore, if there are behavioral differences in the children, are these the outcome or the cause of the adults' developmental expectations? We cannot answer these questions but hypothesize that expectations are both cause and effect of children's behavior. The findings of earlier researchers (reviewed in Goodnow & Collins, 1990; Miller, 1988) have established that parent developmental expectations are a causal factor in development; adults with earlier expectations do tend to pressure children toward earlier performances. However, we also believe that adult beliefs can be an outcome (i.e., shaped by adults' actual experiences with children). Informally we asked many teachers in both Amherst and Pistoia what they were thinking about when they filled out our questionaire: Did they think about what they had learned in child development courses or about real children they knew? They invariably answered that they thought about the children they knew and with whom they worked.

The findings on parent–teacher differences in expectations also raise the obvious questions: Whose expectations are generally more accurate, the parents' or the teachers'? We would hypothesize that because teachers interact with so many more children, day after day, year after year, than do parents, their expectations should be more accurate. In fact, in a previous study using a different questionaire (Edwards & Gandini, 1989), we found that infant teachers in both Amherst and Pistoia were more "accurate" to published developmental norms on those items (such as drinking from a cup) typically achieved during the infant–toddler years, whereas preprimary teachers were more "accurate" on those items (such as counting to 10) typically achieved during the preschool years. In other words, the age group with which the teachers worked predicted their having more accurate knowledge of child behavioral development, according to published norms.

In conclusion, this study suggests the need for of further study of the sources of both parents' and experts' developmental knowledge and goals and raises many questions. How much of adults' personal beliefs about child development is constructed on the basis of such informal experiences as past family and life experiences, current experiences, exposure to mass media, and other meaning-laden communication systems of modern society? How much, in contrast, is constructed on the basis of exposure to such formal knowlege as childrearing literature, courses and meetings, pediatricians' advice, and research reports in magazines or newspapers? And how much are parents and teachers aware of the differences between their perspectives? How much are they changed through contact and interaction with each other? Do parents' and teachers' developmental expectations tend to change systematically over time, as they are exposed to new knowledge and perspectives and have more experiences with real children? Finally, how do cultural differences in parent and teacher expectations relate to actual behavioral outcomes of children? Do children in different cultural communities differ systematically in achievement of developmental milestones, and if so, how do adult expectations play a part in this? And who has most accurate knowledge of children's development, parents or teachers? These kinds of questions, in conjunction with studying the interaction of socialization beliefs, values, and actual behavior, will constitute rich opportunities for those seeking to understand childhood socialization in the contemporary world.

## Acknowledgments

Earlier versions of this chapter were presented at the 1991 biennial meeting of the Society for Research in Child Development, Seattle, Washington, and 1990 lecture to the municipal early childhood department in Pistoia, Italy. The research was supported by a 1988–1989 grant from the University of Massachusetts School of Education Office of Research and Development. We wish to thank Anna Lia Galardini and the Comune di Pistoia Assessorato alla Publica Istruzione for assistance in collecting the Italian data, as well as all the participating schools, teachers, and parents in Amherst and graduate assistants John Nimmo, Hind Mari, and Minaz Bhimani.

## References

Bronfenbrenner, U. (1979). *The ecology of human development: Experiments by nature and design.* Cambridge, MA: Harvard University Press.
Edwards, C. P. (1992). Cross-cultural perspectives on family-peer relations. In

R. D. Parke & G. W. Ladd (Eds.), *Family–Peer relationships: Modes of linkage* (pp. 285–316). Hillsdale, NJ: Erlbaum.

Edwards, C. P., & Gandini, L. (1989). Teachers' expectations about the timing of developmental skills: A cross-cultural study. *Young Children, 44*(4), 15–19.

Edwards, C. P., Gandini, L., & Nimmo, J. (1992). Favorire l'apprendimento cooperativo nella prima infanzia: Concettualizzazioni contrastanti da parte degli insegnanti en due comunita [Promoting collaborative learning in the early childhood classroom: Teachers' contrasting conceptualizations in two communities]. University of Rome: *Rassegna di Psicologia, 9*(3), 65–90.

Edwards, C. P., Gandini, L., & Nimmo, J. (1994). Promoting collaborative learning in the early childhood classroom: Teachers' contrasting conceptualizations in two communities. In L. G. Katz & B. Cesarone (Eds.), *Reflections on the Reggio Emilia approach,* (pp. 81–104). Urbana, IL: ERIC.

Frankel, D. G., & Roer-Bornstein, D. (1982). Traditional and modern contributions to changing infant-rearing ideologies of two ethnic communities. *Monographs of the Society for Research in Child Development, 47*(Serial No. 196).

Gandini, L. (1988). Children and parents at bedtime: Physical closeness during the rituals of separation. Unpublished doctoral dissertation, University of Massachusetts, Amherst (University Microfilms No. 8906282).

Gandini, L. (1993). Apaiser et entormir le nourrison et le petit enfant: Un regard sur l'Italie [Soothing infants and young children to sleep: A look at Italy]. In Helene E. Stork (Ed.), *Les Rituels du Coucher de l'Enfant: Variations culturelles* [Rituals of infant sleep: Cultural variations]. Paris: ESF Editeur.

Goodnow, J. J., Cashmore, J., Cotton, S., & Knight, R. (1984). Mothers' developmental timetables in two cultural groups. *International Journal of Psychology, 19*, 193–205.

Goodnow, J. J., & Collins, W. A. (1990). *Development according to parents: The nature, sources, and consequences of parents' ideas.* Hillsdale, NJ: Erlbaum.

Gorman, K. S. (1987). *The relationship between social structure and beliefs in homes and preschools: A study of mothers and teachers in Peru.* Unpublished doctoral disseration, University of Maryland, College Park.

Gorman, K. S., & Holloway, S. D. (1987). *Peruvian preschool teachers' beliefs about development: Relation to children's social competence.* Paper presented at the biennial meeting of the Society for Research in Child Development, Baltimore.

Hess, R. D., Kashiwagi, K., Azuma, H., Price, G. G., & Dickinson, W. P. (1980). Maternal expectations for mastery of developmental tasks in Japan and the United States. *International Journal of Psychology, 15*, 259–271.

Hess, R. D., Price, G. G., Dickson, W. P., & Conroy, M. (1981). Different roles for mothers and teachers: Contrasting styles of child care. In S. Kilmer (Ed.), *Advances in early education and day care,* (Vol. 2, pp. 1–28). Greenwich, CT: JAI Press.

Holloway, S. D., Gorman, K. S., & Fuller, B. (1988). Child-rearing beliefs within diverse social structures: Mothers and day-care providers in Mexico. *International Journal of Psychology, 23*, 303–317.

Holloway, S. D., & Reichhart-Erickson, M. (1989). Child-care quality, family structure, and maternal expectations: Relationship to preschool children's peer relations. *Journal of Applied Developmental Psychology, 10,* 281–298.

Miller, S. A. (1988). Parents' beliefs about children's cognitive development. *Child Development, 59,* 259–285.

New, R. (1984). Italian mothers and infants: Patterns of care and development. Unpublished doctoral dissertation, Harvard Graduate School of Education, Cambridge, MA.

Nimmo, J. (1992). The meaning of classroom community: Shared images of early childhood teachers. Unpublished doctoral dissertation, University of Massachusetts, Amherst, (University Microfilms No. 9305876).

Ninio, A. (1979). The naive theory of the infant and other maternal attitudes in two subgroups in Israel. *Child Development, 50,* 976–980.

Olmstead, P. P., & Weikart, D. P. (Eds.). (1989). *How nations serve young children: Profiles of child care and education in 14 countries.* Ypsilanti, MI: High/Scope Press.

Spindler, G. D. (1987). The transmission of culture. In G. D. Spindler (Ed.), *Education and cultural process,* (pp. 301–334). Prospect Heights, IL: Waveland.

SPSS, Inc. (1990). *SPSS Reference Guide.* Chicago: SPSS, Inc. 1990

Tobin, J. J., Wu, D. Y. H., & Davidson, D. H. (1989). *Preschool in three cultures: Japan, China, and the United States.* New Haven, CT: Yale University Press.

CHAPTER 12

# Ask the Doctor
## The Negotiation of Cultural Models in American Parent-Pediatrician Discourse

Sara Harkness
Charles M. Super
Constance H. Keefer
Chemba S. Raghavan
Elizabeth Kipp Campbell

One of the most intriguing yet least understood aspects of parental ethnotheories is how cultural belief systems come to be constituted in the minds of individual parents. Goodnow and Collins (1990) have described a basic dichotomy of approaches to this question, corresponding generally to psychological versus anthropological paradigms. In the psychological approach, parents' ideas are seen as deriving from individual experience, which is further assumed to be "neutral" and to be arrived at through a "scientific" process of observation, checking, information seeking, and revising. In the anthropological approach, in contrast, parents' ideas are seen as a group of shared beliefs that may be absorbed in "prepackaged" form, and that in any case are filtered through a cultural lens of more general beliefs, values, and practices. A central feature of parents' cultural belief systems, however, is that they are at once individually constructed and culturally shared. As such, they are the product of integration of a variety of experiences in the wider culture and in the family, dynamically changing in interaction with that experience, reflecting both individual history and dispositions and culturally normative ideas.

Although developmental experience in one's family and community of origin and participation in informal knowledge networks with other parents are important contributors to the construction of parental ethnotheories, culturally appointed "experts" also play an essential role (Harkness, Super, & Keefer, 1992). For many American middle-class parents, this role is best instantiated by pediatricians (Clarke-Stewart, 1978; Young, 1990). As the generation "raised on Spock" has been followed by generations raised on Brazelton, books by pediatricians continue to hold the place of honor in the personal reference libraries of American parents. For parents who are fortunate enough to have access to regular pediatric care, the family pediatrician is also a unique resource—a person who is recognized as an authority on children's development (more so than teachers, for example) and who is relatively available for consultation on individual problems.

Both through the media and in person, thus, pediatricians provide a major source of cultural knowledge about children's behavior and development for American middle-class parents. An indication of just how important these sources may be comes from a study of American parents in the area of Cambridge, Massachusetts (Harkness & Super, 1992a, 1992b; Harkness et al., 1992). A tally of sources of advice mentioned spontaneously by parents in interviews about their children's behavior and development showed pediatricians to be the most frequently used, in nearly half (42%) of the cases. The next most frequent source (20%) was books—many of which were written by pediatricians. Thus, together, pediatricians and books accounted for almost two-thirds of all sources mentioned. In contrast, other sources of advice, such as friends (16%) and family (6%), were less frequently mentioned. Although these parents probably turned to their pediatricians for advice particularly often because of the supportive and accessible pediatric care offered at the health maintenance organization (HMO) through which they were recruited to the study, it seems clear that the Cambridge parents, in consulting with their pediatricians about behavioral and developmental issues, were following a more broadly shared American orientation toward the pediatrician as a source of knowledge about children, parenting, and the family.

Despite their publicly accepted roles as experts on children's development and their importance as a resource for many American parents, most pediatricians lack advanced training in child development. Rather, much of the knowledge and advice that pediatricians offer is culturally constituted, reflecting beliefs and values of the larger society in interaction with their own clinical experience. It can be noted as well that even formal scientific and professional models of child development reflect cultural beliefs of the time (LeVine, 1980). Thus, when a physician is confronted in the clinic with a troubled parent, the diagnostic task is inevitably framed by cultural models of what is appropriate and normal child behavior, and part of the clinician's task is to help the parent to understand the problem from such a frame of reference. Pediatricians, thus, offer a particularly rich resource for the study of how cultural knowledge about children's behavior and development is constituted and communicated.

Given the importance of pediatricians as sources for the construction of parental ethnotheories, it is striking that the growing literature on doctor-patient communication includes virtually no research on this topic. Rather, research on the cultural dimensions of doctor–patient communication has focused primarily on understandings (and misunderstandings) of particular illnesses or disorders among adults (e.g., Kleinman, 1980), whereas studies of the communicative process itself have shed light on the actual linguistic and behavioral patterns involved (e.g., Fisher & Todd, 1983). Among these latter studies, detailed analyses of discourse between parents and pediatricians are especially noteworthy because they document the richness and complexity of communication in this context. As Tannen and Wallat (1983) point out, communication with parents during an examination of the child places multiple communicative demands on the pediatrician. Moreover, the conflicting demands of politeness rules and the need to achieve patient compliance lead, as Aronsson and Rundstrom (1989) show, to the construction of discourse as a negotiated rather than a purely scripted event.

In this chapter, we draw from elements of both cultural and discourse-based approaches to consider how cultural knowledge is co-constructed by parents and pediatricians. We focus particularly on the role of the pediatrician in the construction of parental ethnotheories, through analysis of parent–pediatrician discourse in the context of well child visits in a large HMO, the Cambridge Center of the Harvard Community Health Plan. The seven pediatricians who worked at the plan during the time of the study, including one of the authors (Keefer), participated in the research, along with families who were part of their regular practices. The data to be discussed here come from a sample of 124 well-child visits, including each pediatrician in consultation with parents of children from newborns to 6 years of age (median = 1.3 years).

The pediatricians at the Cambridge Center at the time of the study (1987–1988) varied in age, gender, and cultural background, with three women and four men ranging in age from their mid-thirties to sixties. Six of the pediatricians were American of European background; one was from India. All had been trained at American medical schools and shared a commitment to personal and consistent care of their patients, including attention to normal behavioral and developmental issues. With the exception of Dr. Keefer, however, none of the pediatricians had specialized training in children's psychological development.

The parents at the Cambridge Center included a range of backgrounds, from well-educated professional couples to parents of middle- or working-class background (the fathers' years of education ranged from 9 to 24, median = 18; for mothers, 11 to 25 years, median = 17). They ranged in age from 23 to 52 years (fathers' median = 37, mothers' = 35). Approximately one-third of the parents were from Protestant background, one-third Jewish, and one-quarter Roman Catholic.

Parents in the study were recommended by their pediatricians on the basis of criterion ages of the children at upcoming well-child visits, generally good health status of the child, and absence of major stresses in the home. The great majority of parents contacted agreed to participate in the study, which included filling out questionnaires on children's temperament, on root metaphors of development, and on their own background, as well as having a well-child visit with their pediatrician tape-recorded. With a few exceptions, only children who lived with both parents present were included, and the family size ranged from 3 to 8, with a median of 3.

## Cultural Models and the Structure of Parent–Pediatrician Discourse

In order to understand how cultural models are negotiated in parent–pediatrician discourse, it is necessary to recognize the structure of these conversations. At the formal level, well-child visits are organized by a preestablished set of questions or topics that the pediatrician asks regarding children at any given age. These might include (to take one protocol as an example) the child's physical growth, language development, sleep patterns, sibling relations, diet, and motor skills. The doctor's agenda is to review these topics by asking the parent (usually the mother) questions and making relevant observations of the child, ascertaining that development is normal and providing guidance when it seems to be needed. The doctor also elicits questions or concerns the parent may have. The office visit includes a physical examination, of course, and may end with inoculations or sending the child and parent to the laboratory for tests.

This formal structure is important in its own right, but from the point of view of parent–pediatrician communication, it seems to function as scaffolding on which more or less elaborate conversations are built. In these conversations, we have identified frequently occurring discourse sequences in which explanations of children's behavior are central as a key to understanding the representation and communication of cultural models. These "explanation-centered sequences" consist of five components: (1) introduction of the problem; (2) clarification and elaboration; (3) explanation; (4) advice; and (5) resolution.

## Introduction

The first component signifies the introduction of a new topic. Generally this is done by the pediatrician with a question such as, "How's this little guy's appetite?" The parent may take this question as a cue to introduce her own concern, for example (after answering the doctor's question about the child's diet):

> "He still at lunch has some baby food. He has some meat, vegetable and fruit. He's pretty much rejecting the bottle at this point and I'm not sure how to get enough milk into him."

New topics can also be raised by a parent with permission from the pediatrician, as when the doctor asks the mother, "Well, any particular issues or concerns that you have?" after running through his own list of topics. A notable exception to this typical pattern in which the pediatrician controls the flow of conversation is one doctor who routinely started off office visits with an open-ended greeting and question, "How is [child]?" which led to extended discussions of topics introduced by the parent.

The introduction component of explanation-centered sequences is significant for the communication of cultural models in that it implicitly marks, or indexes, particular topics as ones that parents *should* be concerned with. In addition, the apparently simple form of an introductory question such as, "Does he sleep well at night?" asked by the pediatrician, assumes a shared understanding—in this case, of just what "sleeping well at night" means in behavioral terms. This meaning may be made more explicit in the second component.

## Clarification and Elaboration

This component involves the doctor's elicitation of more information in response to the parent's implicit or explicit indication of a problem. In response to the doctor's question about sleep, for example, the mother says, "He sleeps well at night, but he still tends to want to go to sleep late." The doctor then proceeds with a series of questions, the mother answering each in turn:

DOCTOR: When does he go to sleep?

MOTHER: Well, we try getting him started by about 8:15 or 8:00 and we hope that by 9:00 he'll be more amenable. He could try to stay up until 10:00.

DOCTOR: And when does he wake up?

MOTHER: Usually about 6:00, 6:30, 7:00.

DOCTOR: Does he take a nap?

MOTHER: In day care he'll take a nap. At home he won't always.

As these questions suggest, the doctor's understanding of sleeping well at night centers on the total *amount* of sleep the baby is getting throughout the diurnal cycle. The significance of this information, however, is made most clear in the next component of the sequence, when the doctor states her analysis of the baby's sleep patterns.

## Explanation

As the term "explanation-centered sequences" suggests, we see these segments of parent–pediatrician discourse as organized around propositions or assertions of belief about the nature of the child, of development, and of the child's social environment. For example, in the preceding sequence about sleep, the doctor offers the following explanation after ascertaining information about the baby's sleep patterns:

> "If he's in a good mood and he's healthy, he's getting enough sleep."

Cultural models of child behavior and development—explicitly or implicitly stated—can be constructed from many of these propositions. For example, in the preceding conversation regarding bedtime issues, we find the following interchange:

DOCTOR: So I think it probably is alright and maybe he likes having this time with you. You probably do things together at bedtime.

MOTHER: We've tried to have a lot of together time prior to bedtime so that it's not just the special bedtime. We've tried to really make—that it's his choice as to what he gets before he goes to sleep and have him determine a lot of the conditions except for the bedtime.

The mother's and doctor's talk here includes several related propositions: that there is a need for a definite bedtime; that "special time" is an important component of the parent-child relationship, which can be instantiated at this time; that the child's need for special time is finite and can be satisfied by providing the necessary amount of attention (regardless of its timing); and that autonomy is an important component of child well-being and thus cooperation. Propositions such as these index cultural models of child behavior and development that are generally not fully represented in this discourse but are often shared by parent and pediatrician. Because they share these larger understandings, they can elaborate on each other's statements without a full explanation, as the mother does when she refers to the idea of special bedtime in response to the doctor's mention of doing things together at bedtime.

The explanation component of these sequences can be brief, as above, or elaborate and enriched with narratives of imagined scenarios and metaphors that demonstrate the doctor's understanding of the problem. In response to a father's concern about his young son's reactions to the newly mobile little sister, for example, another doctor creates a whole story that explains the children's behavior as manifestations of their imagined motivations, even adding the parents' possible response, all as a typical example of issues at this age:

> "That's a very common problem. When babies begin crawling or start walking, whatever he's doing, she wants to play. I mean she means well. It's not a question of interfering in the true sense. She just wants to be with him. In general, babies love to be with their older siblings. So she just basically wants to be with him, doing whatever he does, and she wants to emulate him. Obviously she's not as good in terms of playing with some things like Lego pieces or building blocks or whatever it may be. And the end result is that she tends to mess up his game plan. Since he's told not to get angry at her, he's not able to take out his frustrations by pushing or yelling or screaming or hitting her or anything like that. So the end result is he gets very frustrated and upset. What often happens then too is that if she starts crying or if he gets upset and storms out, the tendency is to sort of focus on him. 'What's going on? Why are you upset?' Instead of recognizing maybe she is the source of the problem."

The doctor's explanation leads naturally to—in fact often contains—the fourth component of the sequence.

## Advice

Sometimes advice is implicit, as in the first example concerning sleep behavior, where the doctor's explanation that the child seems to be getting enough sleep implies that the mother should not be concerned about this issue. In other instances, the advice component immediately follows the explanation, as in the previous example in which the doctor continues his imagined scenario with a suggested parental response:

> "Sometimes when he is playing very nicely by himself, what we're dealing with is simply take her away from him. Either take her outdoors—just basically separate the two temporarily. I'm sure there will be times when he wants to play with her, he invites her playing, in which case obviously let them. But when there are times he clearly wants to be alone or he's having fun by himself, doesn't want another person playing along, best thing is really try to keep them separate."

In this example, the advice component is linguistically marked by a transition from a narrative about an imagined sequence of events to a more general statement of principles with use of the imperative form. In other instances, the advice component is enveloped in the same scenario as the explanation. In the following discussion of behavior in a 2½-year-old child, for example, the doctor refers to an apparently favorite metaphor of this period as stormy but ultimately benign. In the process, he offers an explanation of the child's and the mother's behavior as well as advice on her response, recasting difficult 2-year-old behavior as something to regard as "fun":

DOCTOR: They are about the most exciting people around because there is so much going on. I've always said this. Did I ever give you my definition of a 2½-year-old?

MOTHER: Yes, you did. I think I asked for it with Mary. She went through the most. I guess it was my fault. She just went through the most extreme adjustment to society at 2.

DOCTOR: I think it wasn't your fault. I think it was happening and you didn't know quite how to handle it.

MOTHER: I had no idea what to do.

DOCTOR: That's right. And this one is kind of fun because it's like what do you do in a thunderstorm? You let it happen and it gets over.

## Resolution

Having offered an explanation and advice on an issue, the pediatrician is apt to be anxious to move on to the next topic. The last component, resolution, signals the end of the sequence in a correspondingly brief manner. This is sometimes marked by a summary statement, such as the doctor's comment on the child's sleep behavior, "I think this is a reasonably good thing you have." Even more briefly, the doctor may mark the end of the sequence and the transition to the next topic with a single word, as we see from the example of discourse about 2½-year-olds' behavior:

> " . . . And this one is kind of fun because it's like what do you do in a thunderstorm? You let it happen and it gets over. *All right* [emphasis added], is this young woman in any kind of play group or day care?"

Although parents may sometimes provide the resolution component to the sequence by offering their own closing statement, more commonly the doctor controls this transition, as part of a more general pattern of greater control over the content and flow of conversation. The doctor's greater share of control is also indexed by the relative share of propositions made by pediatricians as contrasted to parents: Although they varied considerably, on average the pediatricians stated 81% of the propositions in these interviews.

In summary, the identification of explanation-centered sequences in parent–pediatrician discourse is useful in that it provides a framework for identifying cultural models, as well as for analyzing how they are used or "negotiated" among speakers—a topic to which we will return. Explanation-centered sequences indicate those portions of discourse in pediatric well-child visits in which statements of beliefs and values, understandings of cause and effect, predictions of the future, and related plans of action are most likely to be found. From the indexing of topics of concern in the introduction component to the clarification and elaboration of the dimensions of the problem to the propositions about child behavior and development stated in the explanation component and then to the instantiation of these propositions in advice, and finally to the resolution and transition to the next topic, explanation-centered sequences provide the pediatrician with a variety of ways to communicate cultural knowledge to parents. The fact that this knowledge *is* to a large extent culturally organized becomes evident when we take a closer look at the nature of propositions themselves. As we will suggest, propositions can be seen as expressions of both universal "root metaphors" of development and culturally specific beliefs, for these two dimensions of understanding relate systematically to each other.

## Cultural Models and Root Metaphors

The analysis of root metaphors as expressed in parent–pediatrician discourse is based on the work of the philosopher Pepper (1942), who proposed that these metaphors are the primary basis for abstract thought. Each of the four root metaphors represents a world view that is adequate in its own right but fundamentally irreconcilable with the other orientations. The four root metaphors identified by Pepper are Formism, Mechanism, Organicism, and Contextualism. The Formist orientation approaches understanding through classification of similarities and differences, whereas the Mechanist metaphor explains phenomena through identification of mechanical, causal connections among parts of the whole. Organicism is expressed in recognition of systems aspects of an "organism" of mutually influencing parts, and Contextualism seeks understanding in the context of complete relativism of the historical moment and multiple perspectives. Although Pepper's original formulation concerned systems of philosophy, the metaphors he delineated have been recognized by psychologists to reflect important distinctions in formal theories of human development (Langer, 1969; Moshman, 1982; Super & Harkness, 1995).

Propositions representing all four of the root metaphors are to be found throughout the discourse of both parents and pediatricians. The Formist metaphor, first, occurs in propositions in which the child's behavior is explained in terms of his or her own personality or temperament, as in this mother's description of her 6-month-old daughter in comparison to the child's older brother:

> "She's extremely independent about everything except emotionally. She's just the opposite of him. He's very independent emotionally and doesn't want to do anything by himself—still won't get dressed, refuses to get dressed. Loves to have everyone do everything. But Jacqueline is just the opposite—hates to be abandoned. She's terrified you're going to leave her even though she's never been left. Always wants you to take her along. Doesn't want to be left."

A distinctly different version of the Formist metaphor is manifest in propositions that explain a child's behavior in relation to expectable behavior for all children in this situation, at this age, or at this stage of development. This special case is used twice as frequently by pediatricians as by parents. For example, in discussing the child's eating pattern following recovery from an illness:

DOCTOR: I bet he ate up a storm after he was feeling well.

MOTHER: He was a shark. He absolutely went after everything.

DOCTOR: And that's characteristic. When youngsters have been ill for whatever reason, and they don't feel like eating—it may have been medication. Antibiotics will often take your appetite away. He's up crying at night because he has an earache. He doesn't sleep at night. He sleeps in the day. Doesn't eat much. For whatever reason. When they get better, suddenly they start eating. And he ends up—they eat enough to get them back to where they would have been had they not been sick and then they level off to their usual picky self. And I bet—is he still eating well or did he kind of level off?

MOTHER: He kind of leveled off.

DOCTOR: That's characteristic.

Here, the doctor identifies the child's behavior as belonging to a recognizable category of behavior—thus, normal for children recovering from an illness. In this case, as in many discussions of age-typical behavior, however, the Formist behavior category is embedded in a larger perspective of growth and change. Much as Piaget's developmental stages are conceptualized as qualitatively distinct steps along a path of predictable growth, the doctor's statement that a child's behavior is "characteristic" is part of a larger picture of organically driven development. For this reason, we consider such propositions as fundamentally related to another root metaphor, the Organicist.

The Organicist metaphor is expressed in propositions that emphasize the nature of the child as a growing organism with its own internal forces for development. In the following excerpt, the doctor explains the child's "headstrong behavior" as typical of children who are "going through" a stage of growth. The linguistic metaphor of movement here is an identifier for the underlying root metaphor of growth and change. In contrast, the mother's explanation of the child's behavior seems to evoke only a Formist metaphor—the child's behavior is explained (although paradoxically) in terms of the child's personal disposition as both "easy" and "headstrong."

MOTHER: She seems like, to me she seems like the world's easiest child. She is headstrong, though.

DOCTOR: Well, we expect that. Its doesn't sound like a problem in any sense of the word. You seem to be well in control and certainly she's going to be going through that and has to go through that period. That's fine. It would be abnormal not to be a little headstrong.

A more complex version of the Organicist metaphor is presented in this mother's attempts to interpret her son's behavior relative to toilet training as a response to his own experience of development:

"It seemed like he was sort of identifying that it was one of the last vestiges of babyhood because he was really concerned about would he be a—was he growing up? Was he a little boy now? Was he a baby? Yesterday when he had a poop and it came out of the diaper—it got on the rug, which is something that hadn't happened for maybe a year or so—he really felt like a baby. And he said he felt like a baby. It seemed like he matured so quickly in all these other areas, it was like his last holdout."

In contrast to both the Formist and Organicist metaphors, the Mechanist metaphor is expressed in propositions that link an individual's behavior to an event in the environment, including behavior by another person. For example, a mother describing her child's disrupted sleep patterns says:

"I just spent five days at my parents' house and her crib is in my room there. My husband wasn't with us and I had some terrible nights, but that was because she caught onto the fact that I was going to come in. She would wait for me—she would cry until I came up there. . . . Then she just intermittently all night long kept waking up. But it was my doing. I somehow upset something, anyhow we had some bad nights there."

The Mechanist metaphor can also be used to describe the child's effect on the mother, as in "Well you know it's just that it's funny because it's like this little 2½-year-old knows the right buttons to push to get me upset and I find myself reduced to this game." Here, the Mechanist root metaphor is also expressed in a linguistic metaphor of the mother as a machine that can be turned on or off by her child.

The Contextualist metaphor was rarely used by either parents or pediatricians but occurred sometimes as a way of explaining behavior that explicitly does not tie it to anything beyond the circumstances of the moment, or acknowledges equivalent, multiple viewpoints. In the following case, the pediatrician emphasized the arbitrary conventionality of sleeping position for infants.

MOTHER: I have another question: What about sleeping on her back?

DOCTOR: It's a very cultural thing, sleeping on your tummy or on your back. The Americans like them on their tummy, the Europeans like them on their backs. Other, Third World countries will have the babies sleeping in bed with them and others will tell you . . .

MOTHER: But if you put them on their back they will spit up and choke?

DOCTOR: I don't think that is true at all. However, we are used to them having the babies on their tummies here and I think it is a little bit better . . . but let her choose what she wants.

In summary, four root metaphors of development underlie many of the propositions stated in parent–pediatrician discourse, and these propositions in turn form the building blocks for cultural models of children's behavior and development. The fact that propositions are generally related to cultural models rather than being idiosyncratic productions of either conversational partner is reflected in the observation that most propositions can be easily grouped into a limited set, which appear again and again in multiple conversational contexts. On the frequently discussed topic of sleep, for example, the following four propositions appear, each corresponding to a different root metaphor:

1. The sleep patterns of a particular infant are due to the infant's own personal characteristics (Formist).
2. "Good" or "bad" sleep patterns are caused by proper training or lack thereof (Mechanist).
3. Infant sleep patterns are biologically and developmentally regulated (Organicist).
4. A particular episode of infant sleep behavior is related to the unique circumstances of that moment (Contextualist).

The root metaphor underlying each of these propositions contains not only a way of understanding a certain behavior but also implications for response from the caretakers. As in the above examples, identification with the Formist root metaphor indicates that patience and acceptance may be the most appropriate response. The Organicist metaphor also suggests acceptance but can lead to an active intervention to enhance or "push" development a little faster for the convenience of the parent, or to shape the child's behavior in the immediate context through appropriate responses. The Mechanist metaphor goes further than this and demands an active intervention to shape behavior in desirable ways; in fact, the logic of this metaphor leads to predictions that undesirable behavior in a child may continue indefinitely unless steps are taken to change it. In contrast to the other three metaphors, the Contextualist has no implications for generalizing to other situations, and we suspect that this is the reason it is used so infrequently in parent–pediatrician discourse.

## Parent–Pediatrician Differences
## and the Negotiation of Cultural Models

Insofar as the parents and pediatricians in this study were all members of the same general culture and were studied in joint conversations about child behavior and development, we should expect them to show similar profiles of root metaphor usage. In general, this was the case: Both parents and pediatricians used the Organicist metaphor most frequently during well-child visits, followed by Mechanist metaphors and then Formist metaphors. Contextualist metaphors were used only once in a while, mainly by fathers (who are not shown separately in the figure because there were few of them present in the visits). As Figure 12.1 shows, however, there were also real differences in usage of the

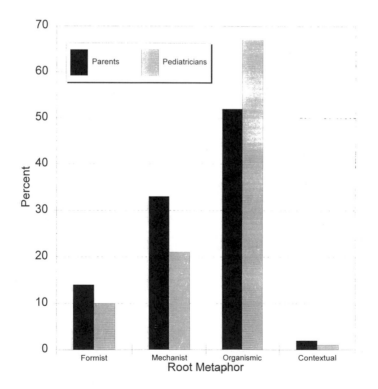

**FIGURE 12.1.** Root metaphor use by parents and pediatricians during well-child visits.

different metaphors by the two groups. In particular, parents used a higher proportion of Mechanist metaphors than did the pediatricians (33% compared to 21%); the pediatricians, conversely, used more Organicist metaphors than did the parents (67% and 52%, respectively). (Approximately one-fifth of the pediatricians' Organicist metaphors included the Formist "typical for this age" nuance, whereas parents used this special version about 10% of the time; the difference is not likely to be a chance finding, $p$ = .01.) Parents used a somewhat higher proportion of pure Formist metaphors than did pediatricians (14% compared to 10%). Taken together, these differences are strongly nonchance findings (chi square = 18.24, $df$ = 3, $p$ = .000), and they suggest systematic subcultural differences between parents' and pediatricians' ethnotheories about children's behavior and development.

The identification of differences in the use of root metaphors and related cultural models in parent–pediatrician discourse is important for our present concerns, first, because it signals moments when cultural models are "negotiated" and possibly reformulated. Second, insofar as differing cultural models with their corresponding root metaphors have differing implications for parents' plans of action, the negotiation of cultural models is of obvious importance for parents themselves, as well as—of course—their children. In this sample, as we have seen, both parents and pediatricians used the different root metaphors in the same rank order, but they differed in their relative preference for the two most frequently used metaphors, Organicism and Mechanism, and in addition they also used the Formist metaphor somewhat differently. These differences are expressed in individual interviews at moments when parents attempt to understand a child's behavior as it is affected either by the individual characteristics of the child or as a result of events in the environment, whereas pediatricians regard the same behavior as the natural expression of growth and development. In fact, it is not an overstatement to say that much of the discourse between parents and pediatricians is *about* these different perspectives as ways of understanding and thus responding to particular examples of behavior. In the following example, we see the mother and pediatrician jointly considering three different metaphors of development (Mechanist, Formist, and Organicist) as explanations for temper tantrums by a 2-year-old boy. The mother suggests both Formist and Mechanist explanations as her own interpretation, while implying that her mother holds a Mechanist view; the doctor, in contrast, proposes an Organicist explanation:

DOCTOR: And is he beginning to get into the 2-year-old syndrome?

MOTHER: Oh, yes.

DOCTOR: Saying no.

MOTHER: Yes. The thing that he does lately is scream. The other little girl I baby-sit for is 5 months younger and she does the same thing. I don't know if it's because I scream a lot, because I do, but Johnny never did it. He just screams when he doesn't get his own way. The other thing he does is he has very bad temper tantrums, very bad. When Johnny did that, when he got mad at me, he'd want me to hold him afterwards. David doesn't want anything to do with me. He has his temper tantrum and I try to calm him down and I say 'Come sit with Mommy,' and he doesn't want anything to do with me. He keeps on screaming and rolling his body on the floor and stuff.

DOCTOR: The important thing about that, none of what you're saying is particularly unusual.

MOTHER: My mother is very upset.

DOCTOR: She's got you upset.

MOTHER: We live in her house. She swears up and down her kids never did that and she had seven kids, and they never, never lost their temper like that to the extent that he does.

DOCTOR: She has seven, including you, seven very atypical, wonderful children. The fact of the matter is it's not at all unusual for youngsters to have temper tantrums. I don't worry about it when a 2-year-old has a temper tantrum and shrieks. I would worry about it when a 7-year-old would do that.

In this example, the mother's Formist explanation of Johnny's temper tantrums as an individual characteristic ("David never did it") is counterposed to a Mechanist explanation ("I don't know if it's because I scream a lot because I do"), which is also by implication the view of her own mother who is "very upset." In response, the doctor offers a humorous vote of confidence in the mother (who is implicitly blamed for her child's behavior according to the Mechanist framework) and states authoritatively ("the fact is") that an Organicist framework provides the correct explanation.

The Mechanist metaphor, as expressed by parents, is also associated with concerns about taking appropriate action, as in this mother's statement about her 3-year-old son (which combines Formist and Mechanist metaphors):

"Actually, he really has kind of a violent temper. I mean I think it's also because Mike beats up on him a lot. He gets into trouble and stuff like that. But I mean—he has potential—I mean like he'll grab onto his father's fingers when his father wants him to do something but he doesn't want to. He'll start squeezing them and Albert said, 'Oh don't. You're hurting me. You're going to make me cry.' And Mark said, 'I'm going to take you into the kitchen and cut them off.' Things like that. Where do you learn those strange things? On TV? Maybe we shouldn't watch as much TV?"

Mechanist metaphors are related to worrying about long-term effects of certain events on children's behavior, as in the following example in a mother's discourse:

"My mother has just left. Is it possible for a 6-month-old to be spoiled in 5 days?"

Or the following:

"One thing, I don't know, kids they have these things that really affect them. They seem to get traumatized by certain events like one thing she hates is a bath. It's such as nightmare for her. It's mainly the hair washing. She hates it. But now, it's gotten to the point, even if she has a bath without hair washing, she just associates it with that and it's this real traumatic thing and I don't know what to do to make her not be so afraid. I keep trying to tell her that it's something everybody does and it's not just her. It doesn't work, I know."

And after some elaboration and exploration of different possible ways of coping, the mother adds:

"It's the kind of thing I don't want that to carry over into her adulthood so that she's not going to always have this bad association with bathing."

Or even the following (related to the concern about the child's violent behavior quoted above):

"You're always wondering who's going to have the kids that grow up and shoot their parents or, you know, mass murders and things like that."

The Mechanist root metaphor is related to the American folk theory of the importance of "consistency" in childrearing, an aspect of parental thinking that has been noted by others (e.g., Reid & Valsiner,

1986) and appears in parent–pediatrician discourse as well. For example, the mother who is worried about how her child "knows how to push the right buttons to get me upset" goes on to castigate herself for not responding with consistent patience:

> "Yeah, unfortunately sometimes I think I'm inconsistent. I know that's a bad thing because sometimes I am able to just let her do her own thing and not let it bother me. And other times I find myself like ranting and raving which I really—I hate that when I get all upset."

In response to mothers' concerns that grow out of a Mechanist paradigm of development, pediatricians frequently offer an Organicist interpretation (sometimes combined with Formist) that takes some of the onus off the parent while offering a more optimistic view of future development for the child, as we saw in the first example of talk about 2-year-old temper tantrums. Likewise, in response to the mother who worries that her child will still hate baths when she is an adult, the doctor says:

DOCTOR: I don't think that at all. This [hating baths] is very common at this age.

MOTHER: Is it?

DOCTOR: Oh gosh. I'm sorry I didn't say that earlier. Sometimes it's a fairly clear event like hair washing that scares them. I think they do get this panic associated with an event or a procedure and they can't unloosen it. Sometimes you can slowly help them to see, yes, it's going to end. Or there won't be hair washing. And sometimes it will go on for months and they can't have a happy bath. But then they leave it. They leave it as they get a little bit older.

The doctor's Organicist perspective on behavior can enable the mother to focus on the positive aspects of development that she sees already, in anticipation of favorable expectations for the future, as in this interchange between the pediatrician and the mother who is worried about her child growing up to be a mass murderer:

DOCTOR: What does he do—because the thing is that you gradually, through your old aggression, is able to be controlled through language or behavior or something. That's why we don't normally end up shooting parents. So do you see him developing some control over it?

MOTHER: Oh, yeah. And we don't—I just kind of don't make a big deal out of it. He's really getting to be more of a—he's just a more manageable child now because he's getting older and you can rationalize with him. I mean this is a great time of life. I really like this age. It's making me wonder whether I should have another.

Recognizing that consideration of alternative root metaphors of development is what some of the discourse between parents and pediatricians is really "about" also allows us to see the logical connections linking sequences of topics that may appear to be unrelated from an outsider's point of view but that are clearly experienced as related from the points of view of the conversational participants. Usually the "real" agenda of conversation is not overtly labeled, but there are such exceptions as the following. Here, the mother has been expressing a series of concerns about how to manage her baby's eating and sleeping behavior. After trying repeatedly to reassure the mother that the behavior she wants to influence is actually not in need of change, the doctor finally makes explicit his Organicist understanding of the child's behavior and development, contrasting it to the mother's Mechanist interpretations:

> "Let me say something to you, Mrs. Harrison. You seem to think you have more control over any of this than you really do. I mean babies give up their naps when they're ready to and this baby—they give up the bottle most of the time when they're ready to, although sometimes we have to take an action. Most babies are napping twice when they're before a year and some time after a year they give up one of those naps. How will you know? Well, he'll wake up more in shorter and shorter periods. And you'll find there will be a transition time when one nap doesn't seem to be enough and yet two naps are more than he wants. And as he gets a little older, he'll give up that nap. So you're right where you want to be. How many teeth does he have?" [And in response to the baby who is babbling, he jokes, "No, I'm not Dada."]

The difference between parents and pediatricians in apparent preference for Mechanist and Organicist root metaphors seems a natural outcome of the different kinds of experience that parents and pediatricians have with children. Parents deal with particular children on a day-to-day basis, and they are concerned about the effects of their own actions on children, as well as the effects of the children's actions on the parents. Pediatricians, on the other hand, have daily contacts with many children of the same age, and they see individual children over a relatively long period of development—at intervals wide enough to notice what has changed between visits. They are thus in a good position to let parents know how age-typical their own children's behavior is and to remind them of a developmental perspective that can sometimes be forgotten in the throes of dealing with particular behavioral issues.

# Conclusion

Fifteen years ago, LeVine (1980), reflecting on contemporary trends in anthropology and child development, pointed to an orientation in both folk beliefs and academic psychology that clearly represents the Mechanistic root metaphor, in the form of a belief in the power of reinforcement:

> One of the most enduring psychological concepts that coincides with American folk belief is reinforcement. Parents who subscribe to the doctrine of encouragement and self-confidence believe that the praise and approval they award a child for desired behavior does some good; they constitute a receptive audience for psychological formulations that emphasize the efficacy of subsequent reward on learning, whether it is called the law of effect or operant conditioning. Of course, behavioristic psychologies have contributed to our folk theories too, and both psychologies and folk theories have been influenced by British empiricist philosophy over the last 250 years. But, at the same time, there are societies where such attitudes play no part in childrearing at all—as, for example, those African groups in which praise is not seen as an aid to learning and reinforcement plays no part in folk psychology. (p. 79)

The evidence reviewed in this chapter suggests that the Mechanist metaphor continues to be a powerful organizer of thinking about children, especially for parents. Among other things, the task of bringing up children includes producing responsible young people who will not refuse to take baths, have tantrums in public, or wake their parents numerous times during the night—not to mention becoming mass murderers. Cultural models based on the Mechanist metaphor provide a basis for a parenting strategy designed to encourage positive behavior while discouraging negative behavior, but exclusive reliance on this metaphor also leads to the logical conclusion that undesirable child behaviors will persist indefinitely unless parental action is taken. In this context, cultural models based on the Organicist metaphor offer a more hopeful prospect centered around recognition of normal growth and development. The Formist metaphor highlights the role of individual differences in shaping children's behavior, and the Contextualist metaphor provides a useful residual category of events and circumstances that need not preoccupy either parent or pediatrician because they have no implications for the future.

Root metaphors and their accompanying cultural models of child development are important both as a resource for members of the culture at a given time and as a source of cultural change across time. For parents in a particular cultural place and time, root metaphors of development, like general all-purpose cultural models, may serve an organizing function, helping to construct a unified approach to understanding and responding to a wide variety of different behavioral and developmental issues in children. For pediatricians, root metaphors offer the complementary function of structuring cultural understandings that provide the basis for advice to parents. It is important to note, however, that whereas the Cambridge pediatricians' preference for the Organicist metaphor appears "natural," earlier generations of pediatricians and other cultural "experts" in American childrearing emphasized the Mechanist metaphor more strongly. In the present study, thus, we see an example of how cultural experts and parents together negotiate new cultural understandings about child behavior and development.

## Acknowledgments

The authors would like to express appreciation to the Spencer Foundation and the Cognitive Studies Seed Grant program at Penn State for their support of the research reported here. An earlier version of this chapter was presented at the meeting of the Society for Research in Child Development, in Seattle, in 1991. All statements made and opinions expressed are the sole responsibility of the authors.

## References

Aronsson, K., & Rundstrom, B. (1989). Cats, dogs, and sweets in the clinical negotiation of reality: On politeness and coherence in pediatric discourse. *Language and Society, 18,* 483–504.

Clarke-Stewart, A. K. (1978). Popular primers for parents. *American Psychologist, 33,* 359–369.

Fisher, S., & Todd, A. D. (Eds.). (1983). *The social organization of doctor–patient communication.* Washington, DC: Center for Applied Linguistics.

Goodnow, J. J., & Collins, W. A. (1990). *Development according to parents: The nature, sources, and consequences of parents' ideas.* Hillsdale, NJ: Erlbaum.

Harkness, S., & Super, C. M. (1992a). The cultural foundations of fathers roles: Evidence from Kenya and the U.S. In B. Hewlett (Ed.), *The father's role: Cultural and evolutionary perspectives.* Chicago: Aldine.

Harkness S., & Super, C. M. (1992b). Parental ethnotheories in action. In I. Sigel (Ed.), *Parental belief systems: The psychological consequences for children and families* (rev. ed.). Hillsdale, NJ: Erlbaum.

Harkness, S., Super, C. M., & Keefer, C. H. (1992). Learning to be an American parent: How cultural models gain directive force. In R. G. D'Andrade & C. Strauss (Eds.), *Human motivation and cultural models.* New York: Cambridge University Press.

Kleinman, A. (1980). *Patients and healers in the context of culture.* Berkeley: University of California Press.

Langer, J. (1969). *Theories of development.* New York: Holt, Rinehart, & Winston.

LeVine, R. A. (1980). Anthropology and child development. In C. M. Super & S. Harkness (Guest Eds.), *Anthropological perspectives on child development* (New Directions for Child Development). San Francisco: Jossey-Bass.

Moshman, D. (1982). Exogenous, endogenous, and dialectical constructivism. *Developmental Review, 2,* 371–384.

Pepper, S. C. (1942). *World hypotheses: A review of evidence.* Berkeley: University of California Press.

Reid, B. V., & Valsiner, J. (1986). Consistency, praise, and love: Folk theories of American parents. *Ethos, 14*(3), 282–304.

Super, C. M., & Harkness, S. (1995). *The metaphors of development.* Manuscript submitted for publication.

Tannen, D., & Wallat, C. (1983). Linguistic analysis of a pediatric interaction. In S. Fisher, S. Todd, & A. D. Todd (Eds.), *The social organization of doctor–patient communication.* Washington, DC: Center for Applied Linguistics.

Young, K. T. (1990). American conceptions of infant development from 1955 to 1984: What the experts are telling parents. *Child Development, 61,* 17–28.

## PART FOUR

# THE INSTANTIATION OF PARENTS' CULTURAL BELIEF SYSTEMS IN PRACTICE

CHAPTER 13

# From Household Practices to Parents' Ideas about Work and Interpersonal Relationships

Jacqueline J. Goodnow

This chapter describes a research effort beginning, however, with some general ideas that reflect my views about work and ethnicity at this point rather than at the start of the journey.

In essence, I propose that all cultures contain ideas about the contributions to the family that each member should make and about the connections, if any, that should exist between what people contribute and what they receive. All cultures also contain practices—in the form of words or deeds—that make these ideas concrete, introduce newcomers to the ideas they should hold, provide rationales for why actions and beliefs take the form they do, and indicate where some flexibility or negotiation is possible or out of the question. Where cultures differ, I suggest, is in the kinds of contribution expected, the connections promoted between what is given and received, the related practices, and the areas of flexibility or negotiation.

Those general proposals have emerged from a series of studies exploring the ideas that parents and children hold about household divisions of labor: ideas about such topics as the possible virtues of household work, why one would turn to one family member rather than another when there is work to be done, what one should do oneself and what one can delegate, what are reasonable and unreasonable ways to assign work or to check that work has been done, what should happen when work is not done, and what is the place of money in relation to household jobs.

The concern in this book is with parental viewpoints. My emphasis is accordingly on the information gathered from parents, with side notes on the points at which the research has branched out to consider children's views or the views of adults who are not parents. The material covers both the content and the quality of parents' ideas. Under content are distinctions, propositions, and principles that parents have in mind. Under quality are features such as the degree of affect or importance attached to particular ideas (some ideas are more firmly held or insisted on than others) and the extent to which parents' ideas display some degree of structure (some form of order, consistency, or hierarchy). To bring out any of these features, we need to consider ideas about both what should be done and what should be avoided (the avoidances—the violations—often bring out most clearly the implicit distinctions or rules). We need also to be concerned not only with actions but also with the words people use when they describe appropriate or inappropriate actions or when they label events and feelings.

In terms of its own structure, the chapter contains a main section and two "bookends." The main section describes studies oriented towards specifying the content and the quality of parents' ideas about household divisions of labor. This description covers both the results and the issues that these raise for the study of parents' ideas in general.

In contrast, the first bookend covers questions of rationale. Why explore parents' ideas? Why use the procedure of starting with a practice and then working backwards to the ideas that may underlie the practice? And why choose household work practices?

The final bookend takes up some unfinished questions, with the major space given to the question: Which ideas about household work are likely to vary across social or ethnic groups? No clear answer can be given; the features that would allow one to predict differences among cultural groups are far from well-known. The chapter ends, however, with the speculation that ideas about tasks and contributions depend on the extent to which a culture emphasizes actions based on choice, willingness, negotiation, and responsiveness to another individual's needs in contrast to actions based on roles and set obligations.

Before I begin the description of studies, a word is needed on the ethnic aspect of the ideas I shall describe. With one exception, the parents interviewed come from a particular ethnic group rather than from comparative research. This group, however, is not easily labeled. Among English speakers in Australia, it is sometimes referred to as Anglo-Australian (my usage here) or Oz, replacing an earlier Old

Australian or Australian, with no qualifying adjective. (Australians for whom English is not the home language undoubtedly use other labels; *kangaruni* is one). The label Anglo in this case does not refer to Australians born in England but to people born in Australia, monolingual in English and with parents for whom English was the home language. The uncertainty about labels reflects the country's history. Currently, one child in four has one or both parents born overseas (a strong immigration program has been in place since the 1940s) and group descriptions are sensitive and unsettled issues. Descriptions of oneself in the U.S. style (Italian-American, etc.) have not yet come into common usage, although Celtic-Australian is emerging as a self-claimed description, and the term ethnic still has immigrant, non-English-speaking overtones. The local Anglos, for instance, would not see themselves as ethnic, although Aboriginal Australians take some pleasure in using this description for them as a way of emphasizing the immigrant status of all groups other than themselves.

My research group concentrated on Anglo parents and children for two reasons. First, we are in a better position to pick up nuances and rhetoric from this group compared with others; we are members of it. Second, once we began to examine their practices and rationales, we found them difficult enough to explain. At times the practices seemed as bizarre to us as those from any "exotic" group. The return to comparative work has accordingly been delayed. A start on that return, however, indicating the direction that this research might take, lies behind the comparative suggestions offered in the final section of the chapter.

## Research Rationale

I begin with a brief comment on reasons for considering the ideas that parents hold and then move to the reasons for concentrating on content related to household labor and for using practices as a basis for working back to expectations and to ideas about what is desirable, acceptable, and unacceptable.

### Exploring Parents' Ideas

This is not a new issue. In essence, the exploration has been argued for on the grounds that these ideas represent (1) an interesting form of adult social cognition and adult development, (2) a way of helping to account for parents' actions, (3) a way of pinning down that amorphous term "social context" and (4) a way of exploring "cultural transmission" or "cultural change" if one considers the ideas held by two generations. That list is a condensation of material from several sources: Goodnow and Collins's (1990) introduction to research on parents' ideas, Quinn and Holland's (1987) introduction to research on cultural models, Molinari, Emiliani, and Carugati's (1992) analysis of parents' ideas as social representations, Reid and Valsiner's (1986) analysis of parents' ideas as folk theories, and Super and Harkness's (1986) extension of Beatrice Whiting's (1980) analysis of the settings or "niches" in which children are located, with one critical component of these being the "psychology" of the people, especially the adults, who form part of the setting.

## Using Practices as a Base

It is possible to explore parents' ideas without starting from what parents do. The study that initiated a concern with household work began, in fact, with questions about expectations that were not specifically grounded in practices. In a study of "developmental timetables" (Goodnow, Cashmore, Cotton, & Knight, 1984), Anglo-Australian and Lebanese-Australian mothers were asked at what age they expected children to be able to carry out a variety of actions such as counting from 1 to 10, naming the primary colors, answering the telephone, resolving a disagreement with siblings without fighting, eating with a spoon without assistance, knowing their surname, and carrying out some regular household task . Such timetable questions have often been asked of parents, and Ninio's (1979) study in Israel was probably the first to use them as a base for comparing ethnic groups.

Research that begins with the ideas that people might hold, rather than with their practices, is perhaps more common among psychologists than among anthropologists or sociologists. Psychologists are accustomed to start by identifying and describing stereotypes, schemas, scripts, or values. They may stop at this point, or they may proceed to ask how far or under what conditions ideas are congruent with actions. This way of beginning, one should note, does not always signal a belief in the view that ideas shape actions, with no reverse direction considered. The popularity of a term such as "doing gender" (West & Zimmerman, 1987), for instance, is one indicator of interest in the idea that practices provide the ways by which people first come to acquire a culture's concepts.[1]

In terms of research strategy, it is as reasonable to start from practices as it is from ideas. Moreover, practices have the advantage of providing a content area which allows an easy flow of talk and, potentially, a point of contrast between groups that can be identified at the start of a study. The challenge is to avoid what Ortner (1985) describes as the "Parsonian" approach of regarding practices as the simple, direct reenactment of rules. Challenge lies also in the problem of how to choose practices that offer a rewarding research base. Priority seems best given to practices that involve some long-term goals, goals that the actors perceive as part of some larger, "developmental project" (Ortner, 1985, p. 152). Priority seems best given also to practices that appear to be "shaped not only by problems being solved, and gains being sought, but by the images and ideals of what constitutes goodness—in people, in relationships, and in conditions of life" (Ortner, 1985, p. 152).

The practices of choice are also those that are not easy to explain. To take a concrete example, the expectation that children will make a work contribution to the household puzzles labor theorists, who point out that the effort extended to get the work done often exceeds the value of the labor contributed (a point taken from Straus, 1962); it is also not well-supported by evidence of its benefits. In fact, the evidence for household tasks giving rise to the expected development of responsibility or sensitivity to other people's needs is decidedly mixed (Goodnow, 1988a). In short, here is a parental practice that compels us to ask: What ideas support it or accompany it?

## The Concentration on Household Practices

The presence of puzzles, I must admit, was not the base from which household practices first came to be chosen. At the time of the study of developmental timetables (Goodnow et al., 1984), I was searching for a content area that would have a number of features. Ideally, it would:

- Elicit differences between ethnic groups.
- Involve some degree of affect, on the grounds that principles or ideals important to the actors would then be more likely to be involved.
- Bring out ideas about the general goals of parenting or the general course of development.
- Be easily talked about by both generations (parents and children).
- Evoke some lack of agreement across generations.
- Enable us to gain some insight into the way parents' concepts or values are conveyed.

Household tasks first stood out as eliciting a sharp difference between two ethnic groups (Goodnow et al., 1984). The content area was then quickly recognized as meeting the other criteria.

In retrospect, it is surprising that household work practices that involve children needed to be recognized in this roundabout way. Psychologists have given them less attention than they deserve (Goodnow, 1988a). This may be because discussions of children's household work have been locked into discussions of altruism or because attention has been focused on gendered divisions of labor between adults. Those perceptions do not hold for all psychologists. Smetana (1988), for instance, sees children's household tasks as an area in which parents and adolescents work through issues of authority and control. More broadly, Belsky and his colleagues have come to argue for all work divisions as critical indicators of family relationships (e.g., Belsky, Lang, & Huston, 1986; Belsky, Rovine, & Fish, 1989). It is nonetheless the case that anthropologists and sociologists have consistently taken a greater interest and a broader view of household divisions of labor, proposing, for instance, that "much of system reproduction takes place via the routinized activities and intimate interactions of domestic life" (Ortner, 1985, p. 156). Reflecting my discipline's bias, I myself have been surprised—and delighted—by the way ideas about household tasks tap into ideas about gender, justice, and the proper nature of family relationships. Each study, as I shall now describe, has opened up new questions and new possibilities.

## Specific Studies: Baseline Descriptions

I begin with two studies that yielded some baseline descriptions of the content of parents' ideas (Goodnow et al., 1984; Goodnow, 1987; Goodnow & Delaney, 1989). These descriptions were in terms both of categories (distinctions among jobs and among relationships) and of propositions (such as "children should be free of work," "everyone should contribute something," or "if you created this problem, it is your job to fix it or to clean it up"). I then take studies dealing with two specific issues. One of these deals with factors considered in the allocation of work to various family members. The other is concerned with the place of money in the family. The order throughout is roughly chronological, but from time to time, I break that sequence in order to show how some of the later material amplified or consolidated some of the earlier results.

The first study is a comparison of Anglo-Australian mothers with Lebanese-Australian mothers (born in Lebanon) for the ages at which they expected their children to display various kinds of competence (Goodnow et al., 1984). The Anglo mothers described their 5-year-olds as expected to do "some regular job." Moreover, they related tasks to chronological age. When asked whether jobs were likely to be the same or to change as the child grew older, these mothers outlined a picture of progressive change with age: from putting pajamas under the pillow, for instance, to putting dirty clothes in the laundry basket, or making the bed (pulling up the duvet). With rare exceptions, the jobs mentioned were all of a type that has been called self-care (White & Brinkerhoff, 1981). The child is expected to look after his or her own body, bed, possessions, and space.

In contrast, the Lebanese-Australian mothers regarded it as laughable that one would expect any regular task of 5-year-olds: "They're still babies" was the frequent phrase. These "babies," however, could be asked to take on a task that few Anglos would assign: look after or amuse a still younger child. Moreover, these mothers did not see age in itself as bringing change. If the mothers' needs changed—if, for instance, another baby was born—then they would ask for more to be done. Otherwise, they considered that children would learn to do household tasks when necessary. That applied to girls as well as boys, with the additional comment made occasionally of girls that they would be "lumbered with all of that soon enough." These mothers did not tell us that "earlier was better" (they might have said this about saying prayers—this was a Catholic sample, as was the Anglo group). Nor did they tell us, as the Anglos did, that these tasks were a way to develop "a sense of responsibility" or to help children realize that "we're a family." The achievement of these goals—a sense of family and of responsibility—was clearly of importance to the "Lebanese," but they presumably had other ways to achieve these same ends and did not see them as jeopardized by not assigning household tasks other than child minding.

How have household tasks come to acquire such value in Anglo eyes? With some sense of amusement that I had not examined my own ideas and practices until this point, I turned to the literature. I looked at a small set of experimental studies that had been designed to check whether children assigned household tasks did in fact develop the expected virtues (reviewed in Goodnow, 1988a). I turned also to some historical material, principally Zelizer's (1985) account of the status of children in the United States from the late 1800s to around 1940. That account brings out the emphasis placed on tasks even for children of the wealthy or for child film stars; their work assignments were presented as proof that they were being brought up "properly". The phenomenon of work expected in the absence of parental need was clearly not new.

In the course of that reading, the way in which children's tasks were being treated as an undifferentiated set first caught my interest. One task, one "chore," I felt was surely not the same as another. The problem then became one of locating the distinctions that people made and the dimensions they used for regarding a task as being of one kind rather than another. At the least, self-care tasks seemed to be different in kind from tasks that I came to call family care (running errands for others, preparing food that others eat, setting the table for a family meal, looking after animals, and fetching food, wood, or water). These are jobs that benefit others and for which there is a clear need.

The vagueness with which parents—and researchers—often described the outcomes they expected also caught my interest. What was meant by terms such as "responsibility" (the effect most often described as expected)? Could one say more specifically what parents expected their children to learn from household tasks or from the interactions and the explanations they involved? Equally challenging appeared to be the sources of the parents' beliefs. Were they perhaps part of some general set of concepts about the nature of children, the obligations of parents, the place of children in the family or—more broadly still—about the way people should treat one another? And would this account for why the tasks often generated so much affect on the part of both parents and children?

With these questions in mind, Susan Delaney and I began a study with Anglo mothers. The children discussed were 9 to 11 years old, old enough to be involved but not so old that their time was eaten into by part-time jobs outside the house. We asked what the children did in the way of household tasks; actually, we asked the mothers to describe a typical day for the child, starting with waking up, and let the activities emerge—with prompts—from that description. We located one self-care and one family-care job and asked what value, if any, mothers saw in their children doing each of these. In addition, we asked mothers for examples of "good" moments and "low" moments, for what they would do if the job were not done, and how they felt about money in exchange for jobs (in the family or from neighbors) and about the acceptability of one sib paying another (Goodnow, 1987; Goodnow & Delaney, 1994).

Throughout these questions, we were looking for central ideas—ideas that might cut across a number of statements and actions—and for the key words in which those ideas were expressed. To compress the data, we emerged with the view that mothers were (1) making distinctions among jobs, (2) making distinctions among relationships, (3) using approaches to work as markers of relationships, and (4) operating from principles that displayed some potential signs of hierarchical order. I comment on each of these in turn, updating what was learned from the Goodnow and Delaney (1989) study with what emerged later (Goodnow & Warton, 1991; Warton & Goodnow, in press).

## Distinctions among Jobs

These distinctions were of two kinds. One was between "regular" and "extra" jobs. The latter were often paid for; the former would seldom be paid for. Payment was in fact regarded by most as "wrong" for regular jobs, except for young children and for children who were highly resistant ("I'd use it as a last resort, if nothing else worked," in the words of one mother).

A second distinction between jobs was made on the basis of causation. To the allocation of jobs, Anglo parents and children often bring a principle that may be called "your mess, your job." If you took these things out, used them, wore them, or created this problem, you should fix it or help to fix it. This distinction emerged most strongly in the mothers' comments on what they would do if a child did not do his or her job. Three possibilities emerged. In one, mothers leave the job in the child's hands, either by insisting that it be done or by waiting until the child reaches a point of discomfort or is pressured by others. In the second, the mother does the job herself. In the third, the mother asks another sibling to do it on more than an occasional, "special favor" basis.

Among our Anglo mothers, family-care jobs were regarded as movable to another sibling. In contrast, self-care jobs were not seen as easily movable, both because "it would not be right" and because "it would be useless." The other child would object that "it's not my bed, not my schoolbag, not my stuff," and so on).[2] A special reason—"a favor," "we all have to do things for one another at times," "she would do it for you," "I need it to be done"—then needs to be invoked to legitimize the transfer of a self-care job.

## Distinctions among Relationships
## and Links between Work and Relationships

At this point, we have two distinctions between jobs—regular versus extra, caused by a specific person or not—that may clearly help account for decisions as to whether tasks can be easily moved from one person to another or whether the move or the request calls for some special legitimation. The two job distinctions, however, do not account for the degree of affect with which distributions of work are often discussed. For this phenomenon, we need to turn to some concurrent distinctions being made among relationships.

One distinction made by the Anglo mothers was between family and nonfamily. Mothers objected, for instance, to one child paying another to do his or her job because "you don't do that in a family."

Also, in reasons offered for children's work, they often referred to family: "We're a family;" "In a family, it has to be give and take; you get a lot, and you have to put in something too."[3] "Family" emerged again in response to questions about some possible ways of allocating jobs, particularly the question: "How do you feel about rosters?" For some mothers, rosters were the ideal way to avoid arguments. For others, rosters were "too managerial." One mother simply stated, "I'm running a family, not a company." (This mother operated mainly on the basis of asking for help as needed, except for some "things they are just expected to do, like cleaning up their own room.")

A subtler distinction—one that underlies many of the references to family—is between relationships that are based on each person's responsiveness to the other's needs and relationships that do not have this basis. Clark (1984) covers part of this contrast in her distinction between "communal" and "exchange" relationships. In her analysis, the former are marked by responsiveness to the other's needs, the latter by norms that allow actions of a more overtly quid-pro-quo type. In exchange relationships, for instance, favors are returned in kind within a short period; open scorekeeping is tolerated; payments for assistance may be in money.

The Anglo mothers did make a communal–exchange type of distinction. In their descriptions of "low moments," for instance, they often referred to the children treating the house as if it were a "hotel, boarding house, guest house, laundromat, and cafeteria." (Fathers, I have since discovered, object to being regarded as operating "a taxi service" or as the equivalent of an automatic banking machine.) Among our Australian samples, such statements about the unacceptability of these commercial-style transactions were made not only to the interviewer but also to the children. In effect, the commercial–non-commercial distinction is one that parents wish their children to know and to respect.

In addition, however, Anglo-Australian mothers make a distinction between relationships that are responsive and relationships that are coercive or demeaning (an exchange relationship need not be coercive or demeaning). Mothers resented being "forced to nag," or "having to act like Simon Legree." They also resented—and were vocal about—any implication that they are "servants" or "slaves" (a position in which they act without choice and are also socially inferior to the person being served or helped).

Why should Anglo mothers be so deeply concerned about being treated as "servants" or "slaves?" Part of the answer, I suggest, is that mothers do often clean up after other people. Mothers violate the rule that at other times they teach: "Your mess, your job." When Anglo mothers do so, however, they expect these actions to be acknowledged as voluntary, as part of a gift relationship. Their "best moments" then come when children recognize that the mothers' actions are gifts (*not* the actions of servants) and when they reciprocate with actions that are also gifts that go beyond obligations or expected tasks.

### A Possible Hierarchy of Principles

Up to this point, I have been describing parents' ideas in terms of categories and dichotomies. For all their importance, however, dichotomies and categories are not likely to represent all that there is to the nature of parents' ideas. One should take into account content in the form of propositions, rules, or scripts.[4] In addition, one should ask about the extent to which there is some degree of structure within the ideas held: some degree of intercorrelation, or some hierarchical order of the kind proposed for scripts (e.g., Shank & Abelson, 1977) or for rules (e.g., Hinde, 1974; Mancuso & Lehrer, 1986; Wertheim, 1975).

What forms of order or structure are likely to be present? And how do we locate these? Basically, the methods reduce to two kinds: asking which ideas cluster and asking whether there is some hierarchical order with one idea being superordinate to another. Palacios (1990) provides an example of a study that uses cluster analysis to yield sets of ideas that he labels "traditional," "modern," and "paradoxical" (a mixture of the first two). Wertheim's (1975) analysis of rules is an example of interest in hierarchy. She distinguishes, for instance, between "ground rules" (e.g., if A is not at home, B does his or her job) and "meta-rules" (e.g., members of a family should help one another). Meta-rules subsume ground rules and can be applied to any situation for which a ground rule has not yet been made clear.

Within research on parents' ideas, the signs used to indicate a hierarchy have been limited so far to noting that some rules are stated in more general terms than others are (Mancuso & Lehrer, 1986; Wertheim, 1975). There is as yet, for instance, no test for subordinate-superordinate status of the kind used in cognitive analyses of categories (e.g., Rosch, 1978). Such analyses are certainly feasible. So also is the generation of vignettes, or descriptions of children's actions, that would allow one to pit one principle against another. One might, for instance, ask parents to rate various actions as more versus less upsetting (e.g., a child who disappears when work needs to be done compared to a child who does the job but complains about having to do it).

Is it possible to suggest a hierarchy of principles that apply to household tasks? The statements of parents often imply a hierarchy (Goodnow & Warton, 1991). When a parent says, for instance, that he or she would pay a child to do a job "as a last resort, if nothing else worked," the implication is that the principle "the child should do this job" has more importance than the principle "children should do jobs willingly."

For Anglo mothers, I suggest, the order of ideas related to "being a family" could be as follows:

The first principle might be stated as "everyone must contribute something." The admonitions to children are then along the lines that "you can't just take and not give something," or "there's no such thing as a free lunch, you know."

Next in the hierarchy would be the principle that "everyone should make a reasonable kind of contribution." For one person to have all the "good jobs." and another all the "dirty work" or all the "dull jobs" is not acceptable. Unacceptable also is a contribution that does not include the jobs that one should do oneself: the self-care jobs, for example, or work that one has caused (especially if there was no need to cause it or to create it).

Third in this possible hierarchy is the principle that "everyone should put in a reasonable amount." Admonitions then are along the lines that "everyone should pull their weight," "you're getting a bit slack, aren't you?" or—more severely stated—"no one gets to play Lord Muck around here" (a reference to one person carrying a lighter load and assuming a higher status than others). We do not, I admit, know how people define "enough," "too much," or "not enough," but at least part of the definition appears to involve comparison with others. Anglo children certainly compare the work they do with the amount that their siblings do.

The fourth principle takes the form that "people should be self-regulating; they should not need continual reminders, money incentives, or the threat of punishment." An 18-year-old said, "You should be able to trust them to do it, especially if they're family."

The final principle has a particular reference to the spirit of a contribution. Ideally, "everyone should make a contribution that is willing and that shows an awareness of the other's need." This principle is "last" in the sense that this is what parents may hope finally to achieve. There will undoubtedly be parents for whom this principle comes first, as in the case of a father who insisted to his children that "if you can't do the job with good grace, don't do it; I'll do it myself," a position the children strongly resented. Most of the parents we interviewed, however, will violate this principle by ignoring complaints. They will also violate the fourth principle—the principle of self-regulation—by using coercion or by paying for jobs if that is needed in order to achieve the first principle (some contribution must be made).

## Implications and Possible Directions

At this point there are several directions in which both concepts and research could move. The possibilities have to do with (1) the specifications of practices, (2) the nature of talk or discourse, and (3) the implications of an ideal, and of what one might settle for as part of the set of ideas that parents bring to family interactions.

### The Specification of Practices

If practices are to provide the base from which we infer or ask about parents' ideas, they need to be described as carefully as possible. Distinguishing among the kinds of jobs that children do in terms of the predominance of self-care or family-care jobs is one step in that direction.

Distinguishing among styles of work allocation is another. For instance, Susan Delaney and I came to group mothers in terms of four predominant styles. (All parents use all styles at some times and with some jobs, but a grouping in terms of predominant styles is nonetheless possible.) One of these styles involved clear, regular assignments with follow through. A second aimed at this way of proceeding but was inconsistent. A third consisted of operating mainly on requests for help as needed (sometimes made easily and openly, sometimes in the form of "heavy hints"). A fourth—we called it "let the tide rise"—let work accumulate until someone's threshold was reached (not always the mother's), and the family then had a "blitz," with everyone doing whatever job came to hand and little or no concern with "whose" job it was (Goodnow & Delaney, 1989).

Each of these parental styles is likely to be associated with particular ideas about what children and parents should do, what "being a family" means, and what the difference is between one job and another. At this point, however, our main source of information about such links is from a study of couples who share household work in a variety of ways: by carving out separate but equivalent areas of responsibility, by trading jobs fluidly as needs or moods change, by following a roster (rare in this group), or by operating on the basis of "I'll do mine, you do yours" (Goodnow & Bowes, 1994).

The ideas that emerge in relation to these styles may certainly be regarded as "ethnotheories," but they are not "parental" in the sense of referring to actions specifically by parents. Accordingly, I shall draw out from this material only two points that confirm the importance of ideas about the nature of the specific job and the links between work and relationships. The first of these has to do with the acceptability of some particular styles as limited to particular jobs. "I'll do mine; you do yours," for instance, occurs mainly with two jobs: ironing and the care of a car. Both may be regarded as forms of self-care. In contrast, cooking only for oneself on other than an occasional basis, or for reasons of shiftwork or diet, is outside the sense of a close relationship. The second point has to do with the nonacceptability of rosters. These were used only at the start of a new work pattern or when a third person was living in the house. Again, the reasons given were in terms of the nature of close relationships: "We know what we each do" in the words of one of the people interviewed; "we can trust each other to do them," in the words of another.

## The Nature of Talk

Part of what people do, and part of the base from which one can explore the associated ideas, consists of the words they use.

One usage that stands out in several of our studies has to do with the word "work." "I don't expect anything of my children," says a mother who denies any allocation of jobs. "I do all the *work* in their rooms and in the house; I vacuum, I dust, and I make their beds; I vacuum their rooms, and change the sheets; all they have to do is keep it tidy after that." To many other mothers (and to children), "keeping it tidy" would count as a regular assigned form of work. The term "work" was also often avoided by many of the mothers who operated on a "request" style. Their children did "little jobs" or "a few things to help," but "work" apparently sounded to these mothers as if an adult obligation was being passed to children. ("You don't have children in order to give your jobs to them;" said one). In contrast, among the more "managerial" mothers, and for those who "let the tide rise;" the terms "work" and "jobs" were used easily. "Work" and "jobs" were what everyone in the house did and was expected to do either regularly or when the need arose. In all groups, however, the word we did not hear in Anglo discussions was "duty" (occasionally "chores," but this is predominantly a U.S. term). "Household duties," one suspects, is a term currently used among Anglos only with reference to adult women, and even for them it sounds a bit quaint, a little old-fashioned. It may well be in wider use, however, in social groups where choice and willingness are less salient issues.

A second aspect of talk or discourse that stands out has to do with the directness or indirectness of what parents say. This aspect been taken up in a collaborative analysis with Judith Becker (Becker & Goodnow, 1991). Mothers in Australia and in the United States, it turns out, are both given to indirect comments. Becker noticed this in her studies of language. Mothers say, for instance, "What's the magic word?"—or "I can't hear you"—when they want the child to say "please." Susan Delaney and I noticed the same phenomenon with regard to children's tasks: "What do you think this is, a hotel?" "Guess we eat with our fingers tonight" (when the table has not been set), "How much do you pay these days?" (when the child has made an inappropriate request). These forms of talk, to both Judith Becker and me, appear to be not only ways of avoiding direct confrontation but also ways of catching the child's attention and transferring some of the cognitive work to the child after a long spell of direct instruction: "You do get to sound like a broken record" were the words of one Australian mother. This is boring for her, not attention grabbing for the child, and, we suspect, occurring when the parent has come to feel that the child should now begin to take some initiative in remembering or noticing what needs to be done.

## The Implications of an Ideal

For many Anglo mothers the ideal appears to be one of help given willingly, without being requested, and with signs of alertness to the other's needs. The cup of tea offered when one is tired is an example that several people give. The job done for you when your day is known to be a busy one, or when you are short of time, is another. My favorite example, however—and one to which Anglo mothers consistently resonate—comes from this description of a "good moment": "When they have a bath, I often warm up their slippers and place them outside the bathroom door so they can just step into them and stay nicely warm. The other day I had a bath and when I came out, there were my slippers all nicely warmed. I felt so happy and I went and hugged them. . . . Of course, I wouldn't expect that to happen every time."

This ideal might well be described as indicating a "gift relationship" (Titmuss, 1970), with the gift tailored to the individual's needs, displaying some signs of choice and thought rather than being based on a routine obligation or duty, or on someone else's initiative. In addition, there is, for Anglo mothers especially, the expectation that the exchange for their "gifts" will *not* be repayment in a distant future (e.g., support in one's old age) but some sign of recognition during childhood that what mothers do is a gift, something that goes "beyond duty," and some reciprocation, by way of a volunteered action that is chosen by the child rather than assigned or suggested by others.

The ideal, I hasten to add, does not mean that Anglo mothers wait patiently and do nothing until their children begin making gifts of work. These mothers, in fact, used a variety of methods to make sure that work was done, while still holding the thoughtful gift as the ideal they might one day see. The ideal, however, sets the stage for hoping that there will be a time when reminders, money incentives, and "nagging" will not be needed; and for disappointment when children get to be of an age at which a parent thinks the ideal might be approximated but is faced with a reality that is uncomfortably distant from it.

Further, this ideal is not limited to Anglo mothers referring to their children. It is a strong theme also in couples' discussions of the way they share work between themselves and of the pleasant and "bumpy" parts of sharing (Backett, 1982; Goodnow & Bowes, 1994). The parental value placed on "voluntarism" (Backett, 1982) or on "gifts of work" seems to grow out of or to be supported by an ideal that applies more broadly.

At this point, however, I am a little ahead of my story with regard to parents. Let me turn then to the directions we chose to follow and that were specifically concerned with the ideas parents expressed or appeared to hold. The first of these took the form of a further exploration of ideas about the movability of jobs from one person to another. From that we learned a great deal about the distinctions drawn among jobs and among family members. The other took the form of exploring parents' ideas about money in exchange for jobs. From that we learned a great deal about the ways in which parents perceive work as linked to the nature of relationships, and about what may be involved when we ask whether parents' ideas display some particular forms of order or structure.

## Factors in the Allocation of Jobs

In the study by Goodnow and Delaney (1989), one of the most rewarding questions had to do with whether a job could be moved from one person to another: whether a mother would ask another child in the family to take over a job left undone by a sibling. It was in discussions of what could be asked of others that the principle of causation—"your mess, your job"—emerged with particular clarity.

In fact, it seemed that one specific way of defining the acquisition of "a sense of responsibility" could be in terms of a child's coming to know the local norms related to the movability of work. In the Anglo world, for instance, one way in which children demonstrate this sense is when they know which jobs can be asked of others and which they should do themselves. On this basis, Pamela Warton and I began to ask about the ages at which Anglo children understood this meaning of responsibility, along with some further meanings. One of these further meanings was in terms of self-regulation (you should not need reminders, and you should not need to be paid). Another was in terms of indirect causation. In this case, the vignette cast the child in the role of having asked a sibling to do a job that the asker normally did. If the job were not done, we asked, "Is it fair that you get into trouble?" Children aged 8 to 14 years were clear about the need to do themselves the jobs that were part of their own space, their own possessions, or their own making. They also accepted the fairness of not being reminded, although they reported that reminders regularly happened. They gave qualified answers, however, about being paid (this depended on the job), and they were strongly against being held responsible for outcomes they had indirectly caused (Warton & Goodnow, 1991).

This prong of research involved a turn toward children with an eye to seeing where age changes might occur and where there might be convergence or divergence between children's views and what we knew, or assumed, were parents' or adults' views.[5]

A great deal still remained to be learned, however, about parents' views of movability. To do so, it seemed best to aim at considerations other than "your mess, your job." What other factors do parents take into account when they consider assigning a task or making a work request to one family member rather than another?

To answer that question, we asked mothers and fathers about possible distributions of work and about their reasons for regarding a particular distribution as comfortable or not (Goodnow, Bowes, Warton, Dawes, & Taylor, 1991). More specifically, we asked parents how they would feel about asking each other or a teenage child (son or daughter) to do a set of 14 tasks, and why they might feel more or less comfortable about making such a request. (We also asked children about the feasibility of asking others in the family—mothers, fathers, a brother, or a sister—but I shall concentrate here on the parental data.)

The answers given by these parents provided a further distinction among tasks. This distinction is in terms of the possible distribution lists that come with a job. Some tasks, for instance, circulated only between fathers and sons (mowing grass, small repairs, washing cars). Some were for mothers only (cleaning a toilet, sewing repairs, regular grocery shopping). A third set could go to mothers or children but were rarely considered distributable to fathers (e.g., vacuuming, ironing, hanging out the wash). The last set (e.g., setting the table, doing dishes) was one likely to have a wide distribution net, although fathers were still seen as the least likely target even for these requests. The sample was deliberately drawn from suburbs where the majority are known to vote in conservative fashion, a strategy used in the hope of gaining a sizable proportion of references to "men's jobs" and "women's jobs."

What kinds of reasons did parents give for feeling comfortable or uncomfortable about a request? We were interested in two aspects. The first was the extent to which reasons could be easily given (more technically, were "accessible"). When a practice has been routinized, reasons may be hard to give. Parents reply, for instance, that they would ask *X* to do a particular job "because that's the job they do." We scored these reasons as "nonreflective" (anthropologists might say "axiomatic"). The second aspect was the kind of reflective reason offered: whether the reference was to the other person's gender, competence, availability, or feelings about the task (likes it, dislikes it, would argue about it).

The surprise result was the scarcity of open references to gender (only 3% of answers) even though gender was clearly a consideration in the distributions of requests and in the reports of the jobs that the children did. Why should this be so? To talk of a "man's job" or "a girl's job" may have become socially undesirable. But what has taken its place? References to competence seemed to be the substitute: "They wouldn't know how"; "they don't have the strength" or "they lack the delicate touch"; "I can do it better."

Competence is an intriguing rationale, all the more so because the assertion of competence or incompetence as a reason for action—both in this and in Goodnow and Bowes's (1994) sample of sharing couples—was often accompanied by laughter or by a qualifier such as "well, that's what she says." Competence, it appears, is sometimes recognized as a cloak that often covers unwillingness. Why not then simply say that one dislikes a job or does not want to do it? The answer goes back to responsiveness and caring as an ideal. When this is the ideal, unwillingness strikes a particularly sour note. So also do answers that may seem "bureaucratic" in style (e.g., "that's not my job" or "not my department"). It is far better to plead that one is "all butterfingers" or that an arrangement would be "inefficient." It is also far better to regard one's child or partner as incompetent than as evading work that he or she is quite happy to see you do.

Do these subterfuges of "competence" and "incompetence" ever give way to more open expressions of likes and dislikes? Among adults, this appears to be most likely when (1) people are already taking a fair share of the work (to say one does not like a particular job can then carry no implication that one is "shirking"), and (2) when there is a clear recognition that something "fair" needs to be done about jobs that both partners dislike. There is then no implication that one person is "using" or "exploiting" the other. The jobs that both dislike may be eliminated, done in turns, or turned over to paid help, but one person does not do them. In the words of one man, "To us fair means that one person does not get stuck with all the jobs we both dislike" (Goodnow & Bowes, 1994). Among these couples, competence may still be a criterion, designed to get the work done most quickly, but "fairness" takes priority and lack of competence is not used as a way to gain a favored position.

## Possible Directions

Once again, the decision to explore ideas about movability brings us to a point where several further studies could branch out. One possibility consists of asking about the legitimacy of children subcontracting work: the legitimacy, for instance, of children passing on a job that is "theirs" to a sibling. Subcontracting and delegation are critical parts of ideas about distributability. We chose, however, to follow up that issue by interviewing children since some of the earlier results with children raised questions about the extent to which children accepted responsibility based on indirect causation, as when a "third party" is involved (Warton & Goodnow, 1991). The results from this follow-up are reported in Goodnow and Warton (1992b).

A second possible direction consists of asking for parents' views about the distribution of jobs to people outside the family: to paid help that comes into the home or to caregivers in family day-care or group-care centers. Informally, caregivers in day-care settings tell us that they avoid proceeding, without permission, to aspects of care that parents may see as "their job only" (e.g., cutting fingernails). Similar actions may also be causes of great dissension when children are in the custody of one parent and visiting the other (M. Steward, personal communication). Each parent apparently sees some actions as marked "for parents only," or "for me only," and the loss of these gives rise to the sense of no longer being in control, no longer being fully a parent or the parent in charge. The identification of the critical features to "feeling like the real parent" (or "like a good mother" or a "good father") has yet to be done. One way forward, however, may lie in identifying features that have to do with what one *must* do oneself or could turn over to others with varying degrees of control or supervision.[6]

A third possible direction takes the form of turning to other cultural groups. We now have procedures that allow us to identify differences among jobs and among family members. The paradigms are easily movable. Would one then expect to find in other cultural groups the same criteria for judging that a job is not movable or is movable only to some particular people? This possible direction is considered in the final discussion.

# The Place of Money

This is the second of the two main lines of research that we chose to work on with parents. (The distribution of jobs was the first). As a practice, giving children money—especially in relation to the work they do—has several of the features listed early in the chapter as indicating content areas that are likely to be rewarding bases for exploring parents' ideas (concrete, likely to be viewed differently by the two generations, likely to vary across social groups). In addition, practices related to money appear to arouse a fair degree of moral feeling. Most Anglo mothers, for instance, felt strongly that there were some jobs that they would *never* pay for. And most regarded it as "wrong" for one child to pay another to do the first child's job. The minority felt that the practice "would not last," that "the child who was being paid would soon find that he or she was being exploited," Goodnow, 1987).

Among Anglo mothers, the objections to money as a reward for jobs seemed to revolve around the sense that this was a violation of what should occur within a family. In effect, we appeared to have here a concrete base from which to explore further a general hypothesis that first emerged in the Goodnow and Delaney (1989) study, namely, that work patterns are used as markers of relationships. The hypothesis is attractive because a link to relationships would provide the large developmental frame within which children's jobs can be placed. Jobs may be regarded then as one of the routes by which children are taught how to be members of a family: how to share work with others and how not to exploit others, what one's place is as a child and what is owed to parents. A link to relationships would also provide a way of understanding the affect that so often surrounds children's performance or nonperformance of work.

In addition, money practices within the family appeared likely to fit neatly with a general opposition that seems to be part of Anglo culture. In the words of a parent educator quoted by Zelizer (1985, p. 198), parents should be careful not to confuse "the principles of the home. . .and the principles of the shop." An allowance for children is acceptable, but the money given them should not be a "wage." The same type of dichotomy appears to operate at the adult level, where the involvement of money, or a concern with money, may be felt to be incompatible with "caring." Teachers or nurses who become vocal about their poor salaries, for instance, are likely to be regarded as "caring" less about their pupils or their patients than they should ("selflessness" is expected to be a mark of these "caring professions") (Warton, Goodnow, & Bowes, 1992). Mothers who "go on strike" make media news, together with discussions of salaries for housewives or the insurance value of wives. "Working" (paid work) and "caring" are somehow entrenched opposites.

If the ideal is that money and household jobs should be separate from one another, however, then everyday life seems to contain several departures from this ideal. We know, for instance, that 50% of an English sample (Newson & Newson, 1976) regard it as acceptable to pay children for "extra" jobs. We also know that the majority of a large U.S. sample regard children as "earning" their pocket money by the regular jobs they do (Miller & Yung, 1990), and we know that the majority of parents in an Australian sample gathered by Feather (1991) answered "sort of automatic" when asked whether the pocket money children were given was linked to the jobs they did or was "automatic."

In effect, ideas about money and jobs seemed to contain some contradictions. The question then becomes: Are parents happily living with a lack of order or clear structure within the ideas they hold? Or are our methods not bringing out the underlying order?

Pamela Warton and I felt that two steps were needed. The first was a more complete description of the practices that involve a link between money and children's household jobs. We could then ask: Which of these do most parents approve of? Where is there variability? The second was for a set of statements expressing some general principles that might underlie practices. We could then ask: Do some of these cluster together?

For the first step, we compiled a list of possible practices, ranging from a tight link between jobs and money (so much for each job, a practice rather like piecework) to a variety of looser links: adding a bonus if regular jobs were done well, reducing pocket money for "bad behavior" or if regular jobs were not being done or not being done properly, paying for specific "extra" jobs, adding a bonus if an extra job is well done (you have, for instance, agreed that a child will wash the car or wash windows, for a set amount), or reducing the amount if the job were not well done (Warton & Goodnow, in press).

We then asked parents (mothers and fathers) of 9- to 16-year-olds to indicate which of these possibilities they practiced and which they would regard in a variety of ways (i.e., feel quite comfortable with, even if they did not do this themselves; regard as reasonable but not ideal; regard as acceptable but only as a last resort; and regard as unacceptable under any circumstances). These options reflected two viewpoints on our part. One is that what parents do is often an incomplete guide to parents' ideas. The actions they adopt may be only one of several options that are compatible with their ideas. The second is that ideas may emerge more clearly from descriptions of what parents would *not* tolerate than from descriptions of what they can live with (a position in common with Garfinkel's (1967) emphasis on locating the violations of rules in order to have these become explicit).

Two practices yielded results that can be dealt with simply. These were links in the form of piecework (so much for each job) and in the form of payment for extra jobs. Piecework was rejected by almost all parents (mothers and fathers). The minority consisted of parents who would accept it as a last resort (several noted that one might also begin this way with very young children). In contrast, payment only for extra jobs was acceptable to most. It was also a practice followed by all but a purist minority—about 10%—who refused to accept any association between children's work and the money they receive. These parents did not accept even indirect links of the kind implied in saying that one might threaten to reduce pocket money if jobs were not done.

In contrast, parents were more divided on the issue of using money as a bonus or a penalty either for regular or for extra jobs. The strongest sign of consistency within the practices endorsed on this score came from finding that the parents who were willing to give extra money were also the parents willing to reduce the amount given. In effect, bonuses and penalties were two sides of the same coin.

It is possible to regard the differences of opinion about bonuses and penalties as stemming from the relative strengths of two or more general principles. When it comes to reducing the amount agreed on for an extra job, for instance, there is a potential tension between the idea that children should learn to "give value for money" and the idea that "we had an agreement." If the former is the stronger principle, the preferred course of action will be to pay less for a job poorly done or to insist that it be done again, to a higher standard. If the latter is the stronger principle, the preferred action will be to pay what was agreed on but keep in mind that next time one should offer less or specify that a better job needs to be done.

The relative strengths of competing principles offer an attractive way of looking at interconnections among parents' ideas. That this is not the only way of looking at interconnections, however, was brought home to us by the results from our second step: asking parents to rate the extent to which they agreed with a set of propositions that we felt might underlie the views held about various practices.

These propositions were taken or adapted from statements that Anglo parents had made to us at various times. Some statements argued for separateness—for example, "Arrangements in the family and in the paid work force are quite separate issues"; "Payment shouldn't be necessary; doing a job well should be its own reward"; or "I don't get paid for what I do around the house, neither should children." Others argued for a link, again in a strong or a weak form: for example, "It's the same as hiring someone else, if I had to bring someone in to do that work, I'd expect to pay for it"; or "If they're getting pocket money anyhow, they should do something in return."

To cut a long story short, we did not find satisfactory clusters among the propositions that parents agree with. Factor analysis, for instance, yielded three factors, but these accounted for less than 40% of the variance. After some thought and a series of increasingly complex statistical analyses, we decided to turn our approach on its head: in effect, to analyze disapprovals rather than approvals. What were the propositions parents disagreed with?

This approach made us realize that some parents agreed with all or most statements. It brought us also to two concepts that offer some amendments to the usual set of proposals with regard to structure within everyday ideas (Goodnow & Warton, 1992a) . One was the concept of a "bottom line." Parents can go along with many viewpoints (and practices) without concern or reflection. At some point, however, they reach their bottom line. At this point, they resist rather than accept or tolerate. Parents' theories may then be poorly structured or ordered once away from the bottom line, in part because there has been little demand for consistency or clarity before the bottom line has been reached.

A certain degree of "waffle" before the bottom line is reached, however, is only part of the story. The other concept that needs to be invoked is "plurality" (the more precise term may be "multiplicity"). All cultures, it has been proposed, contain alternative views of the same event. In "European" culture, for instance, there is an acceptance of both formal and informal medicine, formal and informal education. Intelligence, to take another example, may be defined as social adaptability *and* as manifested in school achievement. Children may be regarded as innocent and basically good, *and* as marked by "original sin." One of these views may be "dominant," the other "recessive" (Salzman, 1981). The two may exist side by side, or there may be friction and little tolerance between the two. Experts may, for instance, display some respect for "lay theories" or may regard them as "rubbish."

Plurality is a feature considered in several accounts of cultural models and of social representations (see Goodnow & Collins, 1990, for one review oriented towards parents' ideas). The parents we interviewed about money fitted the concept very well. Most of them believed both that "jobs and money should be separate" *and* that "as long as they're getting pocket money, they should be doing something in return." Until the need arises to give priority to one view over another (the child, for instance, comes to be seen as not "doing something in return" or "doing enough in return"), the coexistence of both viewpoints presents no problems to the parent.

This view of money does more than fit our data. It is also a useful general way of looking at the theories parents adopt in many content areas. Parents' ideas can accommodate several positions, just as the general culture often does, with the degree of attachment to one or the other shifting from time to time as circumstances change. The same point might also be made with regard to children. Rather than adopting the one position held by their parents, children may be more fruitfully regarded as hearing several messages and taking these over or drawing on them to various degrees at various times.

## Unfinished Questions

One of these certainly has to do with the issue considered at the end of the previous section; namely, *the "plural" nature of ethnotheories*. To start with, some content areas come to be marked as areas in which a rapid shift in position is regarded as undesirable. One may, as Quinn and Holland (1987) point out, readily shift from one theory of how a thermostat works to another. One's view of marriage or parenting, however, is not expected to be so fluid even when a culture contains more than one view of what these commitments should be like. What distinguishes areas where change is more or less easily tolerated? Are the ideas where change is less acceptable the ones that are not only widely shared in a social group but also mark one's membership in the group, that—if not held—would lead to one's being regarded as a marginal member of a group or to being defined as no longer a member? Some ideas, for instance, may carry no sanctions when they are abandoned. Others, however, may carry the implication that one has ceased to be "a Greek," "a Pole," "a real Italian," or "a good parent." The latter may be less open to plural definitions and to easy change than are the former.

A second unfinished issue concerns *the extent to which any set of ideas can be regarded as a "theory."* Theory sometimes implies an alertness to evidence and/or a willingness to change viewpoints if the counterevidence becomes wrong. "Everyday" theories, however, have been noted by several scholars as not having this property to the degree that "scientific" theories may have (e.g., Abelson, 1986 ; Quinn & Holland, 1987). Theory also implies the presence of some interconnections among ideas: some elements of clustering, hierarchy, or structure. The kind of order that may exist within everyday theories, however, and the conditions under which order may be more rather than less present are as yet far from clear, although some interesting possibilities are beginning to emerge. Palacios (1990), for instance, suggests that parents who display inconsistent or "paradoxical" ideas may be those who have moved away from the coherent viewpoint of a village and picked up bits and pieces of alternatives, without the integration that exposure to a coherent, "modern" view of child development might bring.

A third issue concerns the *designation of some ideas as "parental ethnotheories"*. This phrase appears at first to contain a contradiction. "Ethno" implies that an idea will be widely shared among members of a cultural group. "Parental" implies that an idea is likely to be the particular property of a subgroup. What then is the relationship between the views of the subgroup and the majority?

One possibility is that parents, by virtue of their social position, come to articulate an ethnic viewpoint more clearly than nonparents do. The other possibility—and the one I see as more interesting—is that parents may come to emphasize one of the available positions more than another. There is, in fact, some evidence for this type of possibility in Mugny and Carugati's (1985) study of parents' definitions of intelligence. Intelligence can be defined in terms of social skills, adaptability, and what Mugny and Carugati (1985) call "cybernetic" skills (logical problem-solving skills, or skills with abstractions). Before their children enter school, Italian and Swiss parents use all these definitions. Once their children enter schools, however, "cybernetic" definitions become favored. (Once their children leave the world of school examinations and enter the world of paid work, with its demand for interpersonal skills, the definition to which they give most emphasis seems likely to change once more.) It would be unreasonable to regard these parents as varying in the degree to which they are at different times members of their ethnic group. They seem more effectively regarded as simply changing from time to time in the way they sample, appropriate, or emphasize one rather than another of the group's available views. The challenge then is to locate the conditions under which such shifts occur, with one of these being perhaps change in the subgroup to which one belongs (from parents of preschoolers, for instance, to parents of school children).

For all that these are interesting issues, my emphasis in this closing section nonetheless is on the following questions: *Which ideas are likely to be held by most ethnic groups? Which are likely to vary? And why?*

In summary, I propose that all cultural groups face the task of conveying to children—or to newcomers—the nature of their place or their membership in the group. As part of this broad task, all cultures make distinctions among tasks and among relationships. All cultural groups will also use the way a person's work is done or not done as a marker of relationships. All will contain as well some set of propositions or rules about the contributions that children or parents should make to the household, and within this set there is likely to be some form of

hierarchical order. The specific distinctions, the links, and the propositions, however, are likely to vary from one social group to another.

To narrow that broad proposal, let me start by regarding work as
one of the contributions that children or parents may make to a family.
There are others. Children may, for instance, be expected to bring
money into the household, to do well at school, or to bring honor to
the family name by good deeds or acts of holiness outside the home.
The question to ask across cultures, I suggest, is not only which
contributions are expected but also *which contribution substitutes for
another*. In Taipei, I am told, a child who does well at school may be
excused from household jobs; the assignment of work then becomes a
punishment for not doing as well as one should (W. Lin, personal
communication, 1994). In Cameroon, however, the demands of school
do not wipe out the expected work contributions. Instead, children are
expected to become better organized so that they both can fit in (B.
Nsamenang, personal communication, 1994).

The equivalence of contributions of work and of money is a further
aspect of this same type of question. Among "Anglos" in Australia,
there seems to be some difference between generations on this score;
parents often expect that young adults who are contributing money or
"paying board" will continue to make some work contribution, whereas
the younger generation expects that the contribution of money should
lighten their work involvement to some considerable degree. These
questions of equivalence or substitutability, I suggest, are not merely
ways of delineating cultural or ethnic differences. They are also ways
of identifying order within parents' ideas, in the form of what parents
in various groups regard as the more compared with the less important
of the contributions their children can make.

What happens then about distinctions within work contributions?
I have argued for the value of distinguishing between jobs one should
do oneself and jobs that may be asked of others or delegated to others.
That distinction I would expect to apply to all cultural groups. What is
likely to vary, however, are the features used to distinguish between the
more and the less "movable." Among Anglo parents, and their children,
a major issue has to do with causation: Who caused this "mess," this
problem? Who created the need for this work to be done? Special
considerations need to be invoked in order to justify stepping away from
causation: a child is too young, people should help one another, you
might need this kind of help in the future, family members should do
"favors" for one another, mothers should be "kind," and so on.

Attention to causation within Anglo groups is also not confined to
families or households. Outside the household, secretaries object to
cleaning other people's dirty cups (In many an office, one sees the

notice: "Clean up after yourself—your mother doesn't work here!") And all workers object to "picking up the pieces" after another's mistake, to "pulling someone else's chestnuts out of the fire."

A concern with causation, I suggest, is likely to be most marked in societies often labeled as "individualist." What then are the cultures most likely to yield a significant comparison? At the moment I would expect societies in which there is a strong emphasis on the obligations that go with particular roles. In Taiwanese families, for example, mothers are less likely to ask "Who took these things out?" "Who caused this disorder?" than to clean things up themselves, to turn to the amah, or to give the responsibility for cleaning up to the eldest child (who may then command a younger child to do the work) (M.J. Chen, personal communication). Whenever there is a strong age hierarchy or a strong role structure among siblings, this kind of observation suggests, causation as a basis for determining how jobs can be distributed or moved will be given less attention than is otherwise the case.

What is likely to happen then with distinctions among relationships? All cultures seem likely to make distinctions between family and nonfamily, with variations occurring in the nature of what represents behavior appropriate to family compared to nonfamily. All cultures seem likely also to make a distinction between what can be paid for and what should be above money. The specific behaviors or contributions that are "above money," however, may be expected to vary, along with the degree of affect attached to money payments or to arrangements of the type labeled "exchange" or "commercial" in Anglo cultures.

The challenge will be to locate the bases for variations. Let me offer one speculation. Anglo society is one in which the ideal emphasizes choice, willingness, and what Backett (1982), in her analysis of adult work patterns in Scottish households, calls voluntarism. The ideal also views the carefully tailored "gift"—the offer that is not "standard"—as the optimal sign of affection or "caring." The hope is that people will in time decide to be helpful, good, alert to the specific needs of others, and interested in tailoring their offers of work or help to the needs they sensitively perceive. When these views are dominant, there will always be some suspicion that money will undermine the "intrinsic motivation" that should develop. There will also be concern about the moral status of people who do not choose to be helpful, who exploit the degrees of freedom that a system emphasizing choice and flexibility allows.

The viewpoints I have outlined, however, are not the only viewpoints in Anglo society. They are in many ways what would follow from an "enlightenment" position. Anglo society, however, also has a tradition of moral training. In this tradition, certain ways of behaving are regarded as best adopted prior to understanding, usually on the basis of regular procedures that allow for little negotiation and are likely to contain sanctions or cause alarm if they are not followed. This is a minority view among the "Anglo-Australian" parents we interviewed. Even among these, however, there are a few who tell us that they "don't ever discuss how things will be done," who want—in the graphic words of one mother—their children's work behaviors "to be like breathing." The very phrase—a work "contribution," with its implication of a gift that might be negotiable—seemed odd to her.[7] Her viewpoint, I suspect, would be the more likely one to apply in any cultural group in which "choice," "willingness," and the importance of "understanding" are less emphasized than "role," "duty," "obligation," or the importance of "training."

I close this final section with the most general proposal of all. All societies need to find some balance between the interests of the individual and the interests of other members of the group. No unit can survive for long if each of its members pursues an unconstrained policy of self-interest. What children need to learn, and what parents convey, is the particular balance expected among competing interests. What parents seek to convey also is the way in which this balance may vary from one person to another. Older children may be expected to give way, to make "sacrifices" for younger ones. Girls, and mothers, may be expected to place the interests of others above their own. Children's interests may be expected to give way to those of adults. From this general perspective, household work patterns become one way by which the expected relationships between "self" and "others"—the patterns of allowable self-interest, of relative place, of reasonable interdependence—are conveyed, learned, negotiated, and changed. Work patterns are certainly not the only ways by which these relationships are taught. In cultures in which children make some work contribution, however, these contributions provide a set of practices in which the general concepts may be embedded and discovered both by children and by researchers.

## Acknowledgments

The research described in this chapter was supported financially by grants from the Australian Research Committee and the Macquarie University Research Committee. It is part of a project concerned with parents' and children's ideas about parenting and family relationships. I am especially indebted to Jennifer Bowes and Pamela Warton for their involvement throughout this project, and to several others who were particularly involved in the early studies (notably, Judy Cashmore, Lesley Dawes, Susan Delaney, and Rosemary Knight).

# Notes

1. A general review of methods and models in studies of parents' ideas, actions, and affect is offered in Goodnow (1984, 1985a, 1988b).

2. The two types of jobs also attract, in different degrees, the two types of reasons that White and Brinkerhoff (1981) reported for a U.S. sample when parents were asked for reasons for job assignments in general. The reasons were predominantly of two types: (a) "jobs build character or a sense of responsibility," and (b) "we're family." Our Anglo parents, when we asked separately about the value of two specific jobs (one self-care in type, one family care), gave "character and responsibility" answers more often for the self-care job, and "family" answers more often for the family-care job (Goodnow & Delaney, 1989).

3. Comments of this type emerged both in the descriptions of "low moments" and in responses to the following question: "If your child was not doing his or her job—more than just once or twice—what would you say about it?"

4. This point is made especially in Quinn and Holland's (1987) account of cultural models, and in feminist analyses of dichotomies (e.g., male vs. female. public vs. private, and instrumental vs. expressive) as socially constructed rather than as "natural" or "given" (see Goodnow, 1985b; Moi, 1985).

5. The general issue of cross-generation agreement, cutting across several content areas, is discussed in Cashmore and Goodnow (1985) and in Goodnow (1985a, 1992). With the exception of questions about the importance of being "neat" and "obedient" in the Cashmore and Goodnow (1985) study, however, this content does not focus on household tasks. Research on agreement across generations about payment for household jobs is currently under way in conjunction with Pamela Warton.

6. For some identifications from children's points of view, see Goodnow and Burns (1985).

7. In case the question should arise in a reader's mind, this is a well-educated Anglo.

# References

Abelson, R. P. (986). Beliefs are like possessions. *Journal for the Theory of Social Behavior, 16,* 223–250.

Backett, K. C. (1982). *Mothers and fathers.* London: Macmillan.

Becker, J. A., & Goodnow, J. J. (1991). "What's the magic word?" "Were you born in a tent?"—The challenge of accounting for parents' use of indirect forms of speech with children. *Newsletter of Laboratory of Comparative Human Cognition, 13,* 55–58.

Belsky, J., Lang, M., & Huston, T. L. (1986). Sex-typing and division of labor as determinants of marital change across the transition to parenthood. *Journal of Personality and Social Psychology, 50,* 517–522.

Belsky, J., Rovine, M., & Fish, M. (1989). The developing family system. In M. Gunnar (Ed.), *Systems and development, Minnesota Symposium of Child Psychology* (Vol. 22, pp. 119–166). Hillsdale, NJ: Erlbaum .

Cashmore, J., & Goodnow, J. J. (1985). Agreement between generations: A two-process model. *Child Development, 56,* 493–501.

Clark, M. (1984). Implications of relationship type for understanding compatibility. In W. Ickes (Ed.), *Compatible and incompatible relationships* (pp. 119–140). New York: Springer-Verlag.

Feather, N. T. (1991). Variables relating to the allocation of pocket money to children: Parental reasons and values. *British Journal of Social Psychology, 30,* 221–234.

Garfinkel. H. (1967). *Studies in ethnomethodology.* Englewood Cliffs, NJ: Prentice-Hall.

Goodnow, J. J. (1984). Parent's ideas about parenting and development: A review of issues and recent work. In M. E. Lamb, A. L. Brown, & B. Rogoff (Eds.), *Advances in developmental psychology* (Vol.3, pp. 193–242). Hillsdale, NJ: Erlbaum.

Goodnow, J. J. (1985a). Change and variation in parents' ideas about childhood and parenting. In I. E. Sigel (Ed.), *Parental belief systems* (pp. 235–270). Hillsdale, NJ: Erlbaum.

Goodnow, J. J. (1985b). Topics, methods, and models: Feminist challenges in social science. In J. J. Goodnow & C. Pateman (Eds.), *Women, social science, and public policy* (pp. 1–31). Sydney: Allen & Unwin.

Goodnow, J. J. (April, 1987). *The distributive justice of work.* Paper presented at biennial meeting of the Society for Research in Child Development, Baltimore.

Goodnow, J. J. (1988a). Children's household work: Its nature and functions. *Psychological Bulletin, 103,* 5–26.

Goodnow, J. J. (1988b). Parents' ideas, actions and feelings: Models and methods from developmental and social psychology. *Child Development, 59,* 286–320.

Goodnow, J. J. (1992). Parents' ideas, children's ideas: The bases of congruence and divergence. In I. Sigel, A. McGillicuddy-DeLisi, & J. J. Goodnow, (Eds.), *Parental belief systems* (pp. 292–318). Hillsdale, NJ: Erlbaum.

Goodnow, J. J., & Bowes, J. M. (1994). *Men, women, and household work: Couples illustrating change.* Sydney/New York: Oxford University Press.

Goodnow, J. J., Bowes, J. A., Warton, P., Dawes, L., & Taylor, A. (1991). Would you ask someone else to do this task? Parents' and children's ideas about household work requests. *Developmental Psychology, 27,* 817–828.

Goodnow, J. J., & Burns, A. M. (1985). *Home and school: Child's eye views.* Sydney: Allen & Unwin.

Goodnow, J. J., Cashmore, J., Cotton, S., & Knight, R. (1984). Mothers' developmental timetables in two cultural groups. *International Journal of Psychology, 19,* 193–205.

Goodnow, J. J., & Collins, W. A. (1990). *Development according to parents: The nature, sources, and consequences of parents' ideas.* London: Erlbaum.

Goodnow, J. J., & Delaney, S. (1989). Children's household work: Differentiating types of work and styles of assignment. *Journal of Applied Developmental Psychology, 10,* 209–226.

Goodnow, J. J., & Warton, P. M. (1991). The social bases of social cognition: Interactions about work and their implications. *Merrill-Palmer Quarterly, 37,* 27–58.

Goodnow, J. J., & Warton, P. M. (1992a). Contexts and cognitions: Taking a pluralist view. In P. Light & G. Butterworth (Eds.), *Context and cognition* (pp. 157–177). Cambridge: Cambridge University Press.

Goodnow, J. J., & Warton, P. M. (1992b). Understanding responsibility: Adolescents' views of delegation and follow-through in the family. *Social Development, 1,* 87–106.

Hinde, R. A. (1974). *Towards understanding relationships.* London: Academic Press.

Holland, D., & Quinn, N. (1987) (Eds.). *Cultural models in language and thought.* Cambridge: Cambridge University Press.

Holy, L., & Stuchlik, M. (1981). *The structure of folk models.* New York: Academic Press.

Mancuso, J. C., & Lehrer, R. (1986). Cognitive processes during reactions to rule violation. In R. D. Ashmore & D. M. Brodzinsky (Eds.), *Thinking about the family: Views of parents and children* (pp. 67–93). Hillsdale, NJ: Erlbaum.

Miller, J., & Yung, S. (1990). The role of allowances in adolescent socialization. *Youth and Society, 22,* 137–159.

Moi, T. (1985). *Sexual/textual politics: feminist literary theory.* London: Methuen.

Molinari, L., Emiliani, F. & Carugati, F. (1992). Development according to mothers: a case of social representations. In M. von Cranach, W. Doise, & G. Mugny (Eds.), *Social representations and the social bases of knowledge.* Bern: Hans Huber.

Mugny, G. & Carugati, F. (1985). *L'intelligence au pluriel: Les représentations sociales de l'intelligence et de son développement.* Cousset: Editions Delval. (Published in English, 1989, under the title "*Social representations of intelligence*" by Cambridge University Press)

Newson, J., & Newson, E. (1976). *Seven years old in the home environment.* London: Allen & Unwin.

Ninio, A. (1979). The naive theory of the infant and other maternal attitudes in two subgroups in Israel. *Child Development, 50,* 976–980.

Ortner, S. (1985). Theory in anthropology since the sixties. *Comparative Study of Society and History, 26,* 126–166.

Palacios, J. (1990). Parents' ideas about the development and education of their children: Answers to some questions. *International Journal of Behavioral Development, 13,* 137–155.

Quinn, N. & Holland, D. (1987). Culture and cognition. In D. Holland & N. Quinn (Eds.), *Cultural models in language and thought* (pp. 3–42). Cambridge: Cambridge University Press.

Reid, B. V., & Valsiner, J. (1986). Consistency, praise, and love: Folk theories of American parents. *Ethos, 14,* 1–15.

Rosch, E. (1978). Principles of categorization. In E. Rosch & B. B. Lloyd (Eds.), *Cognition and categorization* (pp. 27–48). Hillsdale, NJ: Erlbaum.

Salzman, P.C. (1981). Culture as enhabilmentis. In L. Holy & M. Stuchlik (Eds.), *The structure of folk models* (pp. 233–256). New York: Academic Press.

Schank, R., & Abelson, R. (1977). *Scripts, plans, goals and understanding.* New York: Wiley.

Smetana, J. G. (1988). Adolescents' and parents' conceptions of parental authority. *Child Development, 59,* 321–335.

Straus, J. A. (1962). Work rules and financial responsibility in the socialization of farm, fringe, and town boys. *Rural Sociology, 27,* 257–284.

Super, C. M., & Harkness, S. (1986). The developmental niche: A conceptualization of the interface of child and culture. *International Journal of Behavioral Development, 9,* 546–569.

Titmuss, R. I. (1970). *The gift relationship: From human blood to social policy.* London: Allen & Unwin.

Warton, P. M., & Goodnow, J. J. (1991). The nature of responsibility: Children's understanding of "your job". *Child Development, 62,* 156–165.

Warton, P. M., & Goodnow, J. J. (in press). For love or money: Parents' practices and ideologies related to children's household work. *International Journal of Behavioral Development.*

Warton, P. M., Goodnow, J. J., & Bowes, J. A. (1992). Teaching as a form of work: Effects of teachers' roles and role definitions on working to rule. *Australian Journal of Education, 36,* 170–180.

Wertheim, E. S. (1975). The science and typology of family systems II. Further theoretical and practical considerations. *Family Process, 14,* 285–309.

West, C., & Zimmerman, D. H. (1987). Doing gender. *Gender and Society, 1,* 125–151.

White, L. K. & Brinkerhoff, D. B. (1981). Children's work in the family: Its significance and meaning. *Journal of Marriage and the Family, 43,* 789–798.

Whiting, B. B. (1980). Culture and social behavior: A model for the development of social behavior. *Ethos, 8,* 95–116.

Zelizer, V. (1985). *Pricing the priceless child.* New York: Basic Books.

# How Mayan Parental Theories Come into Play

Suzanne Gaskins

The behaviors that parents exhibit toward their children and expect from them in daily interaction are complexly determined. The immediate physical and social contexts of interaction; the current desires, obligations, and preoccupations of both the parent and child; the history of parent–child interaction built up over both the day and the child's lifetime and the expectations that come with that history—all these local factors contribute to a particular pattern of behavior seen between parent and child. These factors are in turn influenced by more abstract and more general cultural beliefs about *what* the child should become, including such topics as the nature of the self, social interaction, work, and play. Thus, to interpret the ultimate and idealized goal of parents' actions toward their children, one should have a broad understanding of their cultural beliefs as a whole.

But, cultures also provide parents with particular theories about *how* children become functional members of their culture. These include the nature of children, how they develop and learn, and the parents' role in socializing children. Understanding these beliefs, and the priorities thus perceived by the parents, provides the basis for understanding any parent's cultural motivations that underlie the specifics of the way they structure their children's experiences and thus influence the children's development. Without such a foundation, parents' actions toward their children are either uninterpretable or interpretable only by our own cultural system of beliefs and values that we as researchers carry with us. To interpret parents' actions toward and expectations of their children meaningfully, we must first understand their cultural goals as parents.

At the same time, the beliefs themselves do not provide a complete answer to the question of how socialization takes place. Rather, only considering how those beliefs are instantiated in everyday interaction will provide the necessary information. Because every culture's set of beliefs about children and parents will be different, each will be a unique influence on the nature of children's experience. Only by considering the specific details of many such instances can we hope to understand in a more general way how parental ethnotheories influence the more general processes of socialization and development (Mead, 1963).

This chapter provides a case study of how parental theories are applied in a single culture. A brief overview of the Yucatec Maya culture will be followed by a description of the distinguishable phases of children's development. Then, the theories held by Yucatec Mayan parents about how children become adults and the role of parents in that process are discussed. Finally, in order to explore the relationship between theory and practice, the topic of how these theories influence young children's play in everyday interaction is discussed.

Children's play is a behavior often assumed in our own culture to be an example of individual expression, motivated by the child's own cognitive, social, and emotional agendas (e.g., Piaget, 1962; Freud, 1950; Vygotsky, 1967). Given our assumptions, the study of play promises particularly revealing insights into how parents' theories about their children lead to particular structurings of their children's environments, which in turn influence the course of development.

# Ethnographic Overview

The Mayan Indians of Yucatan, Mexico, are historically related to the ancient Mayan peoples whose civilizations flourished during the pre-Columbian era. The Mayan people, in the face of the torture and destruction of their civilization by the conquest, fled to the jungle, taking with them only the knowledge of everyday practices. Many of these practices persist today in traditional remote villages now melded with both colonial Spanish and modern Mexican culture.

The research reported here was conducted over a period of 15 years in a remote, traditional Mayan village in the municipio of Chemax located in the eastern part of the state of Yucatan, Mexico; it reflects an accumulated total of about 4 years of fieldwork in this village. All work has been done in Yucatec Maya, the language spoken in the village.

The village has a population of about 800 inhabitants. The existance of both a colonial church and two good water sources in the village suggest that it has been a population site for at least several hundred years. Almost all the men are subsistence farmers, raising primarily corn, beans and squash for their own family's consumption but also a few cash crops to sell in Valladolid, a large market town about 1 hour away, or in Cancun, a large Mexican tourist development 3 hours away. Yucatec Maya is the language of the village, and most women and young children are monolingual speakers; some men and many teenagers are bilingual to some degree in Spanish.

One of the factors that shapes children's experiences is the physical conditions in which they live. Families in the community studied live in compounds of about 50 x 50 meters square arranged in a grid formation off the main square. Within a compound there are typically one or two houses (depending on a family's wealth and composition), a garden area, a pen for pigs, fruit trees, an area for clothes washing and drying, and an area of bushes used as a latrine. The houses themselves vary in size (from 3 x 4 meters up to 4 x 8 meters), shape (traditional oval with thatch roof or rectangular with laminated cardboard roof), and quality. House floors are usually packed dirt. House walls are constructed of a closely bunched row of posts stuck in the ground and anchored to the house frame, providing a minimal visual, auditory, or psychological barrier between house and yard. There are two doors, on opposite sides of the house, providing most of the light in the house. One end of the house is used as the kitchen area, with three large stones forming a fire pit as the hearth, a small low table with stools for making tortillas and eating, a higher counter for storage and work space, water storage containers, and pots and utensils hung from the sticks of the wall. The rest of the house is used for other daytime activities and becomes the bedroom at night when hammocks are hung throughout the house. Bathing is done in an inconspicuous area of the house or in a small structure in the compound.

Poorer families in the village have few other possessions. Clothes are stored in an old hammock or cardboard box. A few day's supply of corn and beans may be stored in the house, along with a supply of firewood. Wealthier families have many more possessions, including a Western-style table and chairs, a wardrobe, a television, and perhaps a refrigerator for selling soft drinks to their neighbors. But in every household in town, food (whether it is beans or meat) is cooked over a hearth with a wood fire and eaten with tortillas, and everyone sleeps in a hammock. Most families, by working hard and relying on the grace of God, are able to produce enough to be fed, clothed, and sheltered, at least to some minimum standard, and only a few are able to accumulate significant wealth.

Another important factor shaping children's lives is the nature of the culture's social organization and how social relations are structured.

Social organization at the village level is provided by two lines of authority, one in charge of land and production and the other in charge of interpersonal relations. Land is held collectively by the community, and each adult male has the right to cultivate a certain amount of land each year; in exchange, he accepts certain community obligations. Most community decisions are agreed on by the consensus of adult males at town meetings, but most economic, social, and religious activity is organized at the level of the household compound.

Compounds may contain a single nuclear family unit of husband, wife, and offspring (which can number up to 12). But many households are three generational, either because there is a recently married son who has remained with his wife and children in his parents' compound or because there is an elderly parent who is now dependent on his or her children. It is preferred to have both religious and civil ceremonies to begin a marriage, but many couples elope because of financial pressure or their parents' failure to agree to the union. Divorce, or dissolving of an informal union, occurs infrequently; the death of a spouse during the childbearing years is also infrequent now with better health care. Most adults who lose their partner try to remarry if possible, as the division of labor is organized by gender.

Perhaps one of the most important factors influencing children's socialization is the nature of the activities the children will be expected to engage in when they become adults. Both men's and women's work is organized around corn and the associated agricultural and religious practices (see Redfield & Villa Rojas, 1934; and Steggerda, 1941, for good descriptions of traditional agricultural and religious practices). Men are most directly responsible for growing corn (and the other food products eaten with it, such as beans and squash), using a slash-and-burn system that uses almost no modern technology. The fields surround the village and can be as far away as a 2-hour walk. During the periods of the year when cultivation is demanding, men are gone to their fields 6 days a week from sunrise to sunset. Other times of the year they stay home some days to do chores or take care of other business. Many men now also seek wage labor either by working in the neighbors' fields or by going to sell produce and livestock or working at temporary jobs in the nearby Caribbean coast tourist area.

As with the men, corn is the center of daily life for women. Women who are not burdened with young children sometimes help in the fields, but a woman's primary responsibility is to run the house and the yard (see Redfield & Villa Rojas, 1934, for detailed information about food preparation and other women's chores). Two or three times a day the women must prepare corn for grinding, prepare some beans or other side dish, and make tortillas for her family, forming them by hand and cooking them on a griddle over the fire. These tasks take many hours. She also washes her family's clothes by hand and takes care of the livestock and garden. Her work is constantly interrupted by the demands or needs of her children. Besides actually taking care of children herself, she also supervises the work and caretaking responsibilities of the older children.

Men's work is physically demanding, dangerous, solitary, and engaged with nature. To be successful at it, they must be good at timing when to burn and plant, find good plots of jungle to cultivate, anticipate how long a certain task will take, and be diligent about working enough in the face of no immediate pressure. In contrast, women's work is continuous, repetitive, long, and socially focused on the people within the compound. It requires them to have perseverance, to attend to and coordinate the activities of the members of the compound, to anticipate their needs, and to adjudicate when necessary.

Most of the religious practices revolve around corn as well and represent a creative fusion of colonial Catholic and pre-Columbian native beliefs. There are religious beliefs and practices associated with each stage in the agricultural cycle; with various points or periods in the life cycle; with various days of the year associated with patron saints or with anniversaries of recent deaths, and with illness and misfortune. Central to nearly all the religious activities is the theme of inviting the gods to come and share a meal with the participants; hence, food offerings predominate in any religious setting. Events associated with religious observances constitute the bulk of organized recreational social life and, from the native point of view, constitute the highlights of a given day, week, or year.

In addition to one's relations with the gods, one's physical well-being depends on several factors. There are many physical dangers in the environment, from snakes and scorpions to work with big trees and large fires. In addition, one's "soul" must be protected from evil spirits that dwell in the jungle or from the evil eye carried by some people. And a balance must be maintained in one's body between "hot" and "cold," by monitoring one's own intake of foods with these qualities and by limiting exposure to the elements or other people who are temporarily classified as being either one category or the other from their recent activities. For all these types of dangers, children are thought to be particularly vulnerable, and special precautions are taken to protect them.

Children are found everywhere in the Mayan village. Children in great numbers are found in public whenever anything interesting is happening. Except for the very youngest, they are usually found hard at work in their compound, in the field, or nearby jungle, or at school most of the day. Most children attend the local grade school, at least for a few years, where they learn basic literacy and some introduction to Spanish. The quality of the schooling has varied over the years, depending on the political situation and the individual qualities of the school's director and teachers. Few children continue past the sixth grade, because they must leave the village to do so. Children are taken to all social and religious events as there are few adult activities from which they are excluded as onlookers. The villagers are both very fond of and dependent on their children. Most feel that every child is a blessing and a helping hand; few feel that the economic demands of children are greater than their economic contribution.

This ethnographic sketch covers topics of belief and custom that organize the Mayan parents' everyday activities and interactions with their children as well as their expectations and concerns for them. It provides a context for understanding the following description of Mayan beliefs and customs focused on children and parents.

## Beliefs about Children

### Mayan Stages of Development

The following discussion is organized around the developmental distinctions made by men and women in the village. However, these distinctions are not a well-defined set of categories recognized by the culture as formal stages of development. Rather, I derived them from examples of the spontaneous but consistent use of the labels to describe the developmental stage of particular children. The characterizations of each stage are based both on spontaneous references and on interviews with parents about how children grow up. For babies, there are five distinctions made by the Maya which in general recognize some externally visible development in the children. For the rest of childhood, they make only four distinctions, and these reflect the extent to which a child "understands."

### "Very Little Babies"

The youngest of babies are "very little babies." They nurse and sleep on demand. The rest of the time they are laid in the hammock or held. At night they sleep with their mother (and father). Mayan caregivers pay a great deal of attention and are sensitive to the young baby's rhythms and needs. Mothers almost always can get a crying baby to stop, and no small baby cries "for no reason." At the same time, there is little face-to-face interaction. Nevertheless, a mother takes much pleasure in holding and tending to her very young baby and will have someone else attend to the baby only if other responsibilities demand it.

## "Lap Babies"

When babies gain some control of their heads and backs, they are then called lap babies. The younger lap babies still spend most of their time either being held or lying in a hammock. But once children can be held on the hip, they often accompany their sibling caretakers wherever they go, and they are thus exposed to the larger world beyond house and compound. As they become better at sitting up, they will be placed sitting on the floor, sometimes propped up. Babies at this age still sleep with their mother and are nursed on demand day and night. When they cry, they will be changed, nursed, rocked to sleep, bathed, or held by mother or a child caretaker.

## "Scooter Babies"

While sitting on the ground, the baby learns to scoot, sitting up, and thus becomes mobile. With mobility, the dangers of the house and yard become a real concern. The primary physical danger in the house is the open fire pit. Other potentially dangerous items are often within reach of the child as well. In addition, there is an increased danger because of his locomotion that the child's fragile internal balance of "hot" and "cold" will be disturbed by his sitting on damp ground, playing with water, or going outside when it is rainy or cloudy. A mother has only a limited range of options for distracting her mobile infant who is now at risk. Her most effective strategy is simply to monitor the infant's activity closely, moving the infant or removing some undesirable item from him as necessary. Children as young as 3 or 4 are often asked to help with this under their mother's watchful direction.

There is little attention paid to how infants spend their time as long as they are safe. It is thought that infants are learning little, if anything, at this stage. Direct social interaction with infants is usually transitory, often initiated by siblings as part of their own play or by any caretaker in response to the infant's unhappiness. Little speech is directed to infants, although there is often quite a bit of speech about them, especially directions to child caretakers. Scooter babies are never held responsible for their behavior (although their caretakers might be) (see Gaskins & Lucy, 1987, for a discussion of the assignment of blame and responsibility within the Mayan household).

## "Upright Babies"

Sometime after the first birthday, babies learn to stand and then walk, events met with comment and enjoyment by the whole household but little praise or encouragement to the babies themselves. The mothers' new concern about danger is children falling: The unlevel rocky ground found in the house and yard is a challenge and an unforgiving surface for new walkers. The children's roving range is therefore severely limited, and they are still often carried.

It is only in upright babies that parents begin to notice, comment on, and even encourage the infants' behavior, for instance, imitating them at work. Such imitation is seen as a sign that children want to and are trying to learn. Upright babies now have more direct methods of choosing with whom they spend their time. When tired, hungry, or otherwise needy, they usually seek out their mother. But otherwise, they often choose to stay close to their siblings if they are working or playing in the compound. Until they get in the way of work or find something dangerous, they are left on their own. More speech is directed at upright babies who now understand and will obey some directives. They are also now questioned about what they want or where they are going.

## "Talking Babies"

The next major developmental milestone occurs when children begin to talk (at around 18 to 24 months). This is seen as a gradual development, over time, and as something that happens by itself, rather than being taught. Talking babies are not particularly encouraged or even expected to use their new skill. In fact, talking babies still do very little talking in their homes; when they do, it is usually a single word or phrase, often in response to a question by a caretaker.

My own son's language development while in the village was the cause of much discussion initiated by the villagers which provided insights into their theories about language learning. It was generally reasoned that my son spoke English when he arrived at 15 months of age because he had heard English from his parents. I found their interest in explaining his speaking another language surprising because they are frequently exposed to children in the supply town who speak only Spanish; I can only surmise that the exotic nature of English was the source of their amazement that a baby could speak it. They would speculate that if I took one of their babies to the United States, he would return an English speaker. At the same time they would argue that if they went to the United States themselves, it would take them a long time to learn English. Interestingly, they mentioned almost nothing about the influence of environment when my child began to speak only

Mayan after a few months in the village, except for the fact that he could still understand English when we spoke it to him. What they chose to discuss about this peculiar case of language development suggests that behind their claim that a language just "comes out" of children (and the underlying asssumption that it is Mayan that is the language that so emerges), they can indeed credit children as being able to use input from the environment and as being quicker learners than adults.

"Talking children" in the village, continuing the trend begun when they became upright, spend less time with mother and more time out of the house in the company of other children of the compound. They nurse less during the day, until gradually, they are weaned. Nighttime weaning is done somewhat later and is considered a milestone for both mothers and children. Some adult other than the mother tends to the baby during the night until the baby stops waking to nurse. From then on, he or she will sleep with an older sibling.

### "Beginning-to-Start-Understanding Children"

When children can follow simple instructions to do a task and consistently follow directives, it is recognized that they are "beginning to start to understand," and they are no longer called babies. This may happen any time between the ages of 2 and 4 depending on the children's own abilities and the pressures on the household for them to become a productive member. The ability to focus on a task for a while is also taken as evidence of beginning to start to understand. Children also learn to take care of themselves: to feed themselves, follow proper etiquette for elimination, dress themselves, bathe, and go to sleep. Like chores, these are things that they "take up" from time to time, and in partial ways, without explicit instruction from parents or siblings, and without parents or siblings ever expecting the children to try before they know how.

### "In-the-Process-of-Understanding Children"

Children in this stage (beginning usually around age 4 to 6) can now do some things very competently, although they cannot be expected to show much judgment or reasoning ability. They must have chores specifically assigned to them and they usually must be monitored while doing these chores. But they now make significant contributions to chores even though much of their time is still spent in play or idle activity. They spend much of their time "going behind" older siblings on more complex chores and gradually begin to contribute to the chores as well. It is at this age that children's chores and informal learning begin to be determined by sex. Boys begin to go with their fathers to their corn fields, and girls begin to join in on the more complex household chores of food preparation and caretaking of younger siblings. Some time in this stage, depending on the inclination and needs of both the children and their families, they will also begin to go to the local school.

### "Having-Reached-Understanding Children"

Some time between the ages of 10 and 12, children no longer need to do their daily chores under someone else's tutelage. Both the ability to complete the task independently and the recognition and acceptance of responsibility to do so are taken as signs by parents that a child now "understands" and has "learned to work." Their limitations now stem partly from lack of adult physical strength and partly from having adequate understanding of how specific chores fit into an overall scheme for producing a living. Along with this development comes an expectation that children now *will* work, at least a good portion of the day. The locus of parental control is beginning to shift during this period from being shared by both parents (although often expressed by the mother) to being held solely by the same-sex parent.

### "Becoming-Adult Children"

By the time children reach their mid-teens, they finish the transition into adulthood in several ways. They finally take on the most physically demanding or organizationally complex jobs, working side by side with their parents as true partners. They also spend a great deal of time and effort sizing each other up as potential mates. Grooming and personal appearance become important, and dances are especially valued because they offer a chance to interact, even if only for a few moments.

Boys, who now have fields of their own, have many of the responsibilities and privileges of a man. They may now vote at town meetings; they must also give their labor to town projects and serve from time to time as town police. They are free to decide how and where to spend their free time and their own money. Girls have much less freedom of movement granted to them, but they eagerly look for opportunities during their daily chores to discuss their expanding social world with sisters, neighbors, or other friends close in age.

## Beliefs about Development

During both infancy and childhood, children are not usually described as having successfully finished one developmental milestone and being ready to take on the next one. Rather, they are described in terms of being in the process of doing something new; development is seen as an ongoing approximation of a change, so subtle that it is rarely proclaimed that a child has accomplished that change. Linguistically, the expressions used to characterize children's development when parents are talking spontaneously about their children are usually in the progressive—their speech is "coming out" or their understanding is "beginning to come into being." Mothers explicitly stressed how gradual development is, how each new skill is learned "little by little."

Development is seen not only as gradual and continuous but also as largely natural and automatic. In terms of many characteristics, including intelligence, talent, and disposition, children are thought to be influenced almost completely by innate forces that are beyond both their own and their parents' ability to change or control. As a result, Mayans are not particularly concerned about monitoring their children's development in terms of age norms or comparisons with other children. If asked why an individual child is a certain way, the invariable response is, "That's just his way of being." For children, it means they, too, do not feel pressured to change or conform, are not particularly reflective or concerned about either their strengths or shortcomings (although they may be able to list them accurately), and do not compare themselves directly with others.

Because parents believe that development just happens, that children move to a new stage by themselves, they do not feel the need either to take the direct initiative to teach children who fail to meet some developmental ideal or to feel anxiety about their responsibility for it. Parents do recognize that children sometimes respond to such input from the environment as objects on the floor or speech going on around them. But these are characteristics of the environment that are always present and are taken for granted; they do not need to be actively created by a concerned parent. Likewise, there is an understanding that changes in children may lead to changes in the caregiving. They recognize that children will not scoot until they are seated on the floor, but it is assumed that children will no longer be content to lie in a hammock if they are ready to sit and scoot. While they must do something to allow children to learn the new skill, they feel their facilitation is contingent upon the initiation of the babies.

Once development is not tightly connected with age, knowing the age of children becomes relatively unimportant. Frequently, neither the parent nor the child knows offhand how old the child is, especially once the child is beyond being considered a "baby." The primary reason given for keeping track of a child's age is to be able to give the age to government authorities for receiving inoculations or registering the child for school. On such occasions, a child's birth certificate is taken from its safe storage place to prove the child's age; often the mother will look for the birth year with curiosity to find out how old her children are. At the same time, however, the day and month of children's births are remembered very well and celebrated annually.

## Beliefs about Socialization

These beliefs about development do not imply that children are not expected to learn; they are indeed. It is expected by parents that children will learn to perform all the tasks, as well as the motivations behind them, they will need to become good corn farmers and household managers, good citizens within the community, and good servants to God. This is accomplished gradually and continuously, with minimal formal instruction or testing of children's limits or abilities.

It is also expected that children will obey parental authority unquestioningly (see Gaskins & Lucy, 1987). Many parents feel that the only way that they can assert that authority is through the use of threats and the occasional use of force. (Many men feel the same about asserting authority over their wives.) Corporal punishment is therefore quite common, although many parents (especially mothers) express a dislike for hurting their children. The common wisdom is that if your children are not afraid of you, they will not obey you. The ideal method of sustaining their fear is to threaten often and impressively but follow through only when absolutely necessary. This leads to a style of interaction between many parents and their children of testing and asserting limits endlessly (often with loud voices and with great dramatics on the part of the parent) on trivial matters, often ending with the children's inappropriate behavior going unpunished, but virtually complete compliance by the children regarding important rules. A parent who beats his children regularly is not well regarded in the community, but a parent who allows his children to defy his authority on some important issue and go unpunished is even less well regarded.

In seeming contradiction to the strong emphasis on respect for authority, parents give children a lot of control over making decisions that influence their immediate and future well-being. Parents retain authority for making sure that children's work is done and done well, that they demonstrate proper respect for those above them and proper responsibility for those below them, and that they not cause trouble in the larger community. Children, once they are recognized as developing understanding (sometime between the ages of 6 and 8), are given the authority to decide many other issues for themselves, such as whether they continue going to school, whether they want to take medicine when they are sick, whether they will wear their shoes when going out into the jungle, and, when older, whether they will drink too much or how they will spend their money. By virtue of having serious responsibilities, such as caretaking of younger siblings, all children by this age know and understand the value of caution. Their behavior does not usually reflect ignorance or carelessness. While parents may try to influence their children's decisions on these kinds of matters, children going against their parents' wishes are not punished; often parents will simply shrug their shoulders, perhaps laugh, and drop the issue.

## Mayan Children's Play

In order to understand how parental theories influence children's play, one must consider not only the more general theories of development and socialization considered above but also the particular beliefs held about play itself. Mayans do not spend much time reflecting on the meaning or character of play. Adults assume that play is something that children "just do." One way of indicating that an activity has little worth is to characterize it as "just play." Children's efforts to participate in some work task before they have much ability to do it are dismissed as "just playing," even when the efforts appear to be serious. They believe that children play because it is in their nature to do so and because it makes them happy.

Babies are thought to learn how to play on their own, but it is recognized by some that a baby's play can be facilitated by giving the baby objects. The only kind of play for babies that is recognized is play with objects. Some face-to-face social play with babies occurs, usually initiated by a child caregiver, but it is not identified as play. Toddlers begin to become legitimate participants in older children's play. First they watch, then gradually imitate and follow directions from older children, and as they grow older, finally begin to help organize the play themselves. Adults are not involved in children's play, nor in the socialization of it.

Play is generally recognized as being pleasurable for the children: All children like to play, and younger children are eager to become included in their older siblings' play. However, parents differ in their opinions about how much children should play. Women typically permit their children to play some; men usually prefer to see their children engaged in some productive activity. This difference is probably due to the men's absence from the compound during much of the day. Mothers indicate that they like their young children to play because it allows them (the mothers) to get their work done. In some households, there is a particularly high value placed on hard work and evidence of responsibility and initiative. Also, households short of man-, woman-, and child-power do not have the luxury of letting even fairly young children take too much time from chores. In both of these kinds of households, play is not encouraged or even tolerated for any long periods of time. In other households, which are more relaxed either because of outlook or because of surplus person-power, play *is* tolerated to a greater extent, although it is not particularly encouraged, praised, or facilitated.

In all households in the village, the construction of the children's world limits the opportunities for play in two ways. First, play occurs only during those times that are not filled with work or school obligations. Playtime is thus both limited and unpredictable. Second, playmates are usually restricted to the children in the compound. This restriction supports cooperative play, for not only is there likely to be no appropriately aged competitors in the compound group in terms of skill, but the very basis of sibling responsibility (Gaskins & Lucy, 1987) precludes competition as a likely play strategy.

Within these limitations, there are number of ways that children play. Mayan children of all ages play by moving their bodies, learning their capabilities and limitations, and participating with their siblings in informal gross motor games. They also enjoy other kinds of socially focused play, often interacting with or exploring some object or animal they have gained possession of. Older children enjoy a few rule-based games, such as a variation of jacks played with rocks. Preschool children and older children also spend some time in pretend play (Gaskins, 1989), even though there are few props provided or even available to them. Such play, however, does not represent one of the child's primary activities. Even less frequent is play with language, in the forms of jokes or rhymes, reflecting a general cultural norm not to waste words in social interaction.

Certain kinds of dangerous play are never tolerated. For older children, this usually means putting limits on how they play with their bodies: Trees should not be climbed too high; running and other large body movement games should not get out of hand so that they lead to falling down. For babies, there are also physical dangers, like the firepit, from which parents protect their babies. But when asked about "bad kinds of play" in young children, parents focus on health concerns (e.g., eating dirt) or spiritual ones (e.g., playing with water, which is "cold," and would therefore jeopardize the baby's "spirit," which might be "hot," for example, from being in the hot sun or having just awakened from a nap).

In sum, play is not recognized as a valuable activity for children to engage in, beyond giving the mother time to work. Children themselves are needed to work in the compound and in the fields, and many children also go to school, so there is little time when they are free to determine their own activities once they cease to be babies. Play is at best tolerantly accepted by adults, and often it is discouraged or prohibited. As a result, there are few objects available to children for play, and virtually none that are intended to be supportive of or suggestive for play.

## Parental Theory Coming Into Play in Everyday Interaction

The picture of Mayan childhood and the beliefs that lie behind it suggest that from the earliest age, Mayan children receive relatively little intentional input from caregivers about the physical environment or what they should do in it, except for issues of danger. They also receive from adults little or no encouragement to play or guidance on how to play. To explore just how early and profound these influences might be on young children's play, an observational study was made of Mayan infant exploratory play (Gaskins, 1990). We have seen that there is little motivation provided by Mayan beliefs about development, socialization, and play for the construction of an infant-relevant environment or intentional modeling or encouragement of infant-appropriate play behaviors. The observational study looked at how these beliefs come into play through daily interaction and influence the nature of the play expressed by the infants.

A description of 12-month-old Mayan infant exploratory play and social interaction was developed from systematic and detailed observation of eight infants' everyday interactions with objects and people. (see Gaskins, 1990, for the details of this study). Characterizing these observations and comparing them with data available for middle-class U.S. infants allows us to discover whether the behavior observed demonstrates the influence of the cultural beliefs held by the infants' caretakers.

Most generally, the systematic observations revealed that the Mayan infants spend as much time interacting with objects as U.S. infants do. In fact, despite very different physical and social environments, the amount of time Mayan infants spend in a variety of activities is remarkably similar to the amount of time reported for U.S. infants (Clarke-Stewart, 1973), including manipulating (about 35% of their time) and looking at (6%) objects, moving around (6–10%), eating and nursing

(12–13%), looking at people (other than mother) (9–10%) and initiating interaction with them (2%), and crying and fretting (8%). The only general category that showed much difference was the amount of time oriented toward the mother, where Mayan infants spent about 10% of their time and U.S. infants spent about 22% of their time, with most of that time spent looking at mother (4% vs. 15%). These general descriptive data suggest that although socialization patterns in the two cultures do not have an influence on the broadest outlines of infant behavior, they do influence the amount of interest in or dependency on the mother, with Mayan infants demonstrating much less of an orientation toward her.

Although the amount of interaction with objects is about the same in the two cultures, the qualitative nature of the Mayan infants' exploratory play is quite distinctive. Most of the play time is spent in picking up and dropping objects (25%) or manipulating objects in simple ways, such as mouthing or banging (20%). None of these actions takes into account the characteristics of the particular object being used. Very little time is spent in complex exploratory play either of a general sort, such as relating two objects (9%), or of a specific sort, such as attempts to accommodate to the object's particular characteristics or functions (8%). In contrast, one study of U.S. infants at this age (Belsky, Goode, & Most, 1980) estimates that almost 40% of the infants' time is spent on such complex play. It appears, then, that although Mayan infants engage in quite a bit of object play, it is simple, undifferentiated play that yields little information about the nature of the objects played with.

Caregivers' mediation of objects in the environment is also simple and direct. They give objects to the infant and take them away, but they do not interact with the infant with the objects. Objects are rarely (4% of the time) actively mediated by caregivers, either verbally or physically. Comparable data available on U.S. infants (Belsky et al., 1980) suggests that mothers in the United States spend a significant amount of their time mediating objects (39%), most often verbally.

The infants' behavior reflects a division between the social and physical world as well. Most of the time when the Mayan infants are orienting to people around them, either by looking at them or vocalizing to them, they are not simultaneously engaged in interaction with objects (20% of the time vs. 4%). This relationship is reversed for U.S. infants, who spend more time looking at someone while interacting with an object than when not interacting with an object (10% vs. 6%) (McCall, 1974).

Taken as a whole, these data suggest that not only does the form of Mayan infant play differ from that of U.S. infants, but so also does its relation to social life in terms of both orientation and interaction.

These differences suggest that the Mayan infant's motivation for playing is not the same as the U.S. infant's, and that such motivation is not, therefore, universal, as has been assumed by both theorists and practitioners in the West. It appears that the Mayan infant does not engage in object play in order to master the environment or to control or participate in social interactions.

These findings directly reflect the cultural beliefs about the nature of children and play discussed above, as well as the pattern of daily life imposed by reality. Caregivers define their caregiving role in terms of insuring the safety and well-being of the child and in keeping the child content by responding to its needs and desires, not in terms of stimulation or interaction. They believe young children develop and learn largely independently of caregivers' behavior toward them. Moreover, they are involved in many other time-consuming tasks that are necessary for daily life, which gives them little leisure, and they rely on other children to take care of and be responsible for the well-being and happiness of the infant. They do not attribute to play any particular value except distraction or consider their own playful interaction with the infant as socially appropriate or desirable.

It is consistent with these beliefs that the caregiver would have minimal interaction with the infant using objects beyond giving objects to distract the infant and removing objects to protect the infant and that the infant would come to develop an interest in objects that is not mediated by others. The data suggest as well that the complexity seen in object play in U.S. infants may be a result of social mediation that encourages the infant to focus on the properties and functions of objects. It might even be argued that such complexity, along with the motivation to master and explore seen in U.S. infants, but not in Mayan infants, would be considered by Mayan caregivers a negative characteristic for infants to have. Concerns about danger, the workload of adults and older children, and the distribution of caretaking responsibility would lead to a preference for minimal exploratory play, thereby keeping the infant in one place, content, and out of trouble. And that is just the kind of object play found in their infants.

# Conclusion

This example of Mayan infant's exploratory play shows how culturally determined ideas about play can lead to the structuring of children's environments that spawn and support a style of play very different from the one taken for granted in our own culture. The example is particularly interesting because it demonstrates the extent to which the behavior of even very young children, only 1 year old, can be culturally mediated in important ways. It is also significant because this cultural mediation is found in a behavior that is usually considered to be both universal and biologically based.

It appears from pilot work on a wide range of Mayan children's play, which is similarly influenced by the pattern of cultural beliefs described here, that play *in general* has a fairly restricted and limited role in Mayan children's lives (e.g., Gaskins, 1989). More broadly, the cultural nature of play (Haight & Miller, 1992; Haight, 1992; Beizer, 1992; Farver, 1992; Göncü, Mistry, & Mosier, 1992) and the implications of this for theory and research (Gaskins & Göncü, 1992) are beginning to be recognized. But it must also be recognized that to achieve adequate interpretations of both the children's play itself and the parents' mediation of it as culturally constructed behaviors, research must also include an analysis of culturally specific parental theories of play in the context of their more general cultural theories of development and socialization.

More generally, one should consider that many if not all aspects of children's development and behavior may be influenced by culturally based parental theories of children's everyday behavior and on their development itself. This one study serves as an example of how one cannot understand children's development or interpret their daily experiences adequately without first understanding the culturally specific theories about development and learning held by their parents.

## Acknowledgments

The general ethnographic information reported in this chapter was collected as a collaborative effort with John A. Lucy. I especially thank him for his insightful comments on this chapter.

## References

Beizer, L. (1992, April). *Preverbal precursors of pretend play: Developmental and cultural dimensions.* Paper presented at the biannual meetings of the Society for Research in Child Development, Seattle.

Belsky, J., Good, M., & Most, R. (1980). Maternal stimulation and infant exploratory competence: Cross-sectional, correlational, and experimental analyses. *Child Development, 51,* 1163–1178.

Clarke-Stewart, K. A. (1973). Interactions between mothers and their young children: Characteristics and consequences. *Monographs of the Society for Research in Child Development, 38*(6–7, Serial No. 153).

Farver, J. (1992). *Free play activities of American and Mexican mother–child pairs.* Paper presented at the biannual meetings of the Society for Research in Child Development, Seattle.

Freud, S. (1950). *Beyond the pleasure principle.* New York: Liveright.

Garvey, C. (1977). *Play.* Cambridge: Harvard University Press.

Gaskins, S. (1989, February). *Symbolic play in a Mayan village.* Paper presented at the annual meeting of the Association for the Study of Play, Philadelphia.

Gaskins, S. (1990). *Exploratory play and development in Mayan infants.* Doctoral dissertation, University of Chicago.

Gaskins, S., & Göncü, A. (1992). Cultural variation in play: A challenge to Piaget and Vygotsky. *The Quarterly Newsletter of the Laboratory of Comparative Human Cognition, 14*(2), 31–35.

Gaskins, S., & Lucy, J.A. (1987, December). *Passing the buck: responsibility and blame in the Yucatec Maya household.* Paper presented at the annual meetings of the American Anthropological Association, Philadelphia.

Göncü, A., Mistry, J. & Mosier, C. (1992). *Cultural variation in toddlers' play.* Paper presented at the biannual meetings of the Society for Research in Child Development, Seattle.

Haight, W. (1992). *Belief systems that frame and inform middle-class parents' participation in their young children's pretend play.* Paper presented at the biannual meetings of the Society for Research in Child Development, Seattle.

Haight, W., & Miller, P.J. (1992). The development of everyday pretend play: A longitudinal study of mothers' participation. *Merrill-Palmer Quarterly, 38*(3), 331–349.

McCall, R.B. (1974). Exploratory manipulation and play in the human infant. *Monographs of the Society of Research in Child Development, 39*(2, Serial No. 155).

Mead, M. (1963). Socialization and enculturation. *Current Anthropology, 4*(2), 184–188.

Piaget, J. (1962). *Play, dreams and imitation in childhood.* New York: Norton.

Redfield, R., & Villa Rojas, A. (1934). *Chan Kom: A Mayan village.* Chicago: University of Chicago Press.

Steggerda, M. (1941). *Maya Indians of Yucatan.* Washington, DC: Carnegie Institution.

Sutton-Smith, B., & Kelly-Bryne, D. (1984). The idealization of play. In P. K. Smith (Ed.), *Play in animals and humans* (pp. 305–321). New York: Blackwell.

Vygotsky, L. S. (1967). Play and its role in the mental development of the child. *Soviety Psychology, 5*, 6–18.

# Parental Theories in the Management of Young Children's Sleep in Japan, Italy, and the United States

Abraham W. Wolf
Betsy Lozoff
Sara Latz
Roberto Paludetto

The manner in which families in different cultural and ethnic groups manage the sleeping arrangements of their children during infancy and the toddler years has received considerable attention in the anthropological, psychological, and pediatric literature. Such factors as infant survival, climate, house size and room availability, family size, presence of father, privacy, and dependence versus independence have been cited as influencing the proximity of child and parents during the night. Sleep practices in different cultures vary widely, from allowing children to sleep in close physical proximity to parents during the night to placing children in their own room and expecting them to sleep through the night without parental intervention.

Standard pediatric advice in the United States recommends the latter approach, advising that infants should fall asleep alone at bedtime and stay asleep alone during the night. Spock (Spock & Rothenberg, 1992) recommends that "children can sleep in a room by themselves from the time they are born. . . . If they start with their parents, 2 or 3 months is a good age to move them" (p. 212), and that "it's a sensible rule not to take a child into the parents's bed for any reason" (p. 213). Brazelton (1989) states, "A child shouldn't fall asleep in her parent's arms; if she does, then the parents have made themselves part of the child's sleep rituals" (p. 69). These recommendations have also been adopted by Comer and Poussaint (1992), two African-American psychiatrists, who advise in *Raising Black Children*, "If possible, it is a good idea to have your child's crib out of your bedroom by five months. . . . You are asking for trouble if you place him in your bed [in response to crying]" (p. 45). And, "If you must allow him in your bed, remove him to his own as soon as he falls soundly asleep" (p. 46). In our previous work (Lozoff, Wolf, & Davis, 1984) we summarized some of the concerns mentioned in the U.S. literature about the potential ill effects of parents sleeping with children: (1) cosleeping may interfere with a child's independence; (2) sleeping with parents may become a ritual that is difficult to break; (3) children who sleep with parents may be more likely to witness sexual intercourse, a frightening experience for some; (4) intimate body contact involved in cosleeping may be overstimulating to children; (5) cosleeping may reflect disturbances in the mother–child relationship or in the parents' relationships with each other; and (6) children who sleep with parents may develop more sleep problems. The prohibition against adult company at bedtime has proven so strong that in one study of cosleeping (Morelli, Oppenheim, Rogoff, & Goldsmith, 1992), a U.S. mother was reported to have put a pillow over her head to drown out a crying baby rather than comfort the child at bedtime.[1]

Nevertheless, cosleeping is routine in most other cultures and, until the 20th century, was the norm in our own culture. In a review of more than 119 societies, Barry and Paxson (1971) found that 64% of mothers slept in the same bed as their infants, and no other culture expected children to fall asleep in their own beds and stay asleep all night isolated from the parents. Thus, in a representative sample of world societies, the United States was the only one to put young children to sleep in their own room. McKenna (1993) argues that from an evolutionary and cross-cultural perspective, cosleeping may have survival value for the infant insofar as it assists in regulating breathing and, thus, may protect a child from sudden infant death syndrome. Similarly, Super and Harkness (1982), pointing to the widespread pattern of nightly waking and night nursing, suggested that pressuring infants to sleep through the night without parental involvement may be "pushing the limits of infant's adaptability" (p. 52).

Even in the United States, the recommendations against cosleeping are not routinely followed among all groups. African-American families report a high frequency of cosleeping (Litt, 1981; Medansky & Edelbrock, 1990). In our previous work we found that even though all-night cosleeping was rare, some degree of part-night cosleeping was common in white families as well (Lozoff et al., 1984). Another U.S. ethnic group that does not follow pediatric recommendations is the Appalachian. In her study of parent–child cosleeping in eastern Kentucky, Abbott (1992) reported that 71% of children 2 years or younger slept in the same bed or in the same room as their parents, and 47% of children between 2 and 4 years coslept. In this study, cosleeping occurred across all social classes, even though it was least frequent in families with higher occupational and economic status and in households with more rooms. The autobiography of Verma Mae Slone, *Common Folks* (1978), indicates that some ethnic groups in the United States are aware that they differ with pediatric recommendations: "I don't care what doctors say, I believe it is best for the mother and child to be together. . . . These new mothers are losing two of the greatest blessings that God gave mothers—the pleasure of sleeping with the child and letting it nurse. A closeness that cannot be understood unless you have experienced it. . . . How can you expect to hold on to them later in life if you begin their lives by pushing them away" (quoted in Abbott, 1992, p. 60). Elias, Nicolson, Bora, and Johnston (1986) reported that 60% of a group of La Leche League mothers (whose maternal practices resemble those of non-western cultures in that they were still breast feeding at 2 years) coslept with their infants for 1 hour or more during the night. In contrast, only 25% of a group of "standard care" breast-feeding infants who were weaned at 1 year shared their mother's bed. The findings of these studies indicate that sleep management practices even in the United States are heterogeneous, despite the uniformity of child-care recommendations.

Among the earliest reports on cosleeping in other cultures are those of Japanese infants. In particular, Caudill and Plath (1966) emphasize that this practice is not simply a function of lack of space in a densely populated country but reflects parental values regarding childrearing. These values are articulated by Caudill and Weinstein (1962): "In Japan, the infant is seen more as a separate biological organism who from the beginning, in order to develop, needs to be drawn into increasingly interdependent relations with others. In America, the infant is seen more as a dependent biological organism who, in order to develop, needs to be made increasingly independent of others" (p. 15). This suggests that whereas survival and practical factors may influence the practice of cosleeping, the decision to share the parental bed may also be influenced by cultural values regarding interrelatedness and independence.

Studies of Italian childrearing practices also report frequent cosleeping. In their study comparing the use of transitional objects in Italian rural and urban children with a group of foreign, mostly

Anglo-Saxon, middle-class children in Rome, Gaddini and Gaddini (1970) reported that the Italian children were more frequently breast-fed and for longer periods and more frequently slept in the same bed or room as their parents. New (1988) in her field study of a small central Italian town observed that caretaking styles and the infant care environment were marked by a wide range of opportunities for social interaction. Infants typically slept in body contact with the caretaker and would be wakened if someone wanted to play. "Infants commonly slept in the same rooms as their parents regardless of the availability of separate sleeping rooms. It was considered unkind to put an infant to sleep alone in a room" (p. 58).

The aim of the present study was to describe and compare the prevalence and pattern of cosleeping and other sleep practices among families of healthy children in the United States, Italy, and Japan. Although a number of studies have compared samples of U.S. children to either Italian or Japanese children, it has been several decades since some of these studies were performed. Furthermore, the different studies used differing methodologies to collect their data. Our study collected comparable information on five samples. Although information that directly assessed parental theories of child development was not collected, the differing sleep practices observed in this study, combined with parental comments about these practices and the relevant child development literature, will be used to consider parental beliefs about these young children.

# Methods

## Samples

The study included five samples of children: three U.S. samples (a group of white children, a group of African-American children, and a group of white children who were breast-fed for 6 months or more), a sample of Italian children, and a sample of Japanese children. A detailed discussion of methodological considerations of some of these samples is available in our other work (Lozoff et al., 1984).

The same general procedure for subject enrollment was planned in all studies. Healthy children between 6 and 48 months of age were enrolled by contacting families at the time of pediatric well-child-care appointments. The only criteria for inclusion were that a family was scheduled for well-child-care during the hours that the interviewer worked and that the child's primary caregiver was available. Families were chosen in the order of their appointments without input from the health care provider. For families with more than one child less than 4 years of age, the study subject was selected from the two or three qualifying siblings by predetermined random numbers. The pediatric facilities used to obtain the first sample of U.S. children comprised a random sample in the Greater Cleveland area, including private practices, city well-baby clinics, prepaid health plans, and hospital ambulatory services in Cuyahoga County. Because the number of African-American children in this sample was limited, a larger sample of black children was created by enrolling another sample from pediatric facilities that served a predominantly African-American population (again private practices, city well-baby clinics, prepaid health plans, and hospital ambulatory services in Cuyahoga County). To obtain a sample of infants with prolonged breast feeding (more like that in other cultures), a third group of U.S. infants was enrolled in pediatric practices known to advocate breast feeding. The interviews were conducted at the pediatric well-child-care appointment by experienced female health care professionals. An African-American interviewer conducted interviews for the larger sample of African-American children.

The Italian sample was enrolled through the well-baby clinic of a medical school in Naples, using the enrollment strategy and entrance criteria described above. The interviewer was an experienced Italian psychologist.

Although the plan for enrolling the Japanese subjects had been to follow the same procedure, this approach did not prove feasible for several reasons. Time was limited for subject enrollment because the study was undertaken when one of the coauthors was between the second and third year of medical school. In addition, there were special challenges of conducting research in Japan as a foreigner. Therefore, mothers were identified through an informal system of personal introductions from professional contacts in the Tokyo area. The only criterion for inclusion was that the mother have a healthy child in the desired age range. Prior to going to Japan, our coauthor received intensive training in administering and coding the interview. Upon arrival in Japan, she worked with a Japanese interviewer, a trained translator. Participating Japanese mothers were seen in their homes (Latz, Wolf, & Lozoff, 1984).

The demographic characteristics of the five samples are briefly summarized (see Table 15.1). Pair-wise comparisons of the five groups on background variables are reported in Table 15.1 and only the major differences are noted here. The sample of Japanese children was the eldest of the five groups. The mothers of the U.S. breast-feeding sample and of the Japanese sample had the most years of schooling, whereas the Italian mothers had the least; a similar pattern was observed for

**Table 15.1. Demographic Characteristics**

| | United States | | | Italian | Japanese | Significance and pair-wise comparisons[a] |
| | White | Black | Breast feeders | D | E | |
| | A ($n = 90$) | B ($n = 94$) | C ($n = 51$) | ($N = 66$) | ($N = 62$) | |
|---|---|---|---|---|---|---|
| Age (months) | 22.0 (12.1) | 22.9 (12.1) | 20.5 (10.6) | 26.0 (12.0) | 30.3 (10.1) | $F(4,358) = 7.2$*** A–E, B–E, C–E |
| Female (%) | 50.0 | 52.2 | 50.1 | 43.9 | 48.4 | $\chi^2 = 1.63$ (n.s.) |
| Mother's age | 27.6 (5.4) | 26.0 (6.3) | 28.7 (3.9) | 29.2 (5.3) | 32.0 (3.7) | $F(4,358) = 13.2$*** A–E, B–D, B–E, C–E |
| Maternal education (years) | 12.8 (2.9) | 12.6 (2.0) | 14.3 (1.9) | 9.1 (5.1) | 14.6 (1.9) | $F(4,358) = 34.0$*** A–D, A–E, B–C, B–D, B–E, C–D, D–E |
| Father's age | 30.3 (6.3) | 29.7 (7.7) | 30.8 (4.7) | 33.2 (6.3) | 36.6 (6.5) | $F(4,354) = 12.9$*** C–E, A–E, B–E |
| Paternal education (years) | 12.8 (3.5) | 12.9 (2.2) | 14.8 (2.5) | 10.6 (5.7) | 16.0 (2.0) | $F(4,348) = 22.5$*** A–C, A–D, A–E, B–C, B–D, B–E, C–D, D–E |
| Mother employed (%) | 19.2 | 39.8 | 22.0 | 46.2 | 22.6 | $x^2 = 20.5$*** A–B, A–D, D–E |

[a] A one-way analysis of variance was used to test overall differences among means. The Tukey test was used to test for pair-wise comparisons using an alpha level of $p < .01$ to control for experiment-wise error. The chi-square was used to test overall differences among proportions. The Fisher exact test (two-tailed) was used to test pair-wise comparisons using an alpha level of $p < .01$ to control for experiment-wise error.

* $p < .05$; ** $p < .01$; *** $p < .001$.

father's education. African-American and Italian mothers were more frequently employed outside the home.

## Procedure

Data were collected by means of the same structured interview in all samples. The interview protocol focused on actual occurrences in a well-defined, recent period of time, rather than on generalizations. Information on sleep patterns and practices, the child's behavior and development, and family structure was gathered by concentrating on the month preceding the interview. Interviews lasted from 30 to 90 minutes. Caregiver responses to interview questions were subsequently coded by two independent coder–raters. All disagreements were discussed and codes thus agreed on were used in the data analysis. The measures central to the present cross-cultural comparisons are described below.

The parental approaches to sleep management were coded in relation to those practices most frequently recommended in the U.S. child-care literature, typified by Spock (Spock & Rothenberg, 1992). Information was obtained on the following practices: setting a regular time for bed, parental enforcement of bedtime, establishing a bedtime routine, having the child fall asleep alone, handling bedtime protests and night waking firmly, avoiding bottles in bed, locating the child's bed outside the parent's room, and refraining from cosleeping for all or part of the night. For each practice the interviewer determined a family's usual approach in the month preceding the interview.

Cosleeping was defined as parents and children sleeping in body contact with each other. The extent of cosleeping in the month preceding the interview was coded in more detail as follows: unique (an isolated or extraordinary occurrence, such as a thunderstorm or vacation), occasional (more than once a month but less than three times a week), regular part-night (three or more times a week for part of the night), or regular all night (three or more times a week for all of the night). These patterns were dichotomized to compare cosleeping with noncosleeping children within each culture. To make the analyses similar to other studies, children who coslept occasionally or in extraordinary circumstances were grouped with noncosleepers (Schachter, Fuchs, Bijur, & Stone, 1989; Medansky & Edelbrock, 1990).

Coding cosleeping in the Japanese interviews posed special problems and dilemmas due to the widespread use of futons. Futons are Japanese bedrolls that can be taken up and stored in closets when not in use. Thus, a sleeping room can have different functions during the day. For study purposes, however, the use of futons made it harder to know whether a child was sharing the same bed with the parents (i.e., sleeping in body contact) or simply sleeping in the same room. To clarify a family's practice and to evaluate accessibility during the night, the interviewer asked mothers to help sketch the sleeping layout of each family. The sketches guided the coding of cosleeping.

## Statistical Analysis

Statistical comparisons of differences among the five groups used the chi-square test in analyses of categorical variables. The Fisher exact test (two-tailed) was used to test pair-wise comparisons. One-way analysis of variance was used to test differences among groups in analysis of continuous variables. The Tukey test was used for pair-wise comparisons. To control for experiment-wise error, given the large number of pair-wise comparisons involved, a probability value of less than 0.01 was used for both the Fisher exact test and the Tukey test.

## Qualitative Analysis

In addition to the quantitative coding of sleep practices, mothers were given the opportunity to explain their responses and give reasons for how the family approached sleep. Representative examples of these responses are given for each of the five samples.

# Results

## Parental Approach to Sleep Practices

Table 15.2 reports the responses of parents in the five samples to questions regarding their approach to sleep practices. Pair-wise comparisons of the five groups indicated that they varied considerably in how parents put their child to sleep. The white and African-American samples less frequently had a regular time for bed than the other groups; comparatively, the Italians more frequently lacked a bedtime routine. The Japanese were far less likely to have a child fall asleep out of bed, but—similar to the Italians—were more likely to have the child's bed in the parents' room. The breast-feeding and white U.S. samples were less likely than others to have the child's bed in the parents' bedroom. The children in the breast-feeding and white U.S. samples were also less likely to have adult company at bedtime, and the Japanese children were most likely to have adult body contact at bedtime. Although sleeping with a bottle in bed was not common in any of the samples, the Japanese children were less likely to have a bottle in bed.

**Table 15.2.** Sleep Practices

| | United States | | | Italian | Japanese | Significance and pair-wise comparisons[a] |
|---|---|---|---|---|---|---|
| Parental approach[b] | White A ($n = 90$) | Black B ($n = 94$) | Breast feeders C ($n = 51$) | D ($N = 66$) | E ($N = 62$) | |
| No regular time for bed (%) | 20.2 | 36.7 | 11.8 | 5.1 | 8.1 | $\chi^2 = 32.9$*** A–D, B–C, B–D, B–E |
| No bedtime routine (%) | 22.3 | 32.2 | 29.4 | 89.4 | 21.0 | $\chi^2 = 94.5$*** A–D, B–D, C–D, D–E |
| Child falls asleep out of bed | 24.5 | 40.0 | 17.7 | 24.2 | 6.5 | $\chi^2 = 24.1$*** A–E, B–C, B–E, D–E |
| Bed in parents' room (%) | 16.0 | 47.2 | 3.9 | 75.8 | 67.7 | $\chi^2 = 105.4$*** A–B, A–D, A–E, B–C, B–D, C–D, C–E |
| Adult company at bedtime | 36.2 | 70.0 | 19.6 | 54.6 | 66.1 | $\chi^2 = 47.4$*** A–B, A–E, B–C, C–D, C–E |
| Adult body contact at bedtime (%) | 28.7 | 45.61 | 19.6 | 40.9 | 62.9 | $\chi^2 = 28.6$*** A–E, B–C, C–E |
| Protests not firmly handled (%) | 65.4 | 68.4 | 35.7 | 66.7 | 71.4 | $\chi^2 = 6.1$ (n.s.) |
| Bottle in bed (%) | 29.8 | 30.0 | 17.7 | 28.8 | 9.7 | $\chi^2 = 12.2$** A–E, B–E, D–E |
| Regular cosleeping (%)[c] | 19.2 | 57.8 | 16.0 | 42.4 | 58.1 | $\chi^2 = 49.7$*** A–B, A–D, A–E, B–C, C–D, C–E |

*(cont.)*

**Table 15.2.** (*cont.*)

| Parental approach[b] | United States | | | Italian | Japanese | Significance and pair-wise comparisons[a] |
| | White A (n = 90) | Black B (n = 94) | Breast feeders C (n = 51) | D (N = 66) | E (N = 62) | |
| --- | --- | --- | --- | --- | --- | --- |
| Some all-night cosleeping (%) | 17.0 | 56.7 | 5.8 | 34.9 | 53.2 | $\chi^2 = 60.2$*** A–B, A–E, B–D, B–C, C–D, C–E |
| Some part-night cosleeping (%) | 42.6 | 80.0 | 37.3 | 54.6 | 72.6 | $\chi^2 = 41.9$*** A–B, A–E, B–C, B–D, C–E |
| Body contact for night waking (other than cosleeping) (%)[d] | 60.0 | 22.4 | 70.6 | 25.0 | 10.7 | $\chi^2 = 42.3$*** A–B, A–D, A–E, B–C, C–D, C–E |
| Waking not firmly handled | 92.6 | 98.3 | 100.0 | 95.8 | 100.0 | $\chi^2 = 5.9$ (n.s.) |

[a]The chi-square was used to test overall differences among proportions. The Fisher exact test (two-tailed) used to test pair-wise comparisons using an alpha level of $p < .01$ to control for experiment-wise error.

[b]Values represent the percentage of families for whom a given approach was the usual practice during the month preceding the interview.

[c]Regular cosleeping was defined as cosleeping three times a week for the month preceding the interview.

[d]This item assessed body contact other than cosleeping. Hence, black, Italian, and Japanese families are low, because many responded to night waking with cosleeping.

*$p = < .05$; **$p < .01$; ***$p < .001$.

373

**Table 15.3.** Childrearing Environment

| | United States | | | Italian | Japanese | Significance and pair-wise comparisons[a] |
|---|---|---|---|---|---|---|
| | White A (n = 90) | Black B (n = 94) | Breast feeders C (n = 51) | D (N = 66) | E (N = 62) | |
| Breast-feeding duration in months | 7.4 (6.2)[b] | 5.2 (3.7) | 10.3 (3.4) | 4.1 (3.2) | 6.1 (4.1) | $F_{(4,213)} = 16.2^{***}$ A–D, B–C, C–D, C–E, |
| Number of persons in house | 4.1 (1.3) | 4.1 (1.6) | 4.1 (1.0) | 4.7 (1.5) | 4.2 (1.3) | $F_{(4,358)} = 3.1^{*}$ |
| Number of rooms in house | 6.7 (2.0) | 5.9 (1.9) | 7.1 (2.2) | 4.1 (1.4) | 4.9 (1.4) | $F_{(4,358)} = 15.2^{***}$ A–D, A–E, B–C, B–D, C–D, C–E |
| Household density | 0.6 (0.2) | 0.7 (0.3) | 0.6 (0.2) | 1.3 (0.7) | 0.9 (0.2) | $F_{(4,319)} = 37.5^{***}$ A–D, A–E, B–D, C–D, C–E, D–E |
| Father present (%) | 81.9 | 46.7 | 100.0 | 97.0 | 98.4 | $\chi^2 = 105.2^{***}$ A–B, A–C, A–D, A–E, B–C, B–D, B–E |
| Siblings (%) | 58.5 | 51.1 | 68.6 | 78.8 | 61.3 | $\chi^2 = 13.9^{**}$ B–D |
| Grandfather present (%) | 3.2 | 7.8 | 0.0 | 13.6 | 14.5 | $\chi^2 = 14.2^{**}$ C–D, C–E |
| Grandmother present (%) | 6.4 | 24.4 | 2.0 | 16.7 | 19.4 | $\chi^2 = 20.3^{***}$ C–B, C–E |

[a] A one-way analysis of variance was used to test overall differences among means. The Tukey test was used to test for pair-wise comparisons using an alpha level of $p < .01$ to control for experiment-wise error. The Chi-square was used to test overall differences among proportions. The Fisher exact test (two-tailed) was used to test for pair-wise comparisons using an alpha level of $p < .01$ to control for experiment-wise error.

[b] Standard derivation in parentheses

$^{*}p < .05$; $^{**}p < .01$; $^{***}$, $p < .001$

374

The breast-feeding and white U.S. samples were less likely than the other groups to cosleep on a regular basis or to cosleep for part of the night. The African-American and Japanese groups differed from the other groups in terms of their increased likelihood for some all night cosleeping. The breast-feeding and white U.S. children were also more likely to have body contact (other than cosleeping) with children who woke during the night. No differences were observed among groups with respect to how firmly bedtime protests or night waking were handled. These behaviors were not firmly handled in any sample.

## Alternative Factors That Might Influence Sleep Practices

Table 15.3 reports such measures of the childrearing environment as breast feeding and household composition. In the five samples, the children in the U.S. breast-feeding sample, as expected, were nursed the longest, whereas the African-American children were breast-fed for the shortest time.

There were also several differences in household factors. Although none of the groups differed in terms of the total number of persons living in the home, the Italian and Japanese homes had fewer rooms and thus had a greater household density (i.e., the number of persons per room) than those in the three U.S. samples. The African-American sample differed from all groups in having the lowest percentage of fathers living at home. The Italian and Japanese families were more likely to have a grandfather living at home, and the African-American sample was similar to the Italian and Japanese families in terms of having a grandmother present. More than half the children in each sample had a sibling.

## Qualitative Analysis

In the course of the structured sleep interview, mothers were given the opportunity to explain their children's behavior at bedtime and when waking during the night and to give reasons for how the family approached sleep. Although these comments cannot be considered representative of the cultural group as a whole, they do provide an additional perspective on how mothers in the five samples view sleeping arrangements and their children's sleep behaviors.

Mothers in the white U.S. sample tended to focus their comments on their children's bedtime struggles and their children's problems in adjusting to separation at bedtime:

"The child had trouble falling asleep for the first month. Mother felt the nurses in the hospital spoiled the child by holding her too much instead of simply putting her to bed."

"The child will not sleep without its mother. The child is afraid to be alone. The child makes mother nervous and wishes that the child would sleep in her own bed."

"Mother is called back when she leaves her to fall asleep alone because the child just needs to see her and the child is bored. Child settles down right away when mother comes in to see her."

"Child calls mother back because she wants to kiss her one more time or talk about something. Mother says she wants reassurance."

In the U.S. African-American sample, mothers portrayed their children responding to the bedtime situation in an active manner:

"Child gets very active at bedtime and doesn't want to go to bed."

"Bedtime feeding stopped at 10 months when child threw bottle down, he was very eager to use a cup."

"Difficult to settle down at bedtime, at first mom thought she had colic."

In the U.S. breast-feeding sample, mothers cited the practice of cosleeping as a method of managing sleep problems:

"Mother lets child fall asleep in parent's bed, then moves the child to her own bed. If mother tried to put the child in her bed, she would cry and carry on."

"Mother puts child and his older sister in the same room to keep each other company."

"Child woke up and came to parent's bed, returned to sleep in their bed; parents were puzzled and thought maybe he wants more attention."

Mothers of Italian children focused on the use of cosleeping as a response to their child having problems falling asleep alone:

"The child wants his mother when it is time to fall asleep."

"It is difficult for the child to fall asleep without her bottle and being in her father's arms."

One mother directly commented on the cultural aspects of cosleeping, "This child cosleeps with her two brothers because Italian people love to sleep together always."

Mothers of the Japanese children uniformly described cosleeping as a response to night waking and missing their mother:

"He wakes to look for me."

"The child goes to [my] futon and stays until morning [because he misses me]."

"The child wakes twice a night, once for water, and once because he misses mother."

# Discussion

How a child is allowed to fall asleep is one of the earliest forms of culturally determined interaction with the child. Sleep practices are embedded in a set of childrearing behaviors that reflect values about what it means to be a "good" parent and how the parents are to prepare the child for entry into the family and the community. A useful framework for interpreting cross cultural differences is the varying emphases placed on autonomy versus interrelatedness. Caudill and Plath (1966) were among the first to suggest that the practice of cosleeping was not simply due to economic considerations of room availability but reflected a larger societal value of interpersonal interdependency. More recently, Guisinger and Blatt (1994) argued that the values of individualistic self-definition and interpersonal relatedness represent two distinct developmental lines which interact in a dialectical manner. Cultures, with their own unique indigenous psychologies, tend to emphasize one extreme or the other. "Western psychologies have traditionally given greater importance to self-development than to interpersonal relatedness, stressing the development of autonomy, independence, and identity as central factors in the mature personality. In contrast, women, many minority groups, and non-Western societies have generally placed greater emphasis on issues of relatedness" (p. 104). Guisinger and Blatt argue that higher levels of self-development are contingent upon both a well-developed sense of self and a sense of relatedness, which interact in a dialectical fashion at various points in the life cycle.

The distinction between individualistic self-definition and interpersonal relatedness is pertinent to the interpretation of results from the present study. We observed that, in contrast to U.S. white and breast-feeding samples, the Japanese, Italian, and African-American samples more frequently coslept on a regular basis and that grandparents were more frequently present in the household. These findings suggest that the minority and non-North American cultures represented by these samples may be characterized as emphasizing an interpersonal relatedness with regular cosleeping as an example of childrearing practices associated with this value. The cultural groups represented by the samples will be considered in turn.

The Japanese approach to childrearing is characterized by the primacy of the mother–child relationship and the instilling of a sense of interdependency that is later transferred to the child's relationship to the family and, still later, the group. Doi (1963) notes that the concept of *amae*–the feeling of dependency coupled with the expectation of indulgence–is particularly relevant to Japanese values in childrearing.

The Japanese emphasis on interdependency has been contrasted to an American emphasis on independence and autonomy in a number of studies summarized by Fogel (Fogel, Stevenson, & Messinger, 1993):

> The ideal is for the [Japanese] mother to create a relationship in which the infant is naturally drawn into considerate, interdependent, competent interactions with others. The first step is to satisfy the infant's desires for proximity, to accept and respond directly to the infant's proclivities and affectional needs. . . . In the United States, eventual self-reliance and self-assertion are valued. Infants are oriented towards areas in which they can practice and develop autonomy. However, parents attempt to control their children's self-assertion by appealing to their own authority. In this respect, American ideals of child-rearing and actual practice are often inconsistent, such that ideals of autonomy may contribute to parent child conflict. (pp. 48–49)

The emphasis in childrearing in Japan from the earliest stages is on participation with the group rather than on individual assertion.

Reporting on Italian families, New (1988) has commented on the powerful emphasis on family solidarity:

> While there was clear acknowledgement and encouragement of the infant as a member of the family social order, there was little recognition of the infant's increasing capabilities for autonomous behavior. In spite of mother's expressed rationale for infant care based on health and assumed physical needs, actual infant needs were often disregarded in favor of family routines. The unilateral relationship of the child to the family was thus maintained. (p. 60)

This emphasis on *la famiglia* extends beyond the nuclear family to the extended family.

The matriarchal structure of many African-American families suggests that cosleeping in these families may be related to family organization. Bell (1971) suggests that motherhood has traditionally been an important role for African-American women, perhaps even more important than the role of wife. The extended family, especially the grandmother, is a significant source of support and information about parenting (Stevens, 1984; Hale-Benson, 1982; Pearson, Hunter, Ensminger, & Kellam, 1990). In the present study, where fathers were present in less than half of the African-American households inter-viewed and grandmothers were present in nearly 25%, the mother–child relationship with the support of the grandmother may be the primary axis in many families. Furthermore, the high frequency of maternal employment outside the home in the African-American fami-lies in our sample may indicate that mothers do not have much time to spend with their children and use the night for further contact—or cosleep simply because they are too exhausted from working all day long to deal with the bedtime struggles and night waking that follow placing children in their own room to fall asleep.

Although most discussions of childrearing values and sleeping arrangements have tended to associate early separation at bedtime with independence and to associate cosleeping with interrelatedness, researchers on African-American child development have challenged this dichotomy. They note that whereas independence is valued in childrearing practices, interdependence and relatedness are also significant—an approach more consistent with that advocated by Guisinger and Blatt. In her study of African-American family organization and child development, Young (1970) observed that "the infant sleeps next to the mother in the mother's and father's bed, or sometimes with either parent alone" (p. 203). Yet, "The baby is treated as willful and assertive beyond his natural inclination. . . . [and] is highly stimulated and admired for his assertiveness, and his acceptance of authority is expected to be defiant. . . . Strong individuality is paired with strong interpersonal connectedness, not absorption in a group or acceptance of group identity as higher than individual authority, but merely relatedness as distinguished from isolation that characterizes individualism in the Western tradition" (p. 214). Ogbu (1994) also emphasizes the significance of early training for independence in African-American families when he notes that "purposive training in early independence and self-reliance make black children independent and self-reliant much earlier than white middle-class children" (p. 60). Thus, in the African-American family, cosleeping is one component of a set of childrearing practices that emphasize both strong interconnectedness and early independence and autonomy.

Childrearing by American middle-class parents has long been characterized by an emphasis on training for autonomy and independence (Whiting & Child, 1953). Pediatric recommendations that emphasize early separation from parents at bedtime have the effect of encouraging the child to rely on strategies other than the physical presence of the parent to ease the passage into sleep—a passage that is frequently difficult (Freud, 1965). The increased use of self-soothing by "transitional objects" or self-stimulation such as thumb sucking has been associated in several studies with a child being put into bed to fall asleep alone (Wolf & Lozoff, 1989; Gaddini & Gaddini, 1970; Hong & Townes, 1976; Ozturk & Ozturk, 1977). As we have suggested elsewhere (Wolf & Lozoff, 1989), childrearing practices that emphasize separation "may be teaching children not to rely on other people as a way of handling stress, but to rely on objects for comfort" (p. 292).

A rationale for the pediatric recommendations regarding separation at bedtime is that children left to fall asleep by themselves will become less dependent on parents to make the transition to sleep. The ability to fall asleep alone is, presumably, a developmental hurdle the child overcomes to achieve independence and self-reliance. Cosleeping is discouraged because it will encourage attachment to others at bedtime, leading to later dependence. Early cross-cultural reports that compared U.S. and Japanese infants speculated that the early separation of U.S. infants at bedtime facilitated independence, whereas cosleeping in Japanese infants facilitated an interdependence on family and group. Nevertheless, the literature on other cross-cultural groups suggests that these associations may be simplistic. African-American infants cosleep frequently, yet childrearing attitudes emphasize independence and assertiveness. How a child is allowed to fall asleep may be one developmental precursor of independent functioning, but other childrearing practices may modify whatever influence this has on either independence or interrelatedness.

The interaction between pediatric recommendations and childrearing values is not clear. A reliance on medical "scientific" advice could be influencing the manner in which children are managed at bedtime and during the night, particularly among white middle-class families. Alternatively, a cultural emphasis on early separation and individuation toward autonomous functioning may be influencing pediatric recommendations. In this latter alternative, both the practices of white families and the recommendations of experts might be reflections of the same cultural values. The fact that the sleep practices of white families are consistent with pediatric advice may mean that parents have internalized these recommendations to the extent that they represent a set of beliefs and behaviors about sleep management in particular and childrearing in general. In contrast to most other cultures, which rely on the guidance of elder figures in the extended family and community as authority figures regarding childrearing, U.S. culture has a long history (Stendler, 1960) of utilizing varying approaches to childrearing, many with scientific claims. Adherence to "scientific" recommendations appears to replace a reliance on the extended family in the transmission of childrearing behaviors and values. Rather than utilizing elder family figures who are more available in a closely knit extended family, the nuclear organization of white middle-class families and the emphasis on establishing distinct households may contribute to a reliance on expert advice in childrearing. This is consistent with results from the present study in that a greater number of grandparents were present in the households of the African-American, Italian, and Japanese families. Cosleeping may occur more frequently when an elder figure is present in the household and mothers may tend to rely—or be expected to rely—more on the advice of these "elder" figures than on outside expert advise. It is also possible that families try to provide the elder with a separate sleeping place, thus limiting the sleeping space available to the rest of the household.

The qualitative comments made by mothers during the course of the interview are consistent with the quantitative findings. In their comments, white and breast-feeding mothers recognized the difficulties the child had adjusting to nighttime separation as evidenced by bedtime struggles and night waking but seemed certain that adjustment to separation was desirable. In contrast, when the Italian mothers discussed sleep problems, rather than seeing separation as a desired adjustment for the child, they saw bedtime struggles as a need of the child to be with the mother, a need that should be gratified. Similarly, Japanese mothers consistently commented sympathetically on the child's dependency on the mother, feeling that the need to be reunited with her should be satisfied.

The present study is limited both in terms of the interpretation of cultural differences and in determining specific factors that are associated with cosleeping. First, the major differences in the demographic characteristics among the groups may influence the interpretation and generalizability of the findings: Japanese children tended to be older and their parents were older and better educated; Italian and Japanese households had more persons per room; African-American, Italian, and Japanese families had a greater proportion of grandparents in the household; nearly half the African-American families did not have a father present. Interpretation of such cultural differences as those observed in this study are potentially hazardous, prone to stereotyping and superficial explanations. Given the possible confounding with socioeconomic factors and the risk of oversimplification, the preceding discussion of cross-cultural differences is offered with considerable reservations. Second, the focus of this chapter has been on comparing ethnic and cultural groups regarding how they allow children to fall asleep at bedtime and sleep during the night. The presence of differences between samples on specific factors (e.g., greater cosleeping frequency and the presence of grandparents in the household) does not mean that within a specific sample these factors will be significantly associated with each other. The comparison of factors across samples does not permit inferences regarding the covariation of those factors within a sample. However, the comparisons reported in this study do suggest some areas for further analysis and investigation regarding the covariation of some factors.

Whiting (1981) summarizes the model for psychocultural research as follows:

> Features in the history of any society and in the natural environment in which it is situated influence the customary methods by which infants are cared for in that society, which have enduring psychological and physi-

ological effects on the members of that society, which are manifested in the cultural projective–expressive systems of the society and the physiques of its members. (p. 155)

Since its first description among the Japanese, cosleeping has been characterized as a childrearing practice that has enduring psychological effects in terms of facilitating either autonomy or interdependence. The findings of the present study support previous studies that report differences between young children in the United States and those in other ethnic and cultural groups. We suggest, though, that attributing such traits as independence or interrelatedness to cosleeping or separation during the night may be simplistic and ignores other childrearing factors that may encourage individual assertive functioning in groups that practice cosleeping—as in the case of African-American families—, or interconnectedness in groups that separate the child at night. It is not the aim of the present study to advocate for or against the practice of cosleeping. Certainly, the practice of cosleeping has a long history in human evolution and is culturally widespread. Nevertheless, the longitudinal studies to evaluate the risks in separating the child at bedtime or in sleeping with parents are simply not available. As in other childrearing practices, it may not be the specific practice itself, but rather the context and values that are the most important factors.

## Acknowledgments

The authors acknowledge the interviewing of study families by Nancy S. Davis, MSW, and Greta Waugh, M.D., and the coding of interviews by Lois Klaus, Steve Malone, several Case Western Reserve University students, and our Japanese and Italian collaborators. We would also like to thank A. Scott Dowling, M.D., Vonnie McCloyd, Ph.D., and Harold Stevenson, Ph.D., for their careful reading of earlier versions of the manuscript.

## Note

1. The sanctions against mothers sleeping in the same bed as their children is not limited to contemporary pediatric practice. Peiper (1963) notes:
    As late as in the eighteenth century the child slept with his mother. . . . The custom was so widespread—especially because it has ancient origins—and the conditions so bad that legislators many times had to take measures against it. For example, as late as 1817 the general law for the Prussian States decreed, under threat of imprisonment or physical punishment: "Mothers and wet nurses are not allowed to take children under two years of age into their beds at night or to let them sleep with them or others." (p. 611)

# References

Abbott, S. (1992). Holding on and pushing away: Comparative perspectives on an Eastern Kentucky child-rearing practice. *Ethos, 20,* 33–65.

Barry, H. III, & Paxson, L. M. (1971). Infancy and early childhood: Cross-cultural codes 2. *Ethnology, 10,* 466–508.

Bell, R. (1971). The relative importance of mother and wife roles among Negro lower-class women. In R. Staples (Ed.), *The black family: Essays and studies.* Belmont, CA: Wadsworth Press.

Brazelton, B. (1989, February 13). Working parents. *Newsweek,* pp. 66–77.

Caudill, W., & Plath, D. W. (1966). Who sleeps with whom? Parent–child involvement in urban Japanese families. *Psychiatry, 29,* 344–366.

Caudill, W., & Weinstein, H. (1962). Maternal care and infant behavior in Japan and America. *Psychiatry, 32,* 12–43.

Comer, J. P., & Poussaint, A. F. (1992). *Raising black children: Questions and answers for parents and teachers.* New York: Plume.

Doi, L. T. (1963). Amae—A key concept in understanding Japanese personality structure. In R. J. Smith & R. K. Beardsley (Eds.), *Japanese culture: Its development and characteristics.* Chicago: Aldine.

Elias, M. F., Nicolson, N. A., Bora, C., & Johnston, J. (1986). Sleep/wake patterns of breast-fed infants in the first 2 years of life. *Pediatrics, 77,* 322–329.

Fogel, A., Stevenson, M. B., & Messinger, D. (1992). A comparison of the parent–child relationship in Japan and the United States. In J. L. Roopnarine & D. B. Carter (Eds.), *Parent–child relations in diverse cultural settings* (pp. 35–49). Norwood, NJ: Ablex.

Freud, A. (1965). *Normality and pathology in childhood: Assessments of development.* New York: International Universities Press, Inc.

Gaddini, R., & Gaddini, E. (1970). Transitional objects and the process of individuation. *Journal of the American Academy of Child Psychiatry, 9,* 347–365.

Guisinger, S., & Blatt, S. J. (1994). Individuality and relatedness: Evolution of a fundamental dialectic. *American Psychologist, 49,* 104–111.

Hale-Benson, J. E. (1982). *Black children: Their roots, culture, and learning styles* (rev. ed.). Baltimore: Johns Hopkins University Press.

Hong, K., & Townes, B. (1976). Infants' attachment to inanimate objects. *Journal of the American Academy of Child Psychiatry, 15,* 49–61.

Latz, S., Wolf, A. W., & Lozoff, B. (1984). Sleep practices and sleep problems in U.S. and Japan. *Pediatric Research, 18,* 107A (Abstract).

Litt, C. J. (1981). Children's attachment to transitional objects: A study of two pediatric populations. *American Journal of Orthopsychiatry, 15,* 344–353.

Lozoff, B., Wolf, A. W., & Davis, N. S. (1984). Cosleeping in urban families with young children in the United States. *Pediatrics, 74,* 171–182.

McKenna, J. J. (1993). Cosleeping. In M. A. Carskadon (Ed.). *Encyclopedia of sleep and dreaming.* New York: Macmillan.

Medansky, D., & Edelbrock, C. (1990). Cosleeping in a community sample of 2- and 3-year olds. *Pediatrics, 86,* 197–203.

Morelli, G. A., Oppenheim, D., Rogoff, B., & Goldsmith, D. (1992). Cultural variations in infant's sleeping arrangements: Questions of independence. *Developmental Psychology, 28,* 604–613.

New, R. S. (1988). Parental goals and Italian infant care. In R. A. LeVine, P. M. Miller & M. M. West (Eds.), *Parental behaviors in diverse societies* (New Directions in Child Development No.40). San Francisco: Jossey-Bass.

Ogbu, J. U. (1994). A cultural ecology of competence among inner-city blacks. In M. Spencer, W. Allen, & G. Brookins (Eds.), *Beginnings: The social and affective development of minority group children (pp. 45–66). Hillsdale, NJ: Erlbaum.*

Ozturk, M., & Ozturk, O. M. (1977). Thumbsucking and falling asleep. *British Journal of Medical Psychology, 50,* 95–103.

Pearson, J. L., Hunter, A. G., Ensminger, M. E., & Kellam, S. G. (1990). Black grandmothers in multigenerational households: Diversity in family structure and parenting involvement in the Woodlawn community. *Child Development, 61,* 434–442.

Peiper, A. (1963). *Cerebral function in infancy and childhood.* New York: Consultants Bureau.

Schachter, F. F., Fuchs, M. L., Bijur, P. E., & Stone, R. K. (1989). Cosleeping and sleep problems in Hispanic-American urban young children. *Pediatrics, 84,* 522–530.

Slone, V. M. (1978). *Common folks.* Pippa Passes, KY: Alice Lloyd College.

Spock, B., & Rothenberg, M. B. (1992). *Dr. Spock's baby and child care.* New York: Pocket Books.

Stendler, C. (1960). Sixty years of child-rearing practices. In D. Apple (Ed.), *Sociological studies of health and sickness.* New York: McGraw-Hill.

Stevens, J. H. Jr. (1984). Black grandmothers' and black adolescent mothers' knowledge about parenting. *Developmental Psychology, 20,* 1017–1025.

Super, C. M., & Harkness, S. (1982). The infant's niche in rural Kenya and metropolitan America. In L. L. Adler (Ed.), *Cross-cultural research at issue* (pp. 47–55). New York: Academic Press.

Whiting, J. W. M. (1981). Environmental constraints on infant care practices. In R. H. Munroe, R. L. Munroe, & B. B. Whiting (Eds.), *Handbook of cross cultural development* New York: Garland STPM Press.

Whiting, J. W. M., & Child, I. L. (1953). *Child training and personality.* New Haven, CT: Yale University Press.

Wolf, A. W., & Lozoff, B. (1989). Object attachment, thumbsucking, and the passage to sleep. *Journal of the American Academy of Child and Adolescent Psychiatry, 28,* 287–292.

Young, V. H. (1970). Family and childhood in a southern Negro community. *American Anthropologist, 72,* 269–288.

# CHAPTER 16

# Maternal Beliefs and Infant Care Practices in Italy and the United States

Rebecca S. New
Amy L. Richman

The common ground between scholars in the fields of psychology and anthropology is readily apparent in recent attempts to understand the relationship between parental beliefs and caregiving behavior. A growing number of investigators are responding to this challenge by delineating the role of the sociocultural context as it influences adult cognitions and behaviors, particularly as they relate to the parental role. The purpose of this chapter is to contribute to the understanding of the complex and transactional relationship between the sociocultural context, adult ideologies, and strategies of infant care by describing infant caregiving priorities and practices in two contemporary Western societies, Italy and the United States.

## The Study of Parental Beliefs: A History of Benign Neglect

Until recently, the study of parental beliefs and attitudes has been limited in the history of developmental and comparative child development research, and those few studies on the topic have viewed child development outcomes as the dependent variable of interest. This focus—on the consequences rather than the sources or characteristics

of parental cognition—was due at least in part to theoretical orientations to development itself. Both psychoanalytic and behavioristic
orientations to development have emphasized the influence of the
childrearing environment on subsequent personality development. Related research was aimed at identifying critical (and observable) dimensions of child care, with little interest per se in the topic of parental
beliefs.

Early cross-cultural investigations of child care, many conducted
under the tutelage of John and Beatrice Whiting, were also informed
by a psychoanalytic perspective and focused on the relationship between observable childrearing patterns and subsequent child behavior
personality characteristics in various cultural settings (Whiting & Whiting, 1963, 1975). This research offered compelling alternative perspectives to Western theories of optimal child care and development, albeit
with scant attention to the topic of parental beliefs. Yet the cumulative
effect of these and related studies was to contribute to the developing
hypothesis that cultural imperatives of parenting play a major part in
determining both a mother's beliefs regarding her childrearing responsibilities and her strategies and ability to handle them (cf. Minturn &
Lambert, 1964). The classic work by Caudill and colleagues extended
the focus to the infancy period and provided a striking view of culturally
distinct patterns of maternal beliefs as they related to infant care and
development (Caudill, 1973; Caudill & Weinstein, 1969). An interpretation of cultural variablity in the maternal role was in marked contrast
to its contemporaneous counterpoint—that the mother–infant relationship was a result of primary evolutionary instincts (Bowlby, 1969).

The ability to examine the influence of cultural variables on
parental beliefs and role interpretations was facilitated by LeVine's
(1974) comprehensive review of four decades of anthropological research. From this vast data set, a transactional relationship among
culture, ideology, and parental behavior was identified, whereby
broadly construed cultural values as well as past and present environmental pressures play a major role in the determination of parental
goals. Parental goals, in turn, were considered to shape the environments of infancy and early childhood. This theory also provided an
explanation for the apparent inconsistencies found between mothers'
explanations and actual observations of their behaviors; mothers cannot always articulate why they do what they do because they are guided
by cultural imperatives whose function lies "beyond their awareness"
(LeVine, 1974, p. 228).

As the field of infant studies burgeoned throughout the 1970s,
there was a concomitant (albeit more moderate) surge of interest in
cross-cultural investigations of infant care (cf. Leiderman, Tulkin, &

Rosenfeld, 1977; LeVine, 1977; Lozoff & Brittenham, 1972). Even the persisting belief in pan-cultural patterns of maternal behavior (Lewis & Ban, 1977), however, failed to discredit the growing evidence supporting variation in adult perceptions of the tasks and risks of infant care and development as a function of the cultural context (Field, Sostek, Vietze, & Leiderman, 1982; Ninio, 1979; Snow, deBlauw, & van Roosmalen, 1979). Bronfenbrenner's (1977) ecological model of development provided a timely challenge as well as a framework to move beyond the study of observable behavior to consider contextual factors in adult behavior and children's development.

Research of the past two decades has contributed to a more sophisticated conceptualization of the origins, processes, and consequences of parental ideologies (cf. Goodnow, 1980; Goodnow, 1984; Goodnow & Collins, 1990). Yet, there remains a paucity of comprehensive studies on the relationships among and between adult beliefs, goals, and infant-care strategies in culturally diverse populations (Garcia Coll, 1990). In turn, a continuing theme in contemporary discussions of maternal beliefs and parenting behavior is the assumption of a singular maternal role, with a limited and predictable range of behavior (Ruddick, 1982) to be found within the "average expectable environment" (Scarr, 1992, p. 5). Variations in either case are deemed noteworthy only in instances of abuse or neglect.

Support for an assumption of diversity in parenting beliefs and practices can be found in a number of recent sources that challenge the notion of any one "average expectable" [infant-care] environment (Baumrind, 1993; LeVine, 1990, p. 454). Studies on maternal neglect and infant death (cf. deVries, 1987; Scheper-Hughes, 1987, 1990) provide a dramatic contrast to universal theories of "mother love" and emphasize, instead, the consequences of generations of loss on both maternal behavior *and* conceptions of mothering. Less poignant but equally compelling challenges to a pan-cultural model of the mother–infant relationship come from observations of multiple mothering among the Efe pygmies (Tronick, Morelli, & Winn, 1987) and diverse patterns of infant care in a variety of industrialized and nonindustrialized settings (cf. LeVine, Miller, & West, 1988). Infant caregiving among the Gusii of Kenya, Africa, as studied over the course of several decades, reflects distinctly diverse parental interpretations and socially organized means of "cultivating skill, virtue, and personal fulfillment" that take place in accordance with culture-specific goals for human development (LeVine et al., 1994, p. 274).

The cumulative effect of these studies and their related arguments has been to heighten interest in research on the ideological qualities of infant-care environments in contemporary societies and the role of cultural values in the structuring and interpretation of those infant-care environments. This chapter reports on a comparative analysis of two such studies in two Western industrialized settings, with LeVine's parental goals theory (LeVine, 1974, 1988) as the organizing framework for the analysis.

## Variations in Western Values, Beliefs, and Goals of Infant Care

Our findings are based on a comparative study of maternal beliefs and infant care during the first year of life in two contemporary Western settings: central Italy and a suburban New England area in the United States[1] The two studies were influenced by LeVine's (1974) parental goals theory, which views strategies of child care as responsive not only to the infant's biologically based characteristics and behaviors but also to culturally transmitted "prescriptions" for infant care based on environmental pressures and cultural values.

### Purposes and Procedures

The primary objective of the two studies was to delineate the role of cultural values in the determination of maternal goals, beliefs, and strategies of infant care.[2] A related and secondary aim was to consider the role of the sociocultural context in supporting and maintaining these interpretations of parenting. Our discussion covers three points: the long-term goals that mothers in each sample expressed for their infants, their beliefs about the maternal role and typical infant development, and the manner in which key childrearing practices reflect these beliefs and goals. These dimensions of parenting have also been referred to as the *moral direction*, the *pragmatic design*, and *conventional scripts for action*, respectively (LeVine et al., 1994). Our interpretation of diversity in parenting beliefs and practices is facilitated by attention to the physical and social features of each infant-care environment, which—in concert with ideological and behavioral dimensions of caregiving behavior— comprise the "developmental niche" of infants in the two cultures (Harkness & Super, 1983; Super & Harkness, 1986).

### Description of the Studies

Subjects included 40 4- and 10-month-old infants and their families—20 from a small town north of Rome for the Italian sample (*Civita Fantera*) and 20 infants of comparable age from a suburban setting outside of

Boston, Massachusetts ("Eastwood"). In each cultural setting, obstetricians and pediatricians were the source of families with infants of criterion age. All sample infants were healthy, Caucasian, second- or laterborn, from intact two-parent families. Major features of the research design were identical in the two cultural settings and included yearlong data collection for two overlapping age cohorts: 4 through 10 months of age and 10 to 16 months of age. This strategy enabled each study to encompass a 12-month period of infancy from 4 to 16 months. Methods of data collection included naturalistic home observations focused on all interactions that involved the infant,[3] daily routine questionnaires providing a retrospective report of family life and infant care over the preceding 24 hours, and parental attitude interviews regarding mothers' conceptions of norms and processes of child development, the maternal role, and goals and priorities of infant care. The Italian data were interpreted within the framework provided by an ethnographic study of community and family life. Data presented here draw on the 10-month age point, because that period contains pooled data from the entire sample in each of the two studies.

## The Developmental Niche in Two Western Settings

### Social and Physical Characteristics

*Civita Fantera* is a small industrial town approximately 1 hour north of Rome. Residents live in ancient apartments within the crowded historic town center or in suburban homes and condominiums. Community norms include closing down shops so that all family members can be together at the midday meal and full participation (including teenagers and the elderly) during the late afternoon stroll (New, 1984, 1988). This setting is in marked contrast to the suburban community of Eastwood, Massachusetts, where fathers commuted long hours to work in the city and family events were limited to weekends. In spite of these and other salient cultural differences in the two communities, there were also a number of similarities that characterized sample homes in each of the two cultures.

Infants in both cultures resided in nuclear households of comparable family size (mean 4.6), with an average of two children per family. Three of the Italian families included an extended family member, as did two in the U.S. sample. *Civita Fantera* households tended to be slightly more dense, due to a difference in the mean number of rooms per household (Eastwood 5.4 rooms; *Civita* 4.1 rooms). Fathers provided the primary source of income in both settings, with three mothers in each sample employed part-time outside the home. Families in both settings represented a range of socioeconomic status within the middle class, with the *Civita Fantera* families somewhat more heavily represented in the lower middle class (New, 1984; Richman, 1983). These demographic similarities belie differences between other physical and social characteristics of the two cultural groups (see Table 16.1).

The Eastwood infants spent much of their time in settings that were alternately characterized by either intense interaction or isolation. Fully one-third of the time they were observed alone with their mothers in a babyproofed environment that included many objects but few people. It was also common practice for Eastwood infants to have their own rooms, where their toys and other personal possessions were kept. On those occasions when others were present, as in the afternoons when siblings were home from school or when neighbors or friends called, such individuals were observed to greet the infant but rarely if ever shared in his or her care. The belief that infant care was primarily the mother's responsibility was tacitly if not explicitly acknowledged by all the sample mothers, including those who continued to work on a part-time basis (several from within the home). Although siblings were often present, sibling participation in infant care was rare and episodic and primarily took the form of object play or social stimulation. Most nonmaternal care was provided by babysitters (usually unrelated female teenagers) or grandmothers. Mothers reported that fathers helped when possible, although they were rarely observed to do so, even during weekend or evening observations, because infant-care routines often included feeding or bedtime at times other than when the father was at home. Contacts with extended family members varied greatly (ranging from 1 to 56 contacts per week, with an average of 16 across the sample), with visits less likely than telephone calls (Solomon, 1993).

Infants of *Civita Fantera* were also found at home with their mothers, yet that is where the similarity between the two social settings ends. All infants in the Italian sample shared a bedroom with the parents during the first year of life. The Italian infants had virtually no time or space to themselves and were also rarely alone with their

**Table 16.1.** Social and Physical Characteristics

|  | Eastwood | *Civita Fantera* |
| --- | --- | --- |
| Household size | 4.6 | 4.64 |
| Number of children | 2.55 | 2.27 |
| Working mothers | 3 | 3 |
| Number of rooms per household | 5.35 | 4.14 |
| Extended family members in home | 2 | 3 |
| Grandparents within 15 miles | 50% | 95% |

mothers, spending—at 10 months of age—less than 10% of the time in a mother–infant dyad (Miller, New, & Richman, 1982). Rather, these Italian infants were more likely to be found in groups of three or more, observing and interacting with the many different individuals who would come and go through the course of the day. For all but one of the sample infants in *Civita Fantera*, at least one grandparent lived within a short distance, and most mothers reported daily visits with these and/or other extended family members. Home observations supported the finding of a consistent and high level of social activity throughout much of the infant's waking hours, with remarkably little opportunity for solitary activity.

## Parental Values, Beliefs, and Goals

In each of the two cultural settings, mothers were asked a series of open-ended questions about their short- and long-term goals for their infants. They were also asked about their beliefs regarding parental influence in the attainment of these goals. Short-term goals in each group were expressed in terms of their priorities and strategies of infant care related to three common parenting concerns, described below. Clear cultural differences emerged in the parental interviews in the two samples.

Eastwood mothers consistently expressed three long-term goals, the first of which emphasized notions of independence and autonomy. All but one of the Eastwood mothers mentioned (1) the importance of economic and emotional independence—that their children be able to make their own decisions and establish separate lives. Sample mothers acknowledged their role in helping their children achieve a sense of autonomy, noting the value of such feelings for both the child and the parents. (2) Eastwood mothers also valued the attainment of a general sense of well-being in their children, with most expressing the wish that the children be happy regardless of their physical or economic circumstances. (3) The third goal, concerning interpersonal relationships, was mentioned by 17 of the Eastwood mothers. Typically, mothers wanted their children to have honest and respectful relationships with others.

Short-term goals mentioned by the Eastwood mothers included a concern for the child's cognitive and emotional development and highlighted the mother's role in providing a language-rich environment with opportunities for exploration and play. In turn, these mothers evaluated themselves in terms of their ability to provide experiences that contributed to the child's educational and emotional well-being (Welles-Nystrom, New, & Richman, 1994).

*Civita Fantera* mothers' long-term goals explicitly focused on the child's social relations and physical and economic well-being. Family, financial security, and good health were the most often and consistently expressed goals of the 20 mothers in the Italian sample. Mothers went to great lengths to emphasize the importance of their children having a decent family life, which—for most—was a function of finding a "good husband" or wife and being able to have and care for young children. Financial security was explained in terms of having a good job, or steady employment. Although mothers emphasized the importance of education in obtaining steady employment, most indicated that their expectations were modest at best. As one mother noted, "I don't expect him to be an engineer or anything like that." Good health was seen by some as the result of good fortune, whereas others ascribed physical well-being as the result of continuing to eat well. Thus, whereas mothers unanimously agreed on the importance of their children attaining these goals, for the most part they absolved themselves of any direct responsibility should their children "grow up badly." One mother went so far as to declare that although she hoped her son "would not be a juvenile delinquent," there would not be much that she could do about it. *Uno fa quello che puo [One does what one can].*

Mothers expressed more confidence in their ability to control the fate of their children during the infancy period, in contrast to their often explicit disdain for a father's ability to care for an infant (New & Benigni, 1987). Short-term goals related to the care of an infant in the first year of life included protecting the child from the elements, assuring a healthy and adequate diet, and keeping the child clean and well groomed. In spite of the clear maternal responsibilities in reaching these short-term goals, *Civita Fantera* mothers' conceptions of optimal parenting included few of the pressures self-imposed by the Eastwood mothers. In fact, sample mothers were hard-pressed to acknowledge that there *was* such a thing as a bad mother. Some simply declared that "all mothers are good mothers," whereas others ultimately described such a mother as one who consistently kept an eye on the child, "followed" the child in all of his or her activities, and fulfilled the previously mentioned obligations—keeping the child well fed, well groomed, and protected from the elements.

## Child Care Routines and Practices

As described, these social and physical characteristics and adult beliefs regarding infant development and the maternal role contribute to the context in which infants are cared for in these two culturally distinct settings. In this portion of the discussion we consider the relationship between these environmental characteristics as they relate to observed infant-care practices. The discussion focuses on three aspects of infant care that have been identified in previous cross-cultural studies: the avoidance of hazards, sleep arrangements, and the management of eating (LeVine, 1974; Caudill & Plath, 1966). These dimensions of parenting constitute what might be considered the pan-cultural "givens" of infant care, in that the young infant's survival is dependent on the caregivers' ability to respond to his or her basic needs for safety, rest, and nurturance. Because parental responses to these dimensions can none the less vary within the latitudes provided by human tolerances, these three aspects of infant care serve as a useful common ground on which to make cross-cultural comparisons. In particular, the interrelationship among parenting beliefs and practices associated with the three areas highlights the role of cultural values in both the structuring and interpretation of infant care and development.

1. *Motor activity and hazardous exploration of the environment.* To the outside observer, one of the most obvious differences in parental strategies of infant care in the two settings was revealed by the location of the infant over the course of the observation and maternal responses to the potential safety hazards extant in the two settings. In *Civita Fantera*, the vast majority of observations were conducted in the kitchen, in spite of the fact that they rarely co-occurred with mealtimes. Mothers were often engaged in domestic tasks as well as conversations with others; indeed, in many households, kitchens functioned as family rooms for socializing. Perhaps as a result of the number and type of hazards found in the average kitchen, infants were most often found either in some sort of container (walker, stroller, high chair, playpen) or on someone's lap. Yet these locations were also typical for infants who were observed in other settings, both inside and outside of the home. Time on the floor, for 10-month-old infants who were capable of and interested in crawling, represented a scant 26% of the total observation period. Mothers emphasized the risks of placing an active infant on the cold tile floors in terms of both the infant's health and safety and the potential havoc should the baby be allowed to "get into everything." Even in the warm summer months it was rare to see an infant allowed to crawl or attempt to walk outside, and mothers expressed dismay at infants' attempts to get down to the floor. When the adults determined that an infant was ready to learn to walk, two people—often siblings or cousins—would grasp the infant's two outstretched hands and support him or her in taking several steps. Rarely was an infant observed attempting to walk without receiving assistance from another person. There was no concern voiced regarding the extent to which these limitations interfered with the child's ability to

benefit from freely exploring the physical environment. One mother went so far as to brag that all her children had learned to walk without ever crawling on the floor.

The Eastwood homes were no less hazardous than those in *Civita Fantera*, nor were the infants seen as less likely to get into danger. Kitchen appliances, medicines and household chemicals, stairs, and running water are characteristic features of most middle-class U.S. households, and the sample families' homes were no exception. Yet the Eastwood mothers' strategies for dealing with such hazards were quite different from those observed in the Italian homes, despite their acknowledgement of the household dangers. These mothers had several methods for dealing with environmental hazards: childproofing, restricting the child's access to certain areas of the home, and teaching the infant—even at 10 months—what the dangers are. As some mothers put it, the infant "has to learn" where and with what it is safe to play, thus assigning the very young child some responsibility for his or her own safety (Richman, Miller, & Solomon, 1988).

Although 10-month-old Eastwood infants spent most of their time playing and crawling in heavily childproofed and restricted areas of their homes, they also spent time in and with a large variety of baby equipment (wind-up swings, walkers, and playpens) as well as brightly colored toys and stuffed animals, all designated as the infant's personal possessions. Infants were observed in various sorts of "containers" such as high chairs and playpens when their mothers needed or wished to leave them alone (e.g., during meal preparation, housework, or interactions with others). Mothers often left their infants for several minutes while they engaged in activities in an adjacent room. Mothers ascribed positive value to baby equipment such as walkers for their ability to help the prelocomotor child "single-handedly" master the environment, despite acknowledged concerns raised by professionals regarding the risks associated with the use of such paraphernalia. Mothers' intents were clear in each case—to encourage the development of independence and security at being on one's own. Increased motor abilities and heightened curiosity were signs, to the Eastwood mothers, that their infants were capable of moving around and ready to explore the environment. Thus, at 10 months, Eastwood infants were taken out of these high chairs, walkers, and playpens and encouraged to crawl or cruise around the environment. Indeed, at this time the Eastwood infants spent more than half of the observation periods (52%) on the floor. Although mothers acknowledged some of the dangers inherent in this practice, they again underscored the child's need to explore, alluding to its relationship to cognitive and emotional development. They felt confident that their childproofing techniques, in combination with maternal attention and teaching the child about hazards, were sufficient to avoid accidents.

These differences in childrearing practices related to environmental hazards suggest one way in which cultural values shape parental behavior. Allowing the infant freedom of movement within a smaller and safe environment acknowledged Eastwood mothers' goals for hazard prevention *and* mastery of the environment. Preventing such movement enabled the *Civita Fantera* mother to be reassured that the child was kept safe and clean; it also kept the child available for and interested in the social initiatives of others in the immediate environment. Another more striking example of how cultural values influence parental behavior compares the responses of the sample American and Italian mothers to issues of regulating infants' eating and sleeping.

2. *Rock-a-bye baby* . . . In the Eastwood sample, by 4 months of age most infants slept in their own beds and in many cases their own rooms. Several infants shared a room with an older sibling but never with the parents. From 4 to 10 months of age infants were reported to awake at approximately 7 A.M., to nap twice during the day, and to be put to bed at around 8 P.M. About half the infants woke at least once in the middle of the night, a situation that mothers regarded as quite undesirable. Strategies for putting infants to sleep were carefully orchestrated in the Eastwood homes. Bedtime rituals between mother and infant were well established by the second half of the first year and included rocking, feeding, singing, and/or reading a story. At the designated hour, infants were removed from the social stimulation of the dinner table or family room to their own quiet bedrooms. Mothers attached considerable importance to infants getting enough sleep (14 hours a day was seen as adequate), even when the infants showed great resistance to naps and bedtime, including prolonged crying. Mothers' reasons for insisting on keeping to a sleep schedule and routine included the belief that the baby "doesn't know when she's tired," and that children will develop "bad sleeping habits" if they are not put on a schedule during infancy. Many mothers also justified the importance of getting infants to go to bed so that they could have time for themselves or with their husbands (Richman, Miller, & Solomon, 1988). The topic of infant sleep was a common one, and mothers' belief in the importance of infant sleep was shared and reinforced by various pediatric experts (e.g., Ferber, 1985; Sammons, 1989) who offered numerous suggestions to "solve your child's sleep problem" (Ferber, 1985).

Italian sample infants' sleep schedules and related routines were in marked contrast to those observed in the U.S. study. To begin, for many, there was no clear schedule. When mothers were asked to describe when and how much their infants slept at night, several claimed that they did not know. When pressed for information regarding a bedtime, mothers explained that the infants often fell asleep before they were put to bed. Home observations confirmed the practice of keeping very young infants up with other members of the family, often until the adults themselves went to bed. This practice was explained as preferable to putting the infant to bed early—a strategy that one mother referred to as cruel because it limited the infant's opportunity to participate in the family social activity. In the absence of bedtime stories, songs, and other rituals, infants in *Civita Fantera* typically fell asleep in the carriage as it was gently jostled, or in someone's lap—sometimes, but not always, that of a visitor. When infants were finally put to bed, it was typically in the same room in which the parents slept. In most cases, infants shared the same room with the parents until approximately their second birthday.

In spite of this close proximity, mothers also had difficulty responding to the query regarding the infant's period of longest sleep. Many mothers claimed that the infant slept all night, only to remember at a subsequent point in the interview that the infant had, in fact, awakened earlier in the night. Infant naps were also unregulated. Indeed, one mother, who had difficulty describing when and for how long her infant napped during the day, simply explained that "he sleeps when he's tired." What was striking about these conversations with *Civita Fantera* mothers is that none of the mothers appeared concerned or bothered by the child's sleep habits—in marked contrast to the importance attributed to the topic by the Eastwood mothers. Throughout the period of the study, the general impression was that the *Civita Fantera* parents were much less worried about whether their children were getting adequate sleep than were their American sample counterparts. The lack of interest on the part of *Civita Fantera* mothers in their infants' sleep habits, however, was made up for by their keen interest in what and when their infants ate.

3. *Mangia, mangia, fatti grosso . . . [eat, eat, and get fat].*[4] Maternal attitudes toward eating and the resolution of eating difficulties were also culturally specific, and there were a number of differences in the goals and strategies that characterized infant feeding in the two settings. In general, the Eastwood mothers felt that infants can and should regulate their own eating habits. Although all sample mothers recognized the importance of a proper diet for the health and survival of the child, they were hesitant to try to force a change in a child's eating habits before the child indicated an interest in such change. Thus, more than

half of the Eastwood sample continued to breast feed beyond the neonatal period. Regardless of whether infants were breast- or bottle-fed, the Eastwood infants ate "on demand," with approximately six feedings a day throughout much of the first year. As a result of allowing the infants to determine their own feeding times, they were often at variance from family mealtimes. Infant mealtime therefore was typically a dyadic exchange involving the mother, who utilized the occasion as a time to teach and talk with the infant. These mealtimes, with focused mother–infant interactions, none the less precluded opportunities to observe and participate in social exchanges that characterized the family dinnertime. Eastwood infants were typically fed in their high chairs, which, in turn, facilitated self-feeding. Infants were encouraged to eat by themselves with their hands and to use specially designed cups and feeding utensils.

The youngest citizens of *Civita Fantera*, on the other hand, were not only invited but required to be present at all family meals and were offered many supports to assist them in coping with the larger familial agenda. Only two infants in *Civita Fantera* nursed beyond the first few weeks, in spite of the fact that most mothers expressed a preference for breast feeding. Their rationale for switching to formula was based on their claim that they could not produce enough milk. For the most part, the Italian infants were fed on a strict 4-hour schedule from the time they came home from the hospital, which meant that they were often awakened from naps if they had happened to be asleep at a mealtime and/or were offered pacifiers dipped in honey or sugar if hungry before the family mealtime. One mother justified these practices by noting, "The child doesn't know when he is hungry. Only the mother knows." These infants not only had no choice in the matter of when to eat but no choice in what and how much to eat. All infants were placed on solid foods by the fourth month, with the staunch support of the local pediatrician. Infants who resisted the large pasta-spoon servings were often force-fed with a variety of gentle but none the less persuasive techniques, including the alternation of the spoon and the pacifier. After observing one infant cry throughout much of his 4-month feeding, regarding the comment that he "didn't seem to like it very much," the mother noted—with confidence—"he'll get used to it." Indeed, the amount of social stimulation and the conviviality that surrounded family meal times was such that by 10 months most *Civita Fantera* infants responded with enthusiasm to their full inclusion in the social order.

This comparative analysis revealed culture-specific patterns of infant care in each of the two settings, with differences apparent in both maternal beliefs and practices. These differences, in turn, were consistent with the respective goals of child care as well as the cultural norms and ideals of social relationships. In sum, this analysis supports LeVine's conceptualization of the relationship between sample mother's goals (their *moral direction*), their beliefs (the *pragmatic design*), and their practices (*conventional scripts for action*) (LeVine et al., 1994). These dimensions of infant care were all in concert with culturally based interpretations of optimal development. Mothers in the two cultural settings had clearly distinct interpretations of the priorities for the infancy period, and they arranged the infant-care environments in correspondingly different fashions.

Patterns of infant care in the Italian sample reflected an explicit concern for the child's physical well-being, which—as interpreted—was deemed significant to the infant's sense of security as well. In cases of hazard avoidance, sleeping, and eating arrangements, the *Civita Fantera* infant was enmeshed in a dense social setting along with all other members of the family. Although there was little opportunity to establish a sense of independence from others, there was a great deal of support given to the notion of the child's right to participate fully in all family activities. Thus the *Civita Fantera* infants learned to modulate their own needs in coordination with the rituals and routines of the family, and the larger cultural value of social interdependence was both influential and maintained.

The findings from the Eastwood study, in contrast, suggest a major effort on the part of sample mothers to establish a sense of independence between infant and caregiver. Whether sleeping, eating, or playing, the Eastwood infant was often alone and therefore frequently excluded from the activities of the larger family setting. Although interactions with family members were considered vital to the infant's social and cognitive development, priority was given to the infant's independent play and exploration of the environment, the self-determination of feeding habits and schedules, and the ability to learn to sleep alone and away from other family members. The Eastwood infant was clearly and consistently encouraged to accommodate to the culturally sanctioned state of independence in his or her relations with others.

These differences in caregiving priorities and strategies clearly reflect broader cultural aims of independence versus interdependence. In each case, mothers justified their priorities and their practices as essential. Particular strategies of infant care that appeared contrary to infant wishes were deemed necessary, even though the necessity seemed more a function of the mother's own values and beliefs than of the infant's needs or abilities. Thus, Italian sample infants were required to eat along with the rest of the family because "a child doesn't know when he's hungry." Eastwood infants, on the other hand, were required to go to sleep regardless of the amount of their resistance, with an explanation offered about the amount of sleep young children require. In each case, the cultural value of either familial interdependence *or* independence was upheld.

Child-care practices associated with the short-term goals were also in service of these long-term goals. Within the U.S. sample, much that the mothers did within the context of infant care served as training for autonomous behavior as well as later academic success. Within the Italian sample, there was little concern expressed for the infant's intellectual development apart from his social competencies. Issues of autonomous behavior were therefore handled differently in the two cultural settings. Eastwood mothers struggled with the conflicts between hazard avoidance and opportunities for physical exploration, whereas *Civita Fantera* mothers opted for a safe, clean, and typically restrained infant; there was certainly no push for autonomous behavior. Instead, the environment nurtured a dependency between the infant and his or her caregivers, thereby maintaining the status of the family as the essential social unit. Thus, in cultures at relatively the same stage along the demographic transition (at least in terms of family size and nuclear family makeup), mothers saw their differing child-care strategies as the natural course of events.

## Conclusion

Discussions based on cross-cultural and comparative research on parenting and parental cognitions are now increasingly common in the developmental discourse (cf. Bornstein, 1991; Nugent, Lester, & Brazelton, 1989, 1991; Valsiner, 1988) and comparative investigations of the period of early infancy are contributing to social policy considerations as well as research agenda (e.g., to the public and scholarly debate on the merits and pitfalls of nonmaternal or extrafamilial infant care) (cf. Lamb, 1988; Lamb, Sternberg, Hwang, & Broberg, 1992). In this sense, a primary rationale for research on parental beliefs remains pragmatic, with a continuing emphasis on the potential psychological consequences for children (Sigel, McGillicuddy-DeLisi, & Goodnow, 1992). Indeed, some researchers explicitly note the need to better understand the effects of parental beliefs on behavior, in order to *modify* those beliefs—and, by implication, to change parental behavior—as a means of enhancing developmental outcomes (Clarke-Stewart, 1992). Yet there are other and perhaps more critical reasons to study and try to understand the relationship between adult beliefs and their practices with young children.

By "unpackaging" (Whiting, 1976) and then reconstructing the diverse elements of infant care reported from this comparative study, this analysis acknowledges the mutually reinforcing elements and transactional exchange that contribute to maternal behavior in each of the two cultural settings. In addition to revealing complex associations between adult ideologies and patterns of care and development, this analysis has added currency to the belief that culture plays a predominant role in the structuring and interpretation of the parental role. Finally, this study has contributed to our recognition of the extent to which *specific* strategies and patterns of infant care reflect and enhance the subsequent acquisition of cultural values—and makes the issue of "modifying" parental beliefs and practices an ethical as well as a practical dilemma.

An emphasis on cultural values, maternal beliefs, and caregiving practices paves the way for a more thorough understanding of maternal behavior at the individual level, the analysis of which must include recognition of the transactional interplay between cultural models, individual beliefs, and the contributions of the child himself or herself. As research on the psychological dimensions of parenting behavior continues to gain prominence, interest in and methods for studying "cultural models" of adult ideologies will need to expand correspondingly. Of particular relevance will be those studies that can contribute to our growing understanding of socially derived parental "scripts" that are acquired in the course of everyday rituals, routines, and encounters with people (Rogoff & Lave, 1984; Sigel, 1985). Consideration of the development of the individual within this sociocultural context will require creative and thoughtful research and serves as another reminder that we have much to learn about how adults construct their own personal cultures. Comparative research is critical to our understanding of these processes.

# Notes

1. These two studies were part of the Comparative Human Infancy Project, a five-culture examination of parental goals and infant care that also included infants and families from a Gusii community in rural Kenya, a Yucatecan village, and Stockholm, Sweden. (See Richman, LeVine, New, Howrigan, Welles-Nystrom, & LeVine, 1988.)

2. The Boston-based study was conducted from 1979 to 1980. The yearlong ethnographic study in the Italian community took place in 1980–1981.

3. Naturalistic observations in the infant-care environment were conducted with the aid of micro-operated recording equipment, enabling 5-second intervals for lag sequential analyses of criterion events.

4. "Eat, eat, it will make you fat. . ." is the beginning refrain of an oft-heard nursery rhyme cited during the feeding of infants and young children in Civita Fantera.

# References

Baumrind, D. (1993). The average expectable environment is not good enough: A response to Scarr. *Child Development, 64*(5), 1299–1317.

Bornstein, M. H. (Ed.). (1991). *Cultural approaches to parenting.* Hillsdale, NJ: Erlbaum.

Bowlby, J. (1969). *Attachment and loss: Vol. 1. Attachment.* New York: Basic Books.

Bronfenbrenner, U. (1977). Toward an experimental ecology of human development. *American Psychologist, 32,* 513–531.

Caudill, W. (1973). The influence of social structure and culture on human behavior in modern Japan. *Journal of Nervous and Mental Disease, 157,* 240–257.

Caudill, W., & Plath, D. (1966). Who sleeps by whom? Parent–child involvement in urban Japanese families. *Psychiatry, 29,* pp 344–366.

Caudill, W., & Weinstein, H. (1969). Maternal care and infant behavior in Japan and America. In T. S. Lebra & W. P. Lebra (Eds.), *Japanese culture and behavior: Selected readings.* Honolulu. University of Hawaii Press.

Clarke-Stewart, K. A. (1992). Developmental psychology in the real world: A paradigm of parent education. *Early Development and Parenting, 1*(1), 5–14.

de Vries, M. (1987). Alternatives to mother–infant attachment in the neonatal period. In C. Super (Ed.), *The role of culture in developmental disorder.* New York: Academic Press.

Ferber, R. (1985) *Solve your child's sleep problem.* New York: Simon & Schuster.

Field, T., Sostek, A., Vietze, P., & Leiderman, P. H. (Eds.). (1982). *Culture and early interaction.* Hillsdale, NJ: Erlbaum.

Garcia Coll, C. T. (1990). Developmental outcome of minority infants: A process-oriented look into our beginnings. *Child Development, 61,* 270–289.

Goodnow, J. J. (1980). Everyday concepts of intelligence and its development. In N. Warren (Ed.), *Studies in cross-cultural psychology,* London: Academic Press.

Goodnow, J. J. (1984). Parents' ideas about parenting and development: A review of issues and recent work. In M. E. Lamb, A. L. Brown, & B. Rogoff (Eds.), *Advances in developmental psychology* (Vol. 3). Hillsdale, NJ: Erlbaum.

Goodnow, J. J., & Collins, W. A. (1990). *Development according to parents: The nature, sources, and consequences of parents' ideas.* Hillsdale, NJ: Erlbaum.

Harkness, S., & Super, C. (1983). The cultural construction of child development. *Ethos, 11,* 222–231.

Lamb, M. (Ed.). (1988). *The father's role: Cross-cultural perspectives.* Hillsdale, NJ: Erlbaum.

Lamb, M., Sternberg, K., Hwang, C., & Broberg, A. (1992). *Child care in context: Cross-cultural perspectives.* Hillsdale, NJ: Erlbaum.

Leiderman, P. H., Tulkin, S. R., & Rosenfeld, A. (Eds.). (1977). *Culture and infancy: Variations in the human experience.* New York: Academic Press.

LeVine, R. A. (1974). Parental goals: A cross-cultural view. *Teachers College Record, 76*(2), 226–239.

LeVine, R. A. (1977). Child rearing as cultural adaptation. In P. H. Leiderman, S. R. Tulkin, & A. Rosenfeld (Eds.), *Culture and infancy: Variations in the human experience.* New York: Academic Press.

LeVine, R. A. (1988). Human parental care: Universal goals, cultural strategies, individual behavior. In R. A. LeVine, P. M. Miller, & M. M. West (Eds.), *Parental behavior in diverse societies* (New Directions for Child Development No. 40). San Francisco: Jossey-Bass.

LeVine, R. A. (1990). Infant environments in psychoanalysis: A cross-cultural view. In J. Stigler, R. Shweder, & G. Herdt (Eds.), *Cultural psychology: Essays on comparative human development.* New York: Cambridge University Press.

LeVine, R. A., Dixon, S., LeVine, S., Richman, A., Leiderman, P. H., Keefer, C. H., & Brazelton, T. B. (1994). *Child care and culture: Lessons from Africa.* Cambridge, UK: Cambridge University Press.

LeVine, R. A., Miller, P. M., & West, M. M. (1988). *Parental behavior in diverse societies* (New Directions for Child Development No. 40). San Francisco: Jossey-Bass.

Lewis, M., & Ban, P. (1977). Variance and invariance in the mother–infant interaction: A cross-cultural study. In P. H. Leiderman, S. R. Tulkin, & A. Rosenfeld (Eds.), *Culture and infancy: Variations in the human experience.* New York: Academic Press.

Lozoff, B., & Brittenham, G. (1972). Infant care: Cache or carry. *Journal of Pediatrics, 95*(3), 478–483.

Miller, P., New, R., & Richman, A. (1982). *Social ecology of infant development in Italy and America.* Paper presented at the International Conference on Infant Studies, Austin, TX.

Minturn, L., & Lambert, W. (1964). *Mothers of six cultures: Antecedents of child rearing.* New York: Wiley.

New, R. (1984). Italian mothers and infants: Patterns of care and social development. Unpublished doctoral dissertation. Harvard University Graduate School of Education, Cambridge, MA.

New, R. (1988). Parental goals and Italian infant care. In R. A. LeVine, P. M. Miller, & M. M. West (Eds.), *Parental behavior in diverse societies* (New Directions for Child Development No. 40). San Francisco: Jossey-Bass.

New, R., & Benigni, L. (1987). Italian fathers and infants: Cultural constraints on paternal behavior. In M. Lamb (Ed.), *The father's role: Cross-cultural perspectives.* Hillsdale, NJ: Erlbaum.

Ninio, A. (1979). The naive theory of the infant and other maternal attitudes in two subgroups in Israel. *Child Development, 50,* 976–980.

Nugent, J. K., Lester, B. M., & Brazelton, T. B. (Eds.). (1989). *The cultural context of infancy. Vol. 1. Biology, culture and infant development.* Norwood, NJ: Ablex.

Nugent, J. K., Lester, B. M., & Brazelton, T. B. (Eds.). (1991). *The cultural context of infancy. Volume 2. Multicultural and interdisciplinary approaches to parent–infant relations.* Norwood, NJ: Ablex.

Richman, A. (1983). *Learning about communication: Cultural influences on care-taker–infant interaction.* Unpublished doctoral thesis, Harvard University Graduate School of Education, Cambridge, MA.

Richman, A., LeVine, R., New, R., Howrigan, G., Welles-Nystrom, B., & LeVine, S. (1988). Maternal behavior to infants in five cultures. In R. A. LeVine, P. M. Miller, & M. M. West (Eds.), *Parental behavior in diverse societies* (New Directions for Child Development No. 40). San Francisco: Jossey-Bass.

Richman, A., Miller, P., & Solomon, M. (1988). The socialization of infants in suburban Boston. In R. A. LeVine, P. M. Miller, & M. M. West (Eds.), *Parental behavior in diverse societies* (New Directions for Child Development No. 40). San Francisco: Jossey-Bass.

Rogoff, B., & Lave, J. (Eds.). (1984). *Everyday cognition: Its development in social context.* Cambridge, MA: Harvard University Press.

Ruddick, S. (1982). Maternal thinking. In B. Thorne & M. Yalom (Eds.), *Rethinking the family.* New York: Longmans.

Sammons, W. (1989). *The self-calmed baby.* Boston: Little, Brown.

Scarr, S. (1992). Developmental theories for the 1990s: Development and individual differences. *Child Development, 63*(1), 1–19.

Scheper-Hughes, N. (1987). "Basic strangeness": Maternal estrangement and infant death—A critique of bonding theory. In C. Super (Ed.), *The role of culture in developmental disorder.* New York: Academic Press.

Scheper-Hughes, N. (1990). Mother love and child death in northeast Brazil. In J. Stigler, R. Schweder, & G. Herdt (Eds.), *Cultural psychology: Essays on comparative human development.* New York: Cambridge University Press.

Sigel, I. E. (Ed.). (1985). *Parental belief systems.* Hillsdale, NJ: Erlbaum.

Sigel, I. E., McGillicuddy-DeLisi, A. V., & Goodnow, J. J. (Eds.) (1992). *Parental belief systems: The psychological consequences for children* (Vol. 2). Hillsdale, NJ: Erlbaum.

Snow, de Blauw, & van Roosmalen (1979). Talking and playing with babies: The role of ideologies of child rearing. In M. Bullowa (Ed.), *Before speech.* New York: Cambridge University Press.

Solomon, M. (1993). Transmission of cultural goals: Social network influences on infant socialization. In J. Demick, K. Bursik, & R. DiBiase (Eds.), *Parental development.* Hillsdale, NJ: Erlbaum.

Super, C., & Harkness, S. (1986). The developmental niche: A conceptualization of the interface of child and culture. *International Journal of Behavioral Development, 9,* 546–569.

Tronick, E., Morelli, G., & Winn, S. (1987). Multiple caretaking of Efe (Pygmy) infants. *American Anthropologist, 89,* 96–106.

Valsiner, J. (Ed.), (1988). *Children's development within social–cultural structured environments.* Norwood, NJ: Ablex.

Whiting, B. B. (1976). Unpackaging variables. In K. Riegel & J. Meacham (Eds.), *The changing individual in a changing world.* Chicago: Aldine.

Whiting, B. B., & Whiting, J. M. W. (1975). *Children of six cultures: A psychocultural study.* Cambridge, MA: Harvard University Press.

Whiting, J. M. W., & Whiting, B. B. (1963). *Six cultures: Studies of childrearing.* New York: Wiley.

## PART FIVE

# THE CONSEQUENCES OF PARENTS' CULTURAL BELIEF SYSTEMS FOR CHILDREN'S HEALTH DEVELOPMENT

# CHAPTER 17

# My Child Is My Crown
## Yoruba Parental Theories and Practices in Early Childhood

Marian Zeitlin

## Prelude

When I arrived in Nigeria in May 1992, the daughter to whom I had given birth there 25 years earlier had been attending a master's program at the University of Lagos for 8 months, immersed in the culture of her early childhood and supervised by my Nigerian faculty coworkers on a UNICEF-sponsored project. For the 5 weeks that I lived with my daughter while completing my part in the project, our relationship blossomed into an experience that had the quality of an altered state of consciousness, a kind of good dream. Our generational differences were not a rocky battleground, urban wasteland, or Bermuda Triangle but formed a smooth highway as long as the Milky Way that permitted each to travel through the other to the time horizons of our lives, and beyond. This idyll illuminated for me the traditional Yoruba world view that children are the *summum bonum*, or chief good, in life (Babatunde, 1992; Hallgren, 1991; Fadipe, 1970). It provided an experiential frame of reference that I draw on in presenting the data in this chapter on Yoruba traditional beliefs, theories, and practices regarding childrearing. I draw also upon 25 years of intermittent coparenting and conversations with the Yoruba mother of our oldest son—my son by adoption under United States law, her son and the reincarnation of her father, fostered to me according to the laws and customs of Nigeria.

# Introduction

This chapter attempts to illuminate apparent contradictions between traditional Yoruba parental theories, which highly value and celebrate children, and practices that may be viewed by modern standards as child labor, physical abuse, and underfeeding. I hope to show that these contradictions have no presence within the vocabulary of traditional Yoruba parental theories, that lifelong rewards available within the Yoruba paradigms may be undetectable using Western terms of reference, and that cultural adjustment and renewal are needed to assist transition to the socioeconomic standards of the contemporary global economy.

The chapter first presents a general description of Yoruba cosmology and beliefs about the nature of the child, followed by a description of parental practices that train the child in the productive skills and the reciprocal relationships that personify the child's role as the ontological extension of the parents, ancestors, and lineage. It then focuses on economic incentives and social rewards that anchor the traditional economy. These manifest in child feeding practices that employ food restriction to socialize children to respect the leadership and the ethical codes of the community.

# Data and Methods

Some of the data for this chapter come from baseline studies conducted by UNICEF Nigeria in preparation for development of community-based child care and early childhood education projects cosponsored by the Bernard van Leer Foundation. Starting in 1987, the first three of these studies were carried out in households of Yoruba children from 2 to 6 years of age in the following local government areas (LGA): Oyo LGA in Oyo State ($N$ = 249), Oyun LGA in Kwara State ($N$ = 352), Owo LGA in Ondo State ($N$ = 291). These studies used a common questionnaire and a protocol for 3 hours of in-home observation per child to assess health and nutritional status, socialization and stimulation, childcare arrangements, and maternal attitudes toward achievement, formal education, and organized day care. Results for rural and urban samples were presented separately for Oyo and together for the other sites (Wilson-Oyelaran & Ladipo, 1987, 1988, 1989a, 1989b) and were synthesized (Akinware, Wilson-Oyelaran, Ladipo, Pierce, & Zeitlin, 1992).

Additional data come from the Positive Deviance in Nutrition Research Project, which was sponsored by UNICEF New York and the Italian Government through Tufts University in Nigeria, Indonesia, and Nicaragua. The Nigerian study, "Child Development for the Computer Age Project," co-sponsored by UNICEF Nigeria, conducted focus groups, an ethnographic substudy, and a main survey, which included observations and psychological testing among low-income families in the greater Lagos area (Aina et al., 1993). The survey and test sample consisted of 211 children ranging in age from 22 to 26 months in three locations—the Makoko section of central Lagos and semirural and rural areas in Ifo-Ota. In addition to a questionnaire adapted from the UNICEF baseline studies, we collected food frequencies; intrahousehold meat allocation attitudes and rules; the Bayley Scales of Infant Development (Bayley, 1969); interviewer-rated scales of behavior and affect of the mother and child; a modified Caldwell HOME (Home Observation for Measurement of the Environment) Inventory (Caldwell & Bradley, 1984); weights, heights, and mid-upper arm circumference of the children; and weights and heights of the mothers.

Five families from Makoko and five from Ifo-Ota were selected for more than 150 days of intensive ethnographic study. Households were homes of six of the top scorers and four of the bottom scorers on the previously administered Bayley Scales of Infant Development. A less intensive study of a sample of 15 Ifa priests with child apprentices also was conducted to investigate the child teaching practices of the traditional intellectual elite.

Starting in the survey design period and extending through a community-based pilot project phase in the third and fourth years, the project team conducted more than 40 focus groups and in-depth interviews with community leaders, parents and grandparents, social service professionals, and faculty, staff, and students at the University of Lagos.

## The Nature of the Child: Parental Theories and Practices

### Children in the Yoruba World View

The supreme importance of childbearing and proper childrearing among the Yoruba is rooted in the belief that the immortality of the soul flows cyclically through the lineage through the birth of children (Babatunde, 1992; Hallgren, 1991), and not primarily through an afterlife as conceived by Christianity or Islam. According to traditional Yoruba cosmology and religion, the goal of living is to enable the various component parts of the soul to survive eternally in a cycle of three states: the living, the ancestors, and the unborn awaiting reincarnation. Children reincarnate ancestors of their own lineage. Membership in good standing depends on bearing children, living a long and godly life, and being venerated by one's descendants. The merits of one's life are judged after death by the one supreme deity, *Olorun*. Those who lead bad or childless lives and die without funeral rites are like broken crockery. At death they are thrown onto the rubbish heap of the "heaven of potsherds," where they cease their participation in the eternal cycle of rebirth or may be reborn as animals (Hallgren, 1991).

Ancestors continue to appear and interact with the living through dreams and other manifestations during the lives of their descendants who remember them. This permeable boundary between the worlds infuses the Yoruba experience with spirituality; the deceased announce their reincarnation in children about to be born, advise on the distribution of property, help grandchildren with their studies, dictate times for celebration, forewarn the family of dangers, and so on. Newborn children are new emissaries from this other realm. The imminence of the supernatural adds wonder, meaning, and authenticity to a drama centered around intergenerational continuity. Although the majority of Yoruba now practice Christianity or Islam, the Yoruba world view infuses their experience of the value of children.

The good life was actualized here, materially, as part of the eternal, revolving cycle. Earthly success was a main feature of traditional religion. As explained by Hallgren (1991), money was needed to obtain wives, wives were necessary for the birth of children, and children were most important of all. Wealthy and powerful men and women did not stand apart as a separate class but were at the apex of groups consisting of their descendants and other kin, supporters, and disciples (Lloyd, 1966). At the head of a large compound, the successful person led a life in which leisure and sedentarism increased with age (Aronson, 1980). He or she held court to supervise household management, mediate problems, and advise on business activities and also participated in day-to-day politics in the offices of more powerful patrons.

The role of the prestigious, important, virtuous person, *enian pataki*, to which all individuals aspired in life, foreshadowed and prepared the virtuous for a seamless transition to the role of revered ancestor of the lineage after death. The land of the dead was a continuation of the earthly life, with the same social structure (Hallgren, 1991).

The prestigious person possessed *alafia* (Aronson 1980), a word for well-being that includes physical health, peace of mind, material prosperity, harmonious relationships, and a reputation for wisdom. Traditionally, such prestige was not a function of occupation as it is in the West (Aronson, 1980). In colloquial Yoruba, all occupations were classed together in two categories—"clerk" and "trader"—neither with status implications.

The increasing leisure of the elders was made possible by the industry of juniors, with tasks delegated downward. Inherent in the concept of lineage structure was the system of seniority, which established a single hierarchy of reciprocal obligations in all situations (Bascom, 1951; Aronson, 1980). Traditionally, any senior had a right to unquestioned service, deference, and submissiveness from any junior (Lloyd, 1974). Rules assigned age seniority according to order of entry into the lineage, either by birth or by marriage. Seniority also was derived from titles, certification, leadership roles, gender, physical ability, and supernatural endowment (as in the case of the priesthood).

Seniority determined task allocation and resource distribution in the farming, crafts, and trading enterprises of the immediate and extended kinship units. Distinctions defining seniority were, of necessity, elaborate and were expressed in myriad terms by which persons greeted and addressed each other (Fadipe, 1970). In the former non-monetized production system, distinctions among these titles and greetings claimed the same technical importance now attached in the modern sector to job grades and job descriptions. Children staffed the junior ranks of the household production system. Their command of greetings and social distinctions reflected their mastery of the organizational charts of family business and town politics.

## The Milestones of Child Development

The traditional Yoruba believe that before birth, the child chooses or is assigned by God his *ori*, (literally "head," depicted as a clay head, meaning dramatic persona or destiny). Divination on the third day after birth partially reveals this destiny to the parents and elders. Although divination by priests of the old religion has declined, some divinatory revelation regarding the child's psychic identity is common. Certain aspects of the child's character are personally predetermined in the *ori*, and others are acquired through the reincarnation of ancestral or lineage traits. Character weaknesses uncovered by divination may be corrected by prayer and sacrifice and by specific prescriptions for character training. For example, a boy divined as timid may be prescribed to spend more time with his father, or a rascal may be prescribed to be firmly controlled. The child's personal praise song, *Oriki*, (literally "greeting the head") celebrates the lineage origins of the child's *ori*. It is composed by parents and elders and recited to the child.

The infant remains in communication with spirit companions. Its name—*Babatunde* (father returns), *Funmilayo* (brings me honor), *Olaolu* (Glory of God)—describes its origins, circumstances of birth, and role in the family. Children are watched for the unfolding of resemblances to the ancestors they reincarnate.

As the infant grows, parents place high priority on motor development. They encourage infants to support their weight on their legs from birth. From the age of 3 to 5 months, babies are propped in a sitting position in a hole in the ground or with cushions. Agiobu-Kemmer (1984) observed that the Yoruba mothers trained their infants to crawl by repeatedly placing objects just beyond their reach, whereas Scottish mothers in her comparison study did not do so. Yet, in response to interview questions, the Yoruba mothers claimed that they had done nothing special to train their children. The Yoruba parents engaged their infants in social play and motor training for a greater percentage of the time, whereas the Scottish mothers spent more time involving their infants in technical play with objects.

Focus groups with Yoruba mothers and grandmothers found a preference for wiry and agile babies who learned to walk early. Folk wisdom relates that girls and laterborn children walk earlier than do boys and the firstborn, and that spoiled children and children who are carried walk later. It is a important to coax the child to walk with rewards of singing and clapping.

The Yoruba believe that heavy staple foods, such as cassava meal and pounded yam, should be withheld until the child walks out of fear that he will become *wuwo*, a word applied to immobile older infants. This folk diagnosis of the "heavy or clumsy baby" applies both to fat, normally nourished lazy babies and to malnourished starch-fed babies with enlarged stomachs and marginal swelling from *kwashiorkor*.

Focus group discussions revealed that Yoruba parents in Lagos most commonly defined childhood in terms of self-reliance. According to some, children who could talk, walk, dress themselves, and do certain other things around the house were no longer referred to as children. Others defined childhood as the period prior to puberty. Childhood was further defined relative to economic independence: Once a person began to earn a living, he or she ceased to be called a child. The common element in these definitions was dependency on others for care, protection, and development as a result of young age (Aina, Etta, & Zeitlin, 1992).

The expectations regarding normal development set by the parents surveyed in the UNICEF baseline studies included self-care skills, autonomy, providing services, and social interactions. Mean ages for achieving the milestones surveyed are provided in Table 17.1, as are data from a non-Yoruba site, Calabar, in Eastern Nigeria. In the Calabar sample, 94% of fathers had attended school (mothers' schooling was not indicated for Calabar), compared to 21–68% of fathers and 14–54% of mothers in the Yoruba groups. The older ages at which certain milestones were expected in Calabar likely reflect revision in the concept of childhood with exposure to modern education.

The most conspicuous feature of Table 17.1 is the early age at which childhood dependency ends. The child was in many respects a full member of society by age 7. Seven-year-olds were expected to obey and respect their elders, care for themselves and younger siblings, assist in the home, and contribute economically in the workplace. The Oyun survey concluded that "before a child is eight years of age, most mothers expect him or her to be able to contribute to the family economy by providing assistance either on the farm or with trading activities. In addition, children at this age were expected to be able to think for themselves" (Wilson-Oyelaran & Ladipo, 1989b). Parents of 2-year-olds in the Lagos state Positive Deviance survey reported that more than 90% had started to learn how to take things from one place to another, carry water in a small bowl, put their own things away, and wash their own hands and face; 75% to buy things; 39% to wash their own plate or

**Table 17.1.** Mean Age Expectations for Task Achievement in Years

| | Oyo-R[*]<br>(N = 137) | Oyo-U[*]<br>(N = 112) | Oyun<br>(N = 340) | Owo<br>(N = 278) | Calabar<br>(N = 305) |
|---|---|---|---|---|---|
| Stop bedwetting | 2.85 | 2.93 | 2.80 | 2.63 | n.a. |
| Know where to defecate | 2.85 | 2.55 | 2.54 | 2.55 | 2.92 |
| Talk clearly | 3.36 | 3.09 | 2.97 | 3.31 | 3.28 |
| Dress witout assistance | 4.70 | 4.79 | 4.47 | 4.73 | 4.74 |
| Feed self | 3.16 | 2.22 | 2.38 | 2.50 | 2.50 |
| Care for self<br>for 2 hours | 5.17 | 6.20 | 6.15 | 5.87 | n.a. |
| Run errands | 4.44 | 4.10 | 4.23 | 4.35 | 4.77 |
| Care for younger<br>siblings | 6.31 | 6.68 | 6.87 | 6.73 | 7.58 |
| Greet elders | 5.58 | 5.17 | 5.46 | 4.96 | 4.46 |
| Obey elders | 5.73 | 5.69 | 6.02 | 5.33 | 6.45 |
| Think for self | 7.08 | 7.38 | 7.62 | 7.21 | 11.87 |
| Assist with farm | 6.78 | 7.24 | 7.11 | 7.43 | 10.41 |
| Assist with trading | 6.62 | 7.01 | 7.15 | 7.51 | 9.62 |
| Assist with housework | 6.09 | 6.00 | 6.18 | 5.93 | 7.28 |

[*]R = rural; U = urban.

cup; and 28% to learn housework such as sweeping and washing clothes. Fifteen percent of 2-year-olds in the Lagos state sample were reported to actually perform household chores. By age 5, children were expected to have mastered many of these skills, including running errands and greeting elders.

In the UNICEF baseline surveys, children ages 3 to 5 were attentive participants in adult activities. Besides playing, the most frequent activities identified through content analysis of observations of preschool children involved children helping their caregivers by completing errands and spontaneously taking responsibility for tasks. Typically, children were asked to assist in food processing and to retrieve items such as water, bags, chairs, or foodstuffs. Spontaneously helpful activities by preschool children included driving away goats or dogs from foodstuffs, adding wood to the fire, feeding domestic animals, taking care of younger siblings in times of distress, and running to carry an older person's bag without being asked.

The fourth most commonly observed category of activity involved situations in which the children's attention was focused on verbal interactions between adults, where preschoolers displayed a quality of attentiveness expected of adults. These interactions included conversations about foodstuffs, market prices, and the whereabouts of siblings. Several observer notations described children reminding their mothers to watch the fire or attend to a customer, indicating the child's ability to deduce cause-and-effect relationships. For instance, "One little girl who was not quite 3.5 years old commented when she saw a man who worked for the national electricity company that he had probably come to turn off the electricity of a customer who had not paid the bill" (Wilson-Oyelaran and Ladipo, 1989b).

## The Central Role of Errands in Early Childhood Education

The UNICEF baseline studies revealed that the main type of early childhood stimulation activity in Nigeria was the errand—an activity not measured, per se, by Western tests such as the HOME inventory which measures the quality of early child care and the learning environment provided by the home. In answer to the question, "What did your child do that made you proud?" mothers most often responded that they were proud when the child was able and willing to help in the home and, especially, to successfully complete errands. Getting along with others and following directions also were mentioned. Cognitive, artistic, and other expressive skills that are expected among the educated to foreshadow academic performance were not mentioned by mothers in the baseline surveys. In a study of Yoruba mothers, Lloyd (1970) also found that errands were the type of child achievement most valued by their mothers.

At the heart of "baby's first errand" was the task of taking an object from one location and depositing it in another, practiced by 99% of the 2-year-olds in the Positive Deviance survey sample. The earliest observed teaching of this task was with children not yet 1 year old who were repeatedly instructed with the word *gba* (take) to grasp and hold onto an object given. Two-year-olds often were sent on errands and even were given small amounts of money to purchase items from vendors. In most observations, the mother herself requested the task be done and monitored its completion.

The Yoruba acknowledge the rewarding nature of errands and the sense of accomplishment they produce for both parties. Western observers may tend to view errand training as a means of extracting child labor or preparing the child for exploitation through child labor. Yet both the UNICEF baseline reports and the Positive Deviance ethnography record the emotional satisfaction to both mother and child when the mother set a challenging errand and the child completed the task. One little boy was observed to fuss and cry until his mother relented and allowed him to perform an errand. During evening relaxation in the family compound, 4- and 5-year-olds would be sent on comic bogus errands from one family member to another "to exercise them" and entertain the family (V. Oseni, personal communication, 1993). Yet the errand takes shape as a child-stimulation activity only within our frame of reference, in which childhood is a time of learning the components of skills that will much later be integrated into adult performance. Viewed from the perspective of a culture in which childhood ends progressively with the end of the preschool years, errands are similar to on-the-job training that may be given at any age. They are special to early childhood to the extent that "jobs" do need to be specially designed and customized as teaching experiences when those performing them are under the age of 5 or six. Moreover, it inevitably requires more effort to teach and supervise such tasks for the very young than it does to do them oneself.

Errands train the infant child in the prepositions of location (on, under, between). They teach the child to follow sequential instructions, carry and care for objects, and learn the layout of the neighborhood. They also teach the social skills needed for verbal and commercial transactions. In errands and other material transactions, social accountability is stressed. Children are taught to report to their parents any kind gestures of others and to show them any gifts received; they must gradually learn to be honest without being a tattletale (Babatunde, 1992). Thus, all goods entering and activities regarding the household can be confidentially managed according to the household seniority structure. Many of the spontaneous conversations between adults and children recorded in the ethnographic study consisted of the adult making sure that the child had respected the proper social rules and channels within the seniority system for reporting food and other items received by reporting activities to the appropriate senior person and transferring physical objects to appropriate destinations. For example, one child given a ball by the project ethnographer was told to put it away until his father came home and could be informed.

A child who did not focus total attention on mastering and completing errands was perceived to be at high risk. Focus groups affirmed a "spare the rod and spoil the child" attitude. As recalled by Victoria Oseni (personal communication, 1993), "They would tell you once; the next time they would use the switch." Yoruba views regarding the necessity of physical punishment are expressed in two proverbs (Babatunde, 1992):

"When the child behaves foolishly, one prays that he may not die; what kills more quickly than foolishness?"

expresses the understanding that punishment is an act of kindness.

"When we use the right hand to flog him, we use the left hand to draw him back to ourselves,"

expresses the inseparability of the punishment from the need to comfort the child for the pain experienced during punishment.

Early cross-cultural comparisons (Doob, 1965; LeVine, 1963; Lloyd, 1970) characterized Yoruba and other African parenting practices as emphasizing obedience, responsibility, and corporal punishment. More than 92% of the UNICEF baseline mothers said they would use corporal punishment on a child who was misbehaving. The Positive Deviance study of 2-year-olds found that mothers used physical punishment, such as flicking the fingertips against the child's arm, more often than the Caldwell HOME Inventory provided for. We modified HOME item II.15: "No more than one instance of physical punishment during the past week," as follows and found the bracketed response rates: "Child needs spanking: never (17%); more than once a week but less than daily (75%); many times a week, can't remember exactly (8%)."

Errands engage the child in work allocation and task management. Children learn to delegate errands to children junior to them and to perform errands delegated by seniors. According to Fadipe (1970), children in a strictly regulated traditional family had to obey the orders of older siblings as soon as they passed the infancy stage. Handing a switch to the older and instructing him or her to use it on the junior was the common method of teaching this system to resistant youngsters.

Observations in the Oyo urban baseline study (Wilson-Oyelaran & Ladipo 1989a) found that children were sent on many more errands if the mother was the caretaker. Older siblings and other caretakers were less likely to place this type of demand on the children even in a traditional setting.

Errand training yields more rewards to the parents than to others, as the parents are the direct beneficiaries of the child's emerging skills and allegiance. In the mother–child relationship, the child's first errands also represent his or her initiation into society's master plan, into lineage membership, and into a special form of communion with the mother. The proverb *Omo ade iya* (the child is the crown of the mother) expresses the dual role of the crown that extends the power and status of the parents and simultaneously the crown that mobilizes and leads them into the future, their collective will and their immortality (Babatunde, 1992).

## Economic Incentives, Moral Training, and Feeding Practices

### Cultural–Economic Roots

An economic rationale underlies the high value placed on children in Africa (e.g., Caldwell & Caldwell, 1977, 1990). The traditional flow of investment not only in Africa but in industrialized societies through the turn of the 20th century was from child to parent, not from parent to child (Zeitlin et al., 1982). Surveys by Caldwell and Caldwell (1977) indicated that Nigerian children began to contribute substantively to the family's maintenance by the age of 5 or 6 and that each surviving child would remit on the order of 10% of household income, in addition to providing security during old age and disasters. Children also benefited the family at the lineage level. The larger the lineage, the greater its claims on land and other resources, and the greater its chances of surviving in perpetuity (Lloyd, 1974).

When taken literally, the arguments of the "price tag theorists" (Olusanya, 1987)—that parents bear many children because they profit from them financially—are demeaning and inaccurate. These writers miss the inner truth of the Yoruba experience. The religious values of the traditional world view explain why women, to whom Olusanya

(1987) refers as "fertility martyrs," now continue to bear children when further childbearing is not only unprofitable but also places their health and financial security at risk.

Our data support the view that Yoruba childrearing theories are adapted specifically to the African agrarian production pattern, based on communal land ownership, in which autonomous but subordinate female economic subunits extend the land holdings and trade of polygamous male-headed households (Caldwell & Caldwell, 1990). We found that Yoruba theories differ characteristically from those of our study populations in Bangladesh and Indonesia (Zeitlin et al., 1995). Parental theories in the Asian countries protect the survival of heirs to retain possession of privately owned landholdings (Zeitlin et al., 1995); the survival of a legitimate male heir to each father is most important to perpetuate the core unit in Bangladesh. In Nigeria, under communal land tenure, the survival of any individual child is less important to the family unit than survival of the mother.

Under conditions of scarcity, the balance of entitlement to food in the Yoruba system favors the mother over the child (Setiloane, 1995; Zeitlin et al., 1995), whereas in Asian systems, as demonstrated explicitly in Nepal (Gittelsohn, 1991), food distribution often appears to favor the children at the expense of the self-sacrificial mother. Although we had food allocation data, which disfavored children relative to their parents, only for Nigeria, anthropometric measurements of the children and mothers across the positive deviance studies indicated that the Nigerian mothers were much better nourished relative to their children's growth status than were Bangladeshi, Indonesian, and Mexican mothers (Zeitlin et al., 1995). Moreover, the percentage of Nigerian mothers who had ever lost a child (61%) was significantly higher than in the other samples, including the more disadvantaged rural Bangladeshis (44%).

In the Asian and Latin American samples, families who had experienced prior child deaths were more likely to have undernourished children, suggesting impaired caring capacity in these families. In Nigeria, on the other hand, children born to families having experienced child death were on average better nourished (Zeitlin et al., 1995). Allocation shifted to favor the next child if the existing distribution proved insufficient to keep the previous child alive. This interpretation was supported by numerous anecdotes of children favored by their mothers, and thus spoiled, because previous children had died.

The Bangladeshi and Indonesian cultures accorded high value to maternal self-sacrifice in feeding herself last and least (Bangladesh) and to food self-denial as a moral virtue that can be taught even to the infant in the womb (Indonesia). The Yoruba mothers did not express these values. All (99%) in the Yoruba Positive Deviance study were at least partly self-supporting. As independent economic subunits within the larger family structure, these mothers supplied on average 47% of their family's food expenditure from their personal earnings (56% for the small rural subsample). They felt entitled to food as heads of the female subunit, rather than disentitled as nonearning subordinates in male-headed households.

## Prestige Food Distribution and Moral Training

Yoruba parental theories view the distribution of prestige foods to children in terms of the child's moral training. The following economic rationale supports this view. Payment for goods and services often rewarded the provider with a fixed proportion of available resources rather than with fixed quantities in kind or with cash on an item-by-item or contract basis. During times of scarcity, the proportional entitlement system continues to function in the absence of money or surplus stocks for payment. No matter how scarce the resources, they can still be divided proportionally in a manner that recompenses those responsible for provisioning and managing the system. The rules of this proportional distribution system were taught to children through rationed portion sizes of scarce and prized foods such as meat. Changing these portion sizes threatened the integrity of the system.

Yoruba culture appears to lack the concept that children should be favored in food distribution, as shown in the following Yoruba proverbs on ideal parenting behavior (Adewale, 1986). These aphorisms enjoin parents to leave some food for their children, but do not suggest that children require preferential feeding.

> "An elder who consumes everything without leaving a remnant will himself carry his calabash home";

and

> "The dove eats and leaves a remnant for the pigeon. The green wild pigeon eats and leaves a remnant for the mocking bird. I will leave a remnant for my children when I eat."

The ethnographic substudy found that mothers fed their preschoolers portions of fish and meat that were barely visible compared to the portions they gave themselves. Feeding more than "remnants" of these prestige foods was feared to spoil the child's moral character. Apprentices to the Ifa priesthood were given elder status with respect to access to privileged information but were not spoiled with food. The frequent animal sacrifices to the Ifa, however, assured a meat supply to priestly households. Some ceremonies for child apprentices also required them to eat the flesh of the animals whose powers they were to incorporate by ritual means.

During the Positive Deviance survey, mothers were asked to indicate the amounts of meat they would give to family members of different ages by drawing with chalk on a brown wooden board representing meat, marked with a grid of half-inch squares (Setiloane, 1995). The mother was first asked to draw the "right" amount of meat for a child of 2, if the amount of meat available were as large as the 11" x 9" board. The median amount indicated was 0.5 cubic inches. Moreover, 65% affirmed that the child should not have more than the amount they had drawn even if the family could afford it, 31% indicated that more would cause the child to steal, 46% that more would spoil the child, and 66% that more would damage the child's moral character.

As an example of the role of meat in moral training, one grandmother tending a street stall in the Iwaya, Yaba, neighborhood of greater Lagos told the project team a cautionary tale. Her son had married a woman of another ethnic group, who had moved out and left him with their two young children. Her modern son had allowed these children to have as much food as they wanted with the dire result that the children grew accustomed to stealing meat from the family stew without being punished. Soon these children began to take and misuse the property of others. One had even picked the lock on the grandmother's own door when she was out and had raided her room for food and money.

Although more detailed than previous studies, most of our findings were not new. Previous research from Nigeria, reviewed by Setiloane (1995), reported that for preschool children, meat and egg were restricted due to beliefs that too much would cause the child's moral degradation (Ogbeide, 1974; Enwonwu, 1983; Ransome-Kuti, 1972; Vemury & Levine, 1978; Den Hartog, 1972). These studies claimed that such restriction contributes to the high malnutrition rate seen in Nigeria, although no one previously had attempted to quantify and test this contribution. Setiloane (1993) demonstrated that the amount of meat the mother indicated she would allocate to the 2-year-old and her beliefs about spoiling were significantly associated with the child's growth status.

## Distribution Rules for Foods of Animal Origin

Fish, the most frequent animal food eaten by Lagos state children of the Positive Deviance study, was not stated to compromise the child's character. Yet the ethnographic study determined that fish, egg, snail, and other animal source foods were rationed to children, like meat, in small slivers relative to the mother's portion.

Our study population had two styles of meat apportionment. The more traditional style gave the entire amount to the father and awaited his distribution. The more modern and universally practiced style provided for different cooking and eating times and for purchase from vendors. The mother apportioned the pieces according to the family's distribution rules, giving the largest share to the father, who, in turn, could share further with the children. For fish, which was eaten almost daily, apportioning by the mother was the expected form of distribution. In the ethnographic study, many fathers were the providers of snacks and treats, which typically consisted of sweets, sodas, and biscuits.

The distribution rules were affirmed by religious rituals that extended the entitlements and obligations of the human hierarchy beyond the grave. Ancestors and divine beings were seniormost in the hierarchical system. Traditionally, the slaughter of a domestic animal was conducted as a sacrifice preceded by prayers to ancestors or other divine intermediaries. The blood, poured or placed on symbols of these presences, represented the life essence of the animal, whose passage from life to death transacted the communication between the worlds. After the various blessings, the best portions of meat were offered to the male head of household, who was the living representative of the divine authority protecting the lineage and the family. It was then the father's role to apportion the meat to the rest of the family, reserving for himself the largest and best pieces. Feelings about the sacramental entitlement of the father to meat ran deep even among Christian focus group members and are a common theme emerging from focus groups and the ethnographic study.

Once entitlement had been manifested and the lesson of entitlement accomplished, however, adult males could demonstrate their devotion to their children by redistributing their own share of foods. Both the ethnographic study and focus groups repeatedly uncovered a pattern by which fathers "spoil the child with meat." The mother might give the child his or her strictly limited share and then, if the father were available and favorably disposed toward the child, the child would eat again with him. At that time the father would give the child additional meat and fish from his portion. The mothers' official attitude toward this practice was that they disapproved of such spoiling but it was the father's right to do so. However, the tones in which the mothers pronounced this disapproval tended to express veiled pride in having a husband who took such care of her child.

According to Chief S.O. Atanda (personal communication, 1989), the Asiwaju Awo of Lagos, Secretary of the Yoruba Ifa Traditional Healing Association, the sacramental obligations inherent in the male entitlement to animal foods were the grounds through which the father should be motivated to reapportion meat or fish to meet the nutritional needs of younger children. Having received this food as his right, he would be obliged to put the well-being of his children first if he understood their needs for these foods. Some focus group members believed that reallocation of a scarce amount of meat or fish could best occur if the father, mother, and child all ate together, in which case both parents could quietly favor the child if they understood that the food was needed for the child's development. The suggestion that father, mother, and child eat together appeared to blend the traditional presentation of the meat to the father with modern nuclear family values of companionship.

Chief Atande (personal communication, 1989) also related the meat distribution rules to hunting. Meat obtained by hunting involved a risk. A ritual was established whereby the oldest person was given the largest share. Meat was not regarded as an essential food; it was special. Its distribution reflected that value, the biggest share going to the head of the household who presumably protected the household and took the risk of hunting for the meat. Even today, meat distribution to the male household head honors his symbolic role as the hunter/provider. Similar attitudes regarding meat distribution may have existed in Europe and the United States. The author of a novel about second-generation Polish immigrants to the United States in the 1940s relates that the mother was adamant that in her home the "father did not get the lion's share with the children watching hungrily, the way she'd seen meals in other families. In her home they each got one meatball, or one lamb chop or pork chop" (French, 1987).

Chief Atanda noted further that the ritual sacrifices of traditional Yoruba religion rely on animals, birds, and fish to propitiate the "unseen mouths" of those above. Each food has symbolic significance in folk perceptions that correspond to its significance in such sacrifices. For example, cocks are sacrificed to ward off death because they crow at dawn; fish are offered so that they may serve as messengers to the divine by seeking out spirits that reside in the waters. These associations may lend animal foods further resonance even for the majority who now adhere to Christianity and Islam.

Bascom (1951) reported that meat was originally a food for ceremonies and special occasions among the Yoruba, and only the chiefs and wealthy could afford to buy it regularly in the market or to kill a domestic animal simply for food. British colonial influence increased the amount of meat in the average Yoruba diet even though meat was still considered a prestige food.

## Restriction of Staples and Other Foods during Food Scarcity

When food was relatively abundant, as in the Oyo UNICEF baseline sites, restriction for moral training applied only to meat and other taboo foods. Both the Oyo rural and urban studies reported a permissive feeding atmosphere. In Oyo town, where 23 eating events were observed, 11 were snacks, and in almost half, children were fed without having to indicate they were hungry. When food was scarce, however, as at the Oyun UNICEF baseline site (Wilson-Oyelaran & Ladipo, 1989b), the Yoruba appeared to extend the fear-of-spoiling rationale to justify withholding all types of foods from children. In Oyun, 16 children were observed in 45 eating events, of which 45% were unaccompanied carbohydrates, 11% included animal products, and 5% included fruit. Only one instance of a parent offering food without the child's requesting it was observed in Oyun. Only once was a child freely given what he asked for, whereas seven cases of outright refusal were recorded, including requests to have drinking water, to have more food, to eat with the father, to eat what the mother was preparing for sale, to share food with an older sibling, and to be fed anything. It was common for children to ask for food and not receive it until after they cried. Harsh rejecting behavior was observed on four eating occasions when the mother was busy and the child wanted help with eating or a different type of food or complained that the food was spoiled.

In questions regarding their children's feelings, approximately 16% of the Oyun mothers indicated that the child became angry when he or she was hungry, whereas 42% said the child's unhappiness was food related (e.g., caused by not being allowed to eat meat, not receiving as much food as desired, or not being fed on time) (Wilson-Oyelaran & Ladipo, 1989b). Mealtime was reported to be the mother's most stressful time of day. A harsher atmosphere surrounded eating in Oyun than was reported from the other local government areas, and a higher percentage of children also were underweight. In the Oyun observations, children were reported to have clapped, danced, laughed, and sang when they were provided with food.

In the Lagos focus groups, carried out under worsening economic conditions, it was common to hear mothers say of their child, "He is a good baby—he never demands food unless he really needs to eat." Two 2-year-olds in the Lagos ethnographic sample were disciplined for requesting food. The families of petty food vendors confronted these children with the cost of the snacks they demanded. The Lagos mothers repeatedly evaluated their children's social development by the child's ability to control appetite and to go without whining and begging for food. One 2-year-old who frequently cried to be fed an hour or two after eating was the subject of ridicule in his family.

The Positive Deviance project team did not initially recognize the existence of such withholding because mothers did not view themselves as withholding relatively plentiful starchy staple foods from children. Rather they perceived that they generously gave the child all that the child needed of these foods. Several mothers in the focus groups responded to the question of how they would know if their child had eaten enough with such answers as "I know" or "I look at her stomach and I can see."

## Social Change

Negotiating the transition from traditional to modern Yoruba parental theories is of more than theoretical importance. Only 2% of the Positive Deviance survey parents professed adherence to traditional Yoruba religion. When asked their aspirations for their child's future, 90% specified a profession or higher-level business; 86% wanted the child to complete university or professional school. Of the UNICEF baseline sample mothers, more than two-thirds wished their child to have a modern occupation; a fourth, for the child to become a traditional important person (*enian pataki*) in the community; less than 5% to be a farmer, trader, or fisherman (Akinware et al., 1992).

Urban parents in the Positive Deviance study were slowly abandoning traditional beliefs about meat and moral degradation. Many poor urban families paid a sum equivalent to $0.02 per hour (or 2–3% of the average mother's daily disposable income) to send their 3 to 5-year-olds to preschool "lessons" to learn "abc-123." The most animated focus group discussions and interviews centered on discipline and moral training. Some parents described strategies for enforcing manners and ethics to compensate for greater indulgence with food and play. Others expressed helplessness and alienation in the face of new demands and expectations. The Christian Bible and the tracts of the foreign fundamentalist and new African Christian sects were common guidebooks for transition. The Book of Proverbs and the Old Testament rules for animal sacrifice were identified with proverbs and sacrificial rituals of traditional religion (V. Oseni, personal communication, 1993). The New Testament and guidebooks for Christian family life explained ethical issues and prescribed rules of conduct.

New vocabularies and lifestyles are needed to bridge the cultural distance between traditional and new parental theories. Local experts (e.g., Aina et al., 1992, 1993) must be empowered to provide leadership in cultural renewal (Zeitlin et al., 1995) and cultural adjustment (Etounga-Manguelle, 1991) in order to generate new terms, rationales, entitlements, and satisfactions for parents and children.

## Summary and Conclusions

In their own terms of reference, Yoruba parental theories attach supreme value to children. This chapter has attempted to illustrate the fact that the tasks of Yoruba children are not child labor, their discipline is not child abuse, and their underfeeding is for their own good. It is my personal view that the psychological and spiritual rewards of the Yoruba cosmological adventure were more emotionally fulfilling, accessible to parents and children, and harmonious in their evocation of meaning than are the spiritual satisfactions of contemporary Western life. Yet the task of surviving in the world economic order now has placed the traditional village in a state of ontological dissonance with the global village that requires global understanding and assistance to repair.

## References

Adewale, S. A. (1986). Ethics in Ifa. In S. O. Abogunrin (Ed.), *Religion and ethics in Nigeria* (pp. 60–71). Ibadan, Nigeria: Daystar Press.

Agiobu-Kemmer, I. (1984). Cognitive and affective aspects of infant development. In H. V. Curran (Ed.), *Nigerian children: Developmental perspectives* (pp. 74–117). Boston: Routledge and Kegan Paul.

Aina, T. A., Etta, F. E., & Zeitlin, M. F. (Eds.). (1992). *Child development and nutrition in Nigeria: A textbook for education, health and social service professionals* (1st ed.). Lagos: Nigerian Education Research and Development Council and UNICEF Nigeria.

Aina, T. A., Agiobu-Kemmer, I., Etta, E. F., Zeitlin, M. F., & Setiolane, K. (1993). Early Childhood Care, Development and Nutrition in Lagos State, Nigeria, Phase I Survey Results from the Positive Deviance in Nutrition Research Project produced by the Social Sciences Faculty, University of Lagos, and the Tufts University School of Nutrition for UNICEF, New York.

Akinware, M., Wilson-Oyelaran, E. B., Ladipo, P. A., Pierce, D., & Zeitlin, M. F. (1992). *Child care and development in Nigeria: A profile of five UNICEF assisted LGA'S.* Lagos: UNICEF Nigeria.

Aronson, D. R. (1980). *The city is our farm.* Cambridge, MA: Schenkman.

Babatunde, E. D. (1992). *Culture, religion and the self: A critical study of Bini and Yoruba value systems in change.* Lewiston, NY: Edwin Mellen Press.

Bascom, W. A. (1951). Yoruba food. *Africa, 21,* 40–53.

Bayley, N. (1969). *Manual for the Bayley Scales of Infant Development.* New York: Psychological Corporation.

Caldwell, B. M., & Bradley, R. H. (1984). *Home observation for measurement of the environment.* Little Rock: University of Arkansas Press.

Caldwell, J. C., & Caldwell, P. (1990, May). High fertility in sub-Saharan Africa. *Scientific American,* pp. 118–125.

Caldwell, J. C., & Caldwell, P. (1977). The economic rationale of high fertility: An investigation illustrated with Nigerian survey data. *Population Studies, 31,* 5–27.

Den Hartog, A. P. (1972). Unequal distribution of food within the household: A neglected aspect of food behavior. *FAO Nutrition Newsletter, 10*(4), 8–17.

Doob, L. W. (1965). Psychology. In R. A. Lystad (Ed.), *The African world: A survey of social research.* New York: Praeger.

Enwonwu, C. A. (1983). A review of nutrient requirements and nutritional status in Nigeria. In T. Atinmo & O. Akinyele (Eds.), *Nutrition and food policy in Nigeria.* Jos: National Institute for Policy and Strategic Studies.

Etounga-Manguelle, D. (1991). *L'Afrique a-t-elle besoin d'un programme d'adjustement culturel?* Paris: Editions Nouvelles du Sud.

Fadipe, N. A. (1970). *The sociology of the Yoruba.* Ibadan, Nigeria: Ibadan University Press.

French, M. (1987). *Her mother's daughter: A novel.* New York: Summit Books.

Gittelsohn, J. (1991). Opening the box: Intrahousehold food allocation in rural Nepal. *Social Sciences Medicine, 33*(10), 1141–1154.

Hallgren, R. (1991). *The good things in life, a study of the traditional religious culture of the Yoruba people.* Loberod: Botforlaget Plus Ultra.

LeVine, R. A. (1963). Child rearing in sub-Saharan Africa: An interim report. *Bulletin of the Menninger Clinic, 27,* 245–256.

Lloyd, B. B. (1966). Education in family life in the identification of class identification among the Yoruba. In P. C. Lloyd (Ed.), *New elites of tropical Africa.* London: Oxford University Press.

Lloyd, B. B. (1970). Yoruba mothers' reports of child-rearing, some theoretical and methodological considerations. In P. Mayer (Ed.), *Socialization, the approach from social anthropology.* New York: Tavistock.

Lloyd, P. C. (1974). *Power and independence, urban Africans' perception of social inequality.* London & Boston: Routledge & Kegan Paul.

Ogbeide, O. (1974). Nutritional hazards of food taboos and preferences in Mid-West Nigeria. *American Journal of Clinical Nutrition, 27,* 213–216.

Olusanya, P. O. (1987). *Human reproduction in Africa: Fact, myth and the martyr syndrome.*

Ransome-Kuti, O. (1972). Some socioeconomic conditions predisposing to malnutrition in Lagos, Nigeria. *Nigerian Medical Journal, 2,* 111–118.

Setiloane, K. (1995). *Beliefs and practices regarding meat distribution and nutritional status of children in Lagos state, Nigeria.* Unpublished doctoral dissertation, Tufts University School of Nutrition, Medford, MA.

Vemury, M., & Levine, H. (1978). *Beliefs and practices that affect food habits in developing countries.* New York: CARE.

Wilson-Oyelaran, E. B., & Ladipo, P. (1987, August). *Child care and development, a baseline survey of rural areas in Oyo local government.* UNICEF, Nigeria.

Wilson-Oyelaran, E. B., & Ladipo, P. (1988, May). *Child care and development, a baseline survey of preschool age children in Owo local government.* UNICEF Nigeria.

Wilson-Oyelaran, E. B., & Ladipo, P. (1989a, May). *Child care and development, a baseline survey of preschool children in Oyo town.* UNICEF Nigeria.

Wilson-Oyelaran, E. B., & Ladipo, P. (1989b, May). *Child care and development, a baseline survey of preschool age children in Oyun local government.* UNICEF Nigeria.

Zeitlin, M. F., Wray, J. D., Stanbury, J. B., Schlossman, N. P., Meurer, J. J., & Weinthal, P. J. (1982). *Nutrition and population growth: The delicate balance.* Cambridge, MA: Oelgeschlager, Gunn, & Hain.

Zeitlin, M. F., Megawangi, R., Kramer, E. M., Colletta, N. D., Babatunde, E. D., & Garman D. (1995). *Strengthening the family: Implications for international development.* Tokyo: United Nations University Press.

# CHAPTER 18

# Growth Consequences of Low-Income Nicaraguan Mothers' Theories about Feeding 1-Year-Olds

Patrice L. Engle
Marian Zeitlin
Yadira Medrano
Lino Garcia M.

Poor nutrition and inadequate growth continue to be major problems for the developing countries, where the vast majority of the world's children live. According to a 1993 UNICEF report, 35% of these children are underweight; as high to 60% are underweight in southern Asia (UNICEF, 1993). In all countries, underweight peaks during the second year of the child's life, "although the risk of cumulative or chronic malnutrition remains higher from the second year onward" (UNICEF, 1993, p. 14). Inadequate nutrition prenatally and during the first 2 years of life has been causally linked to defects in cognitive functioning in adolescence, particularly among adolescents from poorer socioeconomic strata (Pollitt, Gorman, Engle, Martorell, & Rivera, 1993). Undernutrition should be targeted as a central problem for long-term human investment.

The problem of undernutrition remains difficult to remedy, despite programs that increase income, provide food subsidies, and improve health care (Kennedy, 1989). Increases in income to families with undernourished children have resulted in smaller gains in children's growth than expected (Marek, 1992). Many other factors appear to determine child nutritional status, such as who the income earner is and how the income is translated into food within the household (e.g, Engle, 1993), how food is allocated within the household, healthiness of the environment, breast feeding, and nutrient density of the foods offered to children (summarized in Engle, 1992 and Engle, 1994). Recent work has suggested that not only resource limitations but also the psychosocial aspects of feeding, including encouragement of feeding, frequency of feeding, and maternal beliefs about feeding young children, may contribute to the persistence of the growth stunting. For example, in two samples of undernourished children observed in Guatemala and Mexico, more than half did not eat all the food that was presented to them (Engle, Nieves, La Montagne, & Medrano, 1990; Garcia, Kaiser, & Dewey, 1990). This chapter examines the relation between parental beliefs about child feeding and children's nutritional status in Managua, Nicaragua.

Nutritional researchers tend to focus on issues of food preparation and food availability. Manuals for developing countries describe the kinds of food that should be presented at each age (e.g., Mitzner, Scrimshaw, & Morgan, 1985). Only recently has attention been given to the ways in which this food is presented, particularly to young children (see Myers, 1992). Yet this psychosocial context of feeding may be as important as food availability for adequate nutrition. In developing countries, where malnutrition continues to be a major health problem in young children, sometimes the only resource that can be provided is to enhance the quality of the child's care (Engle, 1992).

One approach to this problem from the perspective of international nutrition has been to identify caregiving behaviors associated with better child nutritional status despite conditions of poverty. Families displaying these behaviors are recognized as positive deviants (Zeitlin, Super et al., 1990), and the behaviors that have contributed to their children's well-being are identified. This strategy identifies strengths within the cultural context instead of failures. Once a strategy or behavior is identified, it is then available to be taught to other families in the same area (Zeitlin, 1991).

Psychological definitions of context help to delineate these psychosocial factors in feeding. Super and Harkness (1986) have introduced the concept of the "developmental niche" of the child as a "theoretical framework for studying cultural regulation of the micro-environment of the child" (p. 552). The environment is considered to have three component subsystems: (1) the physical and social setting in which the child is placed, (2) the culturally regulated customs of child care and childrearing, and (3) the caregivers' individual beliefs about development. Each of these systems has implications for the psychosocial aspects of feeding children under three.

Nonnutritional effects on nutrient ingestion have been found in each of the three subsystems. For example, children under 3 years old fed in the presence of other children were observed to consume more than children fed alone (Engle, Nieves, Zeitlin, La Montagne, & Medrano, 1990), a dimension of the *setting*. Second, cultures frequently have *customs* concerning the order in which family members eat or how family members receive food. In some societies, each person takes food from a single pot, whereas in others the food is distributed by one person to each person's plate (Dettwyler, 1986). These customs may influence intrahousehold allocation of food or the relative amount of food given to various family members. For example, males tend to receive significantly more food than females (Chen, Huq, & De'Souza, 1981; Ravindran, 1986; Van Esterick, 1985; Rogers, 1990; Powell & Grantham-McGregor, 1985). In Guatemala, Engle and Nieves (1993) reported that male heads of household received relatively more protein compared to their recommended need than other family members.

A third subsystem of the developmental niche are caregiver beliefs. *Beliefs* about food and feeding will have significant effects on food allocation. Dettwyler (1989a, 1986) and others (see Engle, 1992, for a review) have suggested that in some cultures mothers assume that young children can and should regulate their own feeding. For example, Dettwyler reported that in Mali, mothers do not begin to feed weaning-age children; rather, the children can take food from the family pot when they are ready. These concepts vary within a culture, but there is little research on the differences. This chapter illustrates some individual differences.

Social cognitive theory provides some structures for thinking about these beliefs. Social cognition is the "way people make sense of other people and themselves" (Fiske & Taylor, 1984, p. 12). One area of investigation is how people make attributions or explain causes in social behavior. Because these judgments are often made in the absence of complete information, they reflect errors and biases that can be systematically studied (Fiske & Taylor, 1984). Another aspect of social cognition is the extent to which people feel they are in control of events or of other agents. Concepts of control may influence the attributional process. Dettwyler (1989b) suggests that cultures differ on a dimension of caregiver–child control of eating. At one end of the scale are cultures in which parents insist that children eat all the food presented (caregiver control), illustrated by force feeding in Nigeria and to some extent by eating encouragement in European and American societies. At the other end of the scale are cultures such as the one described in Mali, in which it is understood that the child will eat when he or she is ready: "The stomach knows." When food is available, eating then becomes under the child's control.

Psychologists have used social cognitive theories to explain how parents account for their children's behavior within the U.S. culture. For example, Himmelstein, Graham, and Weiner (1991) examined parents' perceptions of the importance of childrearing practices versus the child's disposition or the environment as determinants of the child's behavior. The higher the child's level of achievement, the more likely the parents were to attribute the outcome to childrearing; the farther the child from the norm, the more likely the parents were to attribute the outcome to the child's disposition or the environment. Bugental, Blue, and Cruzcosa (1989) distinguished mothers' self-attributions for successful caregiving along a dimension ranging from attributing all variation to caregiving ("self-referent") at one end to attributing all variation to the child's disposition or the environment ("child-referent"). Parents who tended to believe that their children's behavior was related to the child's disposition or to the environment (child-referent) had more negative affect toward their children than those who attributed more of the variance in child behavior to themselves (self-referent) (Bugental et al., 1989). Parents' beliefs or attributions about the causes of their children's behavior may have influences on feeding behaviors that are significant where undernutrition is endemic.

Anthropologists have long argued that parents develop folk theories to explain why their children behave as they do. Second, anthropologists often find that these theories differ from those of American middle-class parents. LeVine (1988) suggests that all parents develop investment strategies and associated behaviors to ensure that their children achieve the parents' goals. The goals will differ according to the cultural and ecological context. These goals may be reflected in feeding behaviors.

Interviews with Nicaraguan mothers during preliminary work (Engle, Nieves et al., 1990) suggested that many held a "maturational" view of their children's development; rather than encourage or push them in a certain path, they trusted that the children would eat according to their needs. For example, when asked, "When a child doesn't finish his meal, is it better to leave him alone, or help him to finish it?" half the mothers responded that it was better to leave the child alone because if the child had been hungry, he or she would have eaten more. This answer seems to attribute the child's failure to eat to the child (child-referent) rather than to maternal caregiving (self-referent). These distinctions may be specific to a particular phase of the child's development. The current study extends this work by examining maternal beliefs about feeding and observations of child behavior from 80 12–19-month-old children living in a poor urban area around Managua, Nicaragua, where undernutrition is endemic. In this study, parents' views about their responsibility versus the child's responsibility for eating were explored, and the association between these opinions and the child's anthropometric status was assessed. It was hypothesized that (1) mothers would vary in their tendency to attribute children's lack of eating to child dispositions (child-referent) or to maternal caregiving (self-referent), (2) mothers with self-referent beliefs would be more likely to have well-nourished children, and (3) mothers with self-referent beliefs would be observed to be more active and encouraging feeders than the more child-referent mothers. This age group was selected for study because nutritional effects may be most evident during the second year of a child's life, typically a period of growth faltering, high rates of illness, and developmental risk, and because children of this age are often not prepared to feed themselves completely. Anthropometric measures assessed include height for age, which tends to reflect long-term nutritional deprivation, and two weight measures—weight for age and weight for height, which reflect wasting or more short-term nutritional effects (ACC/SCN, 1992).

Because those mothers who expressed a greater desire to help their children eat might also be more educated and live in wealthier houses, the analytic design is a multiple regression controlling for these possible confounding variables. In the remainder of this chapter, we describe the setting for the study and the methods used to collect the data and test the three hypotheses initially presented. The purpose of the chapter is to determine whether there are connections between beliefs and behavior that might have an effect on the growth of young children.

# Method

## The Setting

The study location was 10 neighborhoods surrounding Managua, Nicaragua. The barrios were sampled to be representative of a larger UNICEF-funded study of positive deviance (Zeitlin, Bonilla & Medrano, 1991). Half the neighborhoods were established areas and the other half were *asentimeintos*, or settlements built during the decade of the 1980s. The latter were considerably poorer. Given the generally warm tropical temperatures, houses tended to be open. The land around Managua is flat or gently rolling, so that the neighborhoods were rectangular lots with regular streets but with a feeling of openness which permitted some trees. Eighty-five percent of the families had fruit trees.

The most common house had a brick lower half and wood on the upper half, with a roof made of lamina (corrugated material). Half the houses had dirt floors; 27% had tile. Less than half had water available in the home, although potable water was available in the community. Almost all houses had sanitary facilities; 71% had latrines and 25% had flush toilets. Electricity was virtually universal (95%). Most houses were one or two rooms (69%). In terms of household possessions, the most common were a radio (55%), an iron (77%), a clock (46%), and a television (38%). Few owned a refrigerator (7%) or a car (5%).

Although incomes were most likely very low, the research site was not as impoverished as some Latin American shantytowns; families had a plot of land and a house to place on it and some space around them. Under the Sandinistas, land titles were being given to the residents. During the time of the study, the Sandinistas were still in power, and health care, vaccination campaigns, and maintaining health posts in the local neighborhoods were high priorities. Milk subsidies had been provided for some time but were not available at the time of the study. The stress of the war had tremendous effects on family organization.

## Subjects

Eighty children between the ages of 12 months and 19 months were randomly sampled from 10 barrios in which nutritional status had been identified as low. The mean age of the children was 15 months. Half the subjects were girls. More than 28% of the children would be considered undernourished according to World Health Organization (WHO) standards; they were below −2 standard deviations (*SD*) of National Child Health Service (NCHS) standards in height for age. In addition, 21% were below −2 *SD* in weight for age, and 6% were below −2 *SD* in weight for height. Another 22% were between −1 and −2 *SD* in weight for height (WHO, 1983). These three anthropometric measurements are presumed to have different meanings. Height for age generally reflects long-term chronic undernutrition. Weight for height reflects shorter-term acute undernutrition, and weight for age combines both of these measures but in most ages is similar to the weight for height measurements.

The mothers were predominately literate (82%), half had earned at least a 6th-grade education, but only 8% continued beyond 10th grade. Families tended to be nontraditional. Fifty-one percent lived in a consensual relationship with a man, 22% were legally married, and 26% were single mothers. Mothers in relationships did not always live with their partner; 66% lived with the partner full-time, 20% lived with him more than half the time, and 14% lived with him less than half the time, or he was in military service. Not surprisingly, the percentage of families in which the father provided full support for the children was limited; in 54% of the 80 houses, the mother reported full support from the father. Many women were stressed, with 40% reporting having experienced *nervios*, a state of anxiety.

Given the economic situation, it is to be expected that women would work for income. More than half (56%) these mothers of very young children worked for income, on average, 5 days a week and between 4 and 8 hours a day. The most common occupation was street vending (35% of all mothers); only 2 mothers (5%) had technical or professional jobs. Income was not assessed because people are generally reluctant to provide that information and because the rate of inflation was so great that incomes were hard to interpret.

When mothers were working, children were left with another family member (48% older than 13; 7% younger than 13). The other two strategies were to work at home with the child (26% of working mothers) or take the child to the place of work (18%). The effects of these different forms of child care has been explored elsewhere (La Montagne, Engle, & Zeitlin, 1993).

Almost half the children were still breast feeding, although all were receiving supplementary foods. Exclusive breast feeding in the first 6 months was rare; 68% initiated bottle feeding at 1 month or less. The most common foods that the children ate were rice and beans, bread, eggs, milk, and cheese. Common drinks were juices and coffee. On the day of the interview, 20% of the children were suffering from diarrhea.

## Instruments and Procedure

The study occurred in 1989, from July through October. Initial contact with the families was made in the morning. If the family was willing to participate, the observer immediately entered the home, and interviewed the caregiver about the family composition, feeding history, and feeding attitudes. All children under age 4 in the family were weighed and measured. The observer then proceeded to remain in the home quietly observing for an average of 3 hours until lunch was completed. The behaviors surrounding any eating event of the target child were coded onto a standardized coding sheet, and other behaviors were observed for a period of 1 hour. Because the mothers were not warned prior to the visit, they were not able to prepare any special foods for the child or design atypical activities.

At the end of the day, the family was told that the observer would return the following week to visit the family again. However, the day was not specified. On the second visit, observations of behavior and of feeding events were repeated, and the mother was asked her opinions about feeding the child. These questions were reserved for the end of the second day of observation so that the mother would not have been influenced in her feeding behaviors of the child. Observational data were averaged across the 2 days. All families were given gifts at the termination of the study.

The household questionnaire was administered to the mother or other primary caregiver upon entry to the house. The form contained information in four areas: family membership and roles, house quality and possessions, mother's characteristics (education, level of stress, work history, and contraceptive knowledge), and child history (breast feeding, illness, and treatment history).

Event sampling was used to record behaviors during eating events. All feeding events were recorded on standardized forms. For each feeding event, 37 behaviors were coded. For example, the observer noted who fed the child (mother, caregiver, or eating alone), what the child's eating situation was during the eating event (sitting, standing, walking), and with whom the child ate. For the purposes of the questionnaire, it was critical to observe the child's level of interest in the food (did the child ask for more, look at the food consistently, and finish all of the food) and the caregiver's level of encouragement of eating during the eating event. Each observed behavior was coded as either *present* or *absent* for that eating event. The observers estimated the amount of food eaten and the amount of food left.

Snacks, bottles, and lunch were coded separately. Because the observations occurred during mango season, and this was a common food to give to children, it was used as the basis for definition of a snack, the requirement for an observation to occur. The food had to be as large as a piece of mango approximately .5 inches by 1.5 inches, the size of a piece normally cut off of a mango for a child (many times a child was given a whole peeled mango to suck). A smaller nibble given to a child would not be recorded.

Time sampling was used to record the child's activity level and the caregiver's responsiveness. A 1-hour time sample was taken during the morning visit. Every 5 minutes, a series of 13 behaviors of child and caregiver was coded. This assessment was repeated at both visits. If the child ate a snack, bottle, or lunch during the time sample, the sampling was suspended until the eating event was over, and then it was resumed. If the child fell asleep, it was also suspended.

The Eating Attitudes Questionnaire was administered at the end of the second day in order to assess the woman's memory of her child's eating behavior during the day, which could then be compared with the actual behavior as a measure of her recall. The questions also assessed her attitudes toward feeding a reluctant eater and her beliefs about feeding during diarrhea episodes.

The four Nicaraguan observers were physicians or nurses and faculty members at the medical school. Three were doing their social service during this time. All were women. The first author trained each of the observers to an acceptable level of reliability for each of the codes in the time sample form (at least 80%).

## Variables

Nutritional status was assessed with measurements of children's length to the nearest millimeter and weight to the nearest 0.1 kg according to WHO (1983) recommendations. Measurements were made on a Salter scale and a wooden board marked in centimeters, with a headboard and a footboard, which had been constructed specifically for the study for the purpose of measuring length. Children were measured in the horizontal position.

All four testers were trained and standardized in anthropometry by a master's-level nutritionist. All measurements were made in the home. They were then converted into standardized z-scores using the NCHS norms from the United States (Jordan & Staehling, 1986).

## Scale Construction

Three scales were constructed from hypothetically related items. Cronbach's alpha measures were calculated for each scale to measure internal consistency. Those that resulted in higher Cronbach's alpha values (Cronbach, 1984) were retained, and other items were dropped. The final items included and alpha values are shown in Table 18.1. The three scales were (1) the Help Scale, which assessed the mother's responses indicating that she was aware of some actions she could take to increase the amount of food a child would eat and whether or not she helped the child to eat; (2) Active Feeding Scale, reflecting encouragement, threats, serving, or other actions to encourage eating; and (3) the Child Demand Scale, composed of the child's number of food requests prior to eating, his or her appetite during the meal, and his or her requests for additional food. The last two were computed for the lunch meal, snacks, and bottles. Only the lunch score is discussed here because not all children were observed to eat snacks or a bottle, and using these measures would have reduced the sample size. They are discussed in a subsequent paper (Engle, 1995).

Internal consistency measures for the first two scales were low. However, because they were related to other measures as expected, we

**Table 18.1.** Scale Construction: Variables Included and Alpha Values

Help Scale:

1. Number of times mother mentioned mother's responsibility in response to question, "why do you think that some children have little appetite?" (Range 0–3, 58% were 0).
2. Number of times mother mentioned mother's responsibility in response to question, "when your child doesn't want to eat, what do you do?" (Range 0–2, 21% were 0).
3. Mother reports that her child eats with help, rather than on child's own. (59% reports eats with help).
        Alpha = .31

Active Feeding Scale:

| | |
|---|---|
| 1. Mother encourages child to eat during meal. | 56% |
| 2. Mother threatens child if doesn't eat, | 9% |
| 3. Mother serves child more. | 9% |
| 4. Mother offers child more. | 8% |
| 5. Mother orders child to eat more. | 6% |
| 6. Mother demonstrates to child how to eat more. | 7% |
|       Alpha = .40. | |

Child Demand Scale:

| | |
|---|---|
| 1. Food was requested before it was offered. | 14% |
| 2. Number of times child asked for food before receiving it. | *Mean* = 0 |
| 3. Eating enthusiasm at the beginning of meal. | 75% = high |
| 4. Eating enthusiasm at the middle of the meal. | 40% = high |
| 5. Eating enthusiasm at the end of the meal. | 27% = high |
| 6. Child asked for more food. | 9% |
|       Alpha = .67 | |

Child Activity/Motor Development Scale: Mean level of activity observed on 5-minute time samples over a 2-hour period on 2 separate days.

8: running energetically
7: running
6: walking
5: crawling
4: standing
3: sitting
2: lying down
1: being held

felt that they represented a domain of behavior that was measured by a group of unique items.

The average activity level of the children over the 2-hour time sample (24 observations per child on 2 separate days) was computed. Finally, a count of the number of times the child ate during the observer's visit was recorded.

Five groups of variables (15 total) were defined:

1. Help Scale
2. Mother's feeding assistance behaviors: Active Feeding Scale and number of eating events
3. Child characteristics: Activity/Motor Development Level Scale, Child Demand Scale, and the standard demographic variables of age, sex, birth order, and illness on the 2 observation days
4. Mother characteristics: schooling, house quality, and percentage of time she lives with partner (Live With)
5. Outcome measures for children: height for age z-score, weight for age z-score, and weight for height z-score.

# Findings

There is relatively little encouragement of eating in the Nicaraguan sample. When asked whether children who refused food should be encouraged to eat more, 48% replied that children should be left to finish on their own. As another example, 41% of mothers felt that children should be able to eat entirely on their own by 12 months of age, a difficult task for most children. A little more than half the mothers were observed to encourage, verbally or with gestures, their children to eat during a meal, and less than 10% demonstrated how to eat more or offered more food.

## Relations among Attitude Variables

The variable that initially sparked our interest, whether a caregiver would encourage a child who did not finish a meal was related to only one other attitudinal measure of eating: the age at which the mother thought that a child should be able to eat without help. Mothers who said that they would not encourage a child to finish thought that a child should eat without help at 16 months ($SD = 7.2$), whereas those who said that they would encourage a child to finish felt that a child should not be able to eat without help until the much older age of 19.8 months ($SD$

= 6.9). The suggested ages for eating without help differed significantly for the two groups of mothers, $t(77) = 2.14$, $p < .05$.

## Relations of Attitude Variables to Behavioral Variables

Table 18.2 shows the correlations of the Help Scale and the Active Feeding Scale with other variables. The Help Scale (attitude) was unrelated to the Active Feeding Scale (behavior). Correlations with related variables suggested that these two scales are measuring different constructs. The Help Scale scores were higher for mothers living in better houses and with younger and less active children. On the other hand, more active feeding was observed with older children and children who received more feedings (lunch, bottles or snacks).

The Active Feeding Scale was negatively, although not significantly, associated with the Child Demand Scale. Mothers did not encourage children who demanded more; on the contrary, there is a suggestion that they fed children more who demanded less.

## Associations of Help Scale, Active Feeding, and Children's Nutritional Status

Table 18.3 shows simple correlations of the 12 variables and the key dependent measures of height for age, weight for age, and weight for height. As the table shows, the Help Scale is associated with height for age, whereas the Active Feeding Scale is not.

Because the Help Scale was associated with an indicator of socio-

**Table 18.2.** Correlations of Help Scale and Active Feed Scale with Other Measures ($N = 80$)

| Variable | Help Scale | Active Feed Scale |
|---|---|---|
| Mothers' schooling | .15 | .11 |
| House quality | .27** | −.09 |
| Live with father | −.02 | −.07 |
| Self-efficacy scale | .12 | .04 |
| Child's age | −.19[a] | .25** |
| Activity level | −.21* | .18 |
| Birth order | −.10 | -.11 |
| Gender | .03 | −.05 |
| Number of meals | .11 | .22* |
| Child demand | −.10 | -.17 |
| Illness during observation | −.06 | .01 |

*$p < .05$; **$p < .01$; [a]$p < .10$.

economic status and child activity variables that were also associated with anthropometric status, a multiple regression of the Help Scale on anthropometric status was performed controlling for these variables. Four measures were dropped from the regression because they were consistently not significant and had no other conceptual reason for being included. Variables dropped were Illness on the day of the observation, percentage of time mother lived with partner, Active Feeding Scale, and number of eating events. The resulting regression model is shown in Table 18.4.

For the Help Scale, the slopes were significant for the height for age and marginal for weight for age. The model for weight for height was not significant. Other variables that were also associated with height for age were schooling of the mother, Activity/Motor Development Scale for the child, gender (girls lower than boys), and the Child demand score (negative). For weight for age, there were also significant associations for schooling of the mother, birth order, and activity level.

The anthropometric status variables are standardized by age and gender. The lower height for age for the girls reflects differences not observed in the standardization sample (U.S.). One possibility is that they are receiving less care than the boys. They did receive significantly less encouragement (active feeding) to eat snacks than boys, $M = 1.73$ for boys, $M = 1.28$ for girls, $t(59) = 2.06$, $p < .05$, although no differences by gender were found for the noon meal.

In these regressions, child demand (or appetite for lunch) was

**Table 18.3.** Correlations of Help Scale, Active Feeding Scale and Other Measures with Eight for Age, Weight for Age, and Weight for Height Scores ($N = 80$)

| Variable | Ht./Age | Wt./Age | Wt./Ht. |
|---|---|---|---|
| Mothers' schooling | .28** | .19[a] | .00 |
| House quality | .17 | .18[a] | .11 |
| Live with father | .12 | .10 | −.01 |
| Self-efficacy scale | −.05 | −.06 | .00 |
| Child's age | −.05 | .07 | .02 |
| Activity level | .27** | .39** | .23* |
| Birth order | −.13 | .03 | .19[a] |
| Gender | −.22* | −.17 | −.01 |
| Number of meals | .16 | .28** | .22* |
| Child demand | −.22* | −.17 | −.01 |
| Active feeding | .11 | .10 | −.02 |
| Help scale | .25* | .15 | .01 |
| Illness during observation | −.09 | −.15 | −.15 |

*$p < .05$; **$p < .01$; [a]$p < .10$.

negatively associated with height for age and weight for age. In other words, it appeared that the less hungry the child, the better his or her nutritional status. This association may be a function of the type of meal. Child demand for snacks and for bottles was positively associated with the anthropometric measures, significantly for weight and for height (Engle, 1995) as expected. It is possible that a child who has received enough food between meals, and is better nourished, may be less interested in lunch.

# Discussion

This project was searching for "positive deviants," families who managed to rear healthy children despite poverty and lack of resources (Zeitlin, Mansour, & Boghabi, 1990). We hypothesized that believing that it is important to encourage young children to eat more might be a positive deviant belief, and that it might be associated with better growth among the children living under conditions of poverty.

The first hypothesis, that mothers would vary in their attitudes toward their responsibility for ensuring that young children eat (the Help Scale), was supported. Some mothers expressed more concern about helping children to eat and were more likely to take responsibility for the children's lack of eating than were others.

Our second hypothesis, that these variations in the mother's beliefs about responsibility would be associated with growth, was also supported. It appears that the mother's belief that if her child does not eat, she can do something about it is associated with better growth for her

**Table 18.4.** Regression Analysis of Help Scale on Nutritional Status Indicators Controlling for Contextual Variables ($N = 80$) ($b$ values)

| Variable | Ht./Age | Wt./Age | Wt./Ht. |
|---|---|---|---|
| Help Scale | .24[**] | .15[a] | .02 |
| Age of child | −.09 | −.04 | −.05 |
| Gender of child | −.40[a] | −.27 | −.00 |
| Birth order | −.00 | .10[a] | .13 |
| Child demand | −.14[*] | −.10[a] | −.02 |
| House quality | −.00 | .02 | .04 |
| Mother's schooling | .07[*] | .05[a] | .01 |
| Activity/motor | .41[**] | .45[**] | .26[*] |
| $F$ of model | 4.01[**] | 4.20[**] | 1.89[a] |
| $R^2$ | .31 | .32 | .18 |

[*]$p < .05$; [**]$p < .01$; [a]$p < .10$.

12–18-month old children, even controlling for a number of socioeconomic measures. An attitude that if a child does not eat, the mother can take some action is a self-referent perspective and contrasts with the view that the child's failure to eat is a function of his or her characteristics (child-referent).

The third hypothesis, that mothers with self-referent beliefs would be more active feeders than those with child-referent beliefs, was not supported. The behaviors that link a self-referent perspective with improved anthropometric status are not clearly evident from this study. No association between the Active feeding score and the Help Scale was found. It appears that active feeding as measured here occurs in response to child refusal. One aspect of low child demand—failure to finish a meal—was associated with active feeding for both snacks and bottles (Engle, 1995). Thus, parents' encouragement for children to eat seemed to be a response to a perceived problem rather than a proactive effort for most mothers.

Feeding encouragement could be based on two different goals: compensation for a lack of eating or enhancement of the child's growth. Engle (1992) draws a distinction between those behaviors intended to return a child to a previously accepted state of health or development (compensatory care) and those that serve to enhance further development (enhancement care). Examples of compensatory care are taking an ill child to a health care center to bring the child back to health or encouraging an anorexic child to eat until the child achieves a normal appetite. Enhancement care could include stimulating a child in play and language, encouraging a well-eating child to finish the last bite, or taking a child to the health center for preventive care or vaccinations.

It appears in the Nicaraguan sample that children who received more eating encouragement were those who tended to refuse food (compensatory care), a finding also reported by Bentley, Stallings, Fukmoto, and Elder (1991) in Peru. However, other studies have found examples of active feeding which appear to be enhancement care. Two studies by Zeitlin et al., one in Mexico (Zeitlin, Houser, & Johnson, 1989), the other in Bangladesh (Zeitlin, Super et al., 1990), found that when the mother/caregiver's feeding behavior was measured quantitatively (e.g., the amount of time spent preparing food or the number of spoonfuls given to the child), active feeding *was* associated with better nutritional status. The measure of Active Feeding constructed here may reflect behaviors that occur too late in the eating event to have an effect on ingestion. Therefore, we may have been measuring compensatory feeding, not enhancement feeding. It is likely that enhancement feeding would be positively associated with the Help Scale (self-referent attitudes), whereas our measures were unrelated to either self- or child-referent attitudes.

Caregivers who expressed child responsibility may assume that unless the child appears to have a problem, the child should determine the amount of food eaten. This observation is consistent with the previous finding of more active feeding in response to lower demand. Unfortunately, low child demand plays an important role in the creation of malnutrition (Bentley, Dettwyler, & Caulfield, 1993). When a child begins to refuse food, perhaps due to illness, food quality or timing, it may be the extra efforts of the caregivers' insistence on eating that bring the child out of the vicious circle of illness, loss of appetite, and loss of energy. These efforts could be associated with the mothers' self-referent attitudes.

Self-confidence of the mother has been linked to the ability to encourage active feeding of a malnourished child (Gibbons & Griffiths, 1984). In a related analysis of these data, mothers who reported higher self-esteem also showed some evidence of increased eating encouragement (Engle & Davidson, 1991); the higher-self-esteem mothers were more likely to help their children to eat than the lower-self-esteem mothers. Although self-esteem and self-referent attitudes are positively associated here, the level was not significant.

In sum, these data clearly link maternal attitudes about child and self-responsibility for eating with child nutritional status during this crucial period in the children's lives. On the other hand, behavioral encouragement to eat as observed here did not reflect the sense of responsibility of the mother about feeding. Further work is needed to determine the ways in which mothers translate their belief in helping children to eat into feeding behaviors.

## Acknowledgments

An earlier version of this chapter was presented at Society for Research in Child Development, Seattle, Washington, April 1991. Support for this project was provided under a contract to the second author by UNICEF New York and the Joint Nutrition Support Fund of the Italian Government.

## References

Administrative Committee on Coordination/Subcommittee on Nutrition (1992). *Second report on the world nutrition situation.* Geneva: United Nations (ACC/SCN).

Bentley, M. E., Dettwyler, K. A., & Caulfield, L. E. (1993, March 14–19). *Child anorexia and its management in developing country settings: Review and recommendations.* Paper prepared for the Workship and Expert Meeting on Guidelines for Nutrition and Feeding of Children 0-5 years in the Latin American Region, Porlamar, Venezuela.

Bentley, M. E., Stallings, R. Y., Fukumoto, M., & Elder, J. A. (1991). Maternal feeding behavior and child acceptance of food during diarrhea, convalescence, and health in the central Sierra of Peru. *American Journal of Public Health, 81,* 43–47.

Bugental, D., Blue, J., & Cruzcosa, M. (1989). Perceived control over caregiving outcomes: Implications for child abuse. *Developmental Psychology, 25,* 532–539.

Chen, L., Huq, E., & De'Souza, S. (1981, March). Sex bias in the family allocation of food and health care in rural Bangladesh. *Population Development Review, 7,* 55–69.

Cronbach, L. (1984). *Essentials of psychological testing* (4th ed.). New York: Harper & Row.

Dettwyler, K. A. (1986). Infant feeding in Mali, West Africa: Variations in belief and practice. *Social Science and Medicine, 23,* 651–664.

Dettwyler, K. A. (1987). Breastfeeding and weaning in Mali: Cultural context and hard data. *Social Science and Medicine, 24,* 633–644.

Dettwyler, K. A. (1989a). Interaction of anorexia and cultural beliefs in infant malnutrition in Mali. *American Journal of Human Biology, 1,* 683–695.

Dettwyler, K. A. (1989b). Styles of infant feeding: Parental/caretaker control of food consumption in young children. *American Anthropologist, 91,* 696–703.

Engle, P. L. (1992). *Care and child nutrition.* Theme paper for the International Nutrition Conference (ICN). New York: UNICEF.

Engle, P. L. (1993). Influences of mother's and father's income on children's nutritional status in Guatemala. *Social Science and Medicine, 37*(11), 1303–1312.

Engle, P. L. (1994). *An interactive model of child care and nutrition and implications for programs.* Ithaca, NY: UNICEF/Cornell Lecture Series on Food and Nutrition Policy, Cornell Food and Nutrition Policy Program, Cornell University.

Engle, P. L. (1995). *Active feeding behavior: Nicaragua and Guatemala.* Manuscript submitted for publication.

Engle, P. L., & Davidson, K. (1991, November). *Maternal self efficacy: Nicaragua.* Paper presented at the Association for Women in Development, Washington, DC.

Engle, P. L., & Nieves, I. (1993). Intra-household food distribution among Guatemalan families in a supplementary feeding program: Behavior patterns. *Social Science and Medicine, 36*(12), 1605–1612.

Engle, P. L., Nieves, I., Zeitlin, M., La Montagne, J., & Medrano, Y. (1990). *Active feeding behavior: Guatemala and Nicaragua.* Paper presented at the Society for Cross-cultural Research, Claremont, CA.

Engle, P. L., Zeitlin, M., La Montagne, J., Medrano, Y., & Bonilla, J. (1990).

*Infant feeding and behavioral observation study* (Submission 2, Tufts/UNAN Positive deviance in Nutrition Project), Tufts University, Medford, MA.

Fiske, S. T., & Taylor, S. E. (1984). *Social cognition.* New York: Random House.

Garcia, S. E., Kaiser, L. L., & Dewey, K. G. (1990). Self-regulation of food intake among rural Mexican preschool children. *European Journal of Clinical Nutrition, 44,* 381–387.

Gibbons, G., & Griffiths, M. (1984). *Program activities for improving weaning practices.* (Report prepared for UNICEF). Washington, DC: American Public Health Association.

Harvey, J. H., & Weary, G. (1981). *Perspectives on attributional processes.* Dubuqe, IA: Brown.

Himmelstein, S., Graham, S., & Weiner, B. (1991). An attributional analysis of maternal beliefs about the importance of child-rearing practices. *Child Development, 62,* 301–310.

Jordan, M., & Staehling, N. (1986). *Anthropometric statistical package, version 3* (statistical program). Atlanta: Centers for Disease Control.

Kennedy, E. (1989, December). *The effects of sugarcane production of food security, health, and nutrition in Kenya: A longitudinal analysis* (Research Report No. 78). International Food Policy Research Institute. Washington, DC.

La Montagne, J. F., Engle, P. L., & Zeitlin, M. F. (1993). *Maternal employment and nutritional status of 12-18 month-old children.* Manuscript submitted for publication.

LeVine, R. A. (1988). Human parental care: Universal goals, cultural strategies, individual behavior. In R. A. LeVine, P. M. Miller, & M. M. West (Eds.), *Parental behavior in diverse societies* (pp. 3–12). (New Directions for Child Development No. 40). San Francisco: Jossey-Bass.

Marek, T. (1992). *Ending malnutrition: Why increasing income is not enough.* The World Bank Africa Technical Department, Population Health and Nutrition Division, Technical Paper No. 5, October.

Mitzner, K., Scrimshaw, N., & Morgan R. (Eds.). (1985). *Improving the nutritional status of children during the weaning period. A manual for policymakers, program planners and field workers.* Washington, DC: USAID.

Myers, R. (1992). *The twelve who survive.* London: Routledge.

Pollitt, E., Gorman, K. S., Engle, P., Martorell, R., & Rivera, J. (1993). Early supplementary feeding and cognition: Effects over two decades. *Monographs of the Society for Research in Child Development, 235*(58), No 7.

Powell, C. A., & Grantham-McGregor, S. (1985). The ecology of nutritional status and development in young children in Kingston, Jamaica. *American Journal of Clinical Nutrition, 41,* 1322–1331.

Ravindran, S. (1986). *Health implications of sex discrimination in childhood: A review paper and annotated bibliography.* Geneva: World Health Organization/UNICEF/FHE 86.2.

Rogers, B. L. (1990). The internal dynamics of households: A critical factor in development policy. In B. L. Rogers & N. P. Schlossman (Eds.), *Intra-household resource allocation.* Tokyo: UNU University.

Super, C. M., & Harkness, S. (1986). The developmental niche: A conceptualization at the interface of child and culture. *International Journal of Behavioral Development, 9,* 545–569.

UNICEF. (1993). *Child Malnutrition: Progress toward the world summit for children goal.* New York: Statistics and Monitoring Section, United Nations Children's Fund.

Van Esterick, P. (1985). *Intra-family food distribution: Its relevance for maternal and child nutrition* (Cornell Nutritional Surveillance Programme, Working Paper No. 31). Cornell University, Ithaca.

World Health Organization. (1983). *Measuring change in nutritional status.* Geneva: Author.

Zeitlin, M. F. (1991). Nutritional resilience in a hostile environment: Positive deviance in child nutrition. *Nutrition Reviews, 49*(9), 259–268.

Zeitlin, M., Bonilla, J., & Medrano, Y. (1990). *Nicaraguan positive deviance in nutrition research project.* (Phase I Reports and First Phase II Product. Report submitted by Tufts University School of Nutrition to UNICEF and the Italian Government).

Zeitlin, M. F., Houser, R., & Johnson, F. C. (1989, April). *Active maternal feeding and nutritional status of 8-20 month old Mexican children.* Paper presented at the meeting of the Society for Research in Child Development, Kansas City, MO.

Zeitlin, M., Mansour, M., & Boghani, M. (1990). *Positive deviance in nutrition.* Toyko: United Nations University.

Zeitlin, M., Super, C., Beiser, M, Gulden, G., Ahmet, N., Zeitlin, J., Ahmed, M., & Sockalingam, S. (1990, January). A behavioral study of positive deviance in young child nutrition and health in Bangladesh. (Report to Office of International Health and USAID).

# The Three R's of Dutch Childrearing and the Socialization of Infant Arousal

Charles M. Super
Sara Harkness
Nathalie van Tijen
Ellen van der Vlugt
Marinka Fintelman
Jarissa Dijkstra

New parents in all societies face the challenge of meeting their infants' demands for both rest and stimulation, at the same time integrating that cycle of activity with their own needs as adults. Cultures have derived a variety of customary methods for meeting this challenge, depending, presumably, on a combination of pragmatic and ideological factors. To any particular parent faced with a hungry, fussy baby at 2 a.m., however, the task may seem a solitary one that requires thought and conviction as well as love. Less a challenge, perhaps, but equally universal, is the question of regulating the flow of activities and personal interaction throughout the day, for young children as well as infants. The resulting patterns form a substrate for the looking and doing and listening and talking, for all the learning that is the very stuff of development in the opening years. More or less deliberately, parents create the shape of daily life for their children, routines that reflect larger cultural patterns and prepare the next generation to participate in them.

The socialization of arousal states, like other domains of socialization, is poised at the enigmatic interface between individual development and cultural functioning, with personal concreteness on the one side and intangible systematics on the other. Unlike a number of other socialization domains, however, it is curiously understudied. On the cross-cultural side, there has been occasional scrutiny of some relevant topics such as bedtime routines (Wolf, Lozoff, Latz, & Paludetto, Chapter 15 this volume) and cosleeping (Abbott, 1992; Caudill & Plath, 1966; Morelli, Rogoff, Oppenheim, & Goldsmith, 1992), but there are virtually no studies of the larger patterns of engagement and respite (one exception is Super & Harkness, 1982).

At the level of individual organisms, arousal state and particularly the growth of self-regulation have been of keen interest to researchers and clinicians in several ways. The literature is scattered, however, reflecting in part its diverse conceptual roots. Three traditions of research are relevant.

First, the larger organismic view includes substantial work on the normative ontogeny of sleep and sleep–wake differentiation and patterning (Parmalee, Wenner, & Schultz, 1964) and on the physiological concomitants of these developments (Berg & Berg, 1979). The role of environmental contribution to this developmental phenomenon, however, has not been given much attention, except in a few discrete studies (Elias, Nicolson, Bora, & Johnston, 1986; Sander, 1987; Super & Harkness, 1982). Second, the role of short-term changes in arousal has also received considerable study with infants, and recognition of the importance of state organization marked a turning point in infant research (e.g., Korner, 1972; Als, Tronick, Lester, & Brazelton, 1979). In this tradition, researchers have examined state as both a response and a platform for other behaviors. Infant arousal as indexed by smiling, vocalization, and physiological measures has been shown to vary contingently with maternal response. This is true both positively, as high interaction leads to increased infant arousal (Symons & Moran, 1987), and negatively, in that deliberate simulation of non-responsive maternal behavior has been shown to result in disrupted infant arousal and affect (Cohen & Tronick, 1983). Beyond these transient effects, state of arousal is also a potent mediator of further experience, determining opportunities to engage in social activity, demonstrate competence, and acquire new skills. For this reason, arousal regulation has been seen by some to be a central task of early development, with possible links to later accomplishments across the domains of physical, social, and cognitive growth (Sroufe, 1979). Empirical support for long-term effects, however, is minimal. One exception is Gable and Isabella's (1992) report that maternal activity and arousal in early infancy (1 month) have a direct effect on later (4-month) infant arousal behaviors. Third, the literature on temperament and emotions includes substantial consideration of arousal and regulation, using concepts such as "intensity," "emotionality," "regularity," and "inhibition." However, these terms are typically used to refer to relatively stable, biologically based characteristics of the individual, and environmental influences are not well elaborated.

Thus, by and large, the empirical and theoretical literature has focused on inborn individual differences, on short-term regulation by environmental stimulation, and on prototypical changes over the course of development in Western industrial societies. Absent from these three paradigms is consideration of long-term, environmentally induced variations, including organismic adaptations that contribute to their maintenance. This kind of phenomenon is exactly what cultural regulation is known to produce. Understanding the mechanisms of enculturation remains a continuing challenge to the developmental sciences, and the present study was undertaken to explore the possible role of enculturation in the emergence of arousal patterns.

The theoretical framework of the "developmental niche" (Super & Harkness, 1986a) has proven useful for understanding the dynamics of enculturation for a wide range of developmental topics, including motor skills (Super, 1976), emotional expression (Harkness & Super, 1985), literacy and mathematical skills (Harkness & Super, 1993; Pellegrini & Stanic, 1993), the "goodness of fit" between child temperament and environmental demands (Super & Harkness, 1986b; Super & Harkness, 1993), the construction of developmental dysfunction (Super, 1987), and the household production of health (Harkness & Super, 1994). In this framework, the physical and social settings of development, the customary methods of child care, and the psychology of the caretakers are seen as three componental subsystems of the niche, and environmental effects are most pronounced when these components press toward the same behavioral outcome.

Parents' ethnotheories are accorded a special significance in this framework. They are a mediating mechanism between the cultural past, current possibilities, and the actual environments for children. Parental ethnotheories contribute to the organization of children's early experience through the choice of settings, the instantiation of customary caretaking behaviors, and guiding of moment-to-moment interaction (Harkness & Super, 1992; Harkness, Super, & Keefer, 1992). It is easy to imagine that each of these mechanisms plays a role in the regulation of arousal states in the opening years of life. The present study is a preliminary attempt to describe in two diverse settings the culturally integrated niches in which infant arousal develops and to examine in turn the patterns of arousal that arise there.

## Bloemenheim and Cambridge

The infants and parents studied here reside in metropolitan areas of the Netherlands and the northeastern United States. Bloemenheim (a pseudonym) is a peri-urban community that lies in the heart of a densely populated area stretching from Amsterdam to the Hague. It is a small town, surrounded by the famous Dutch bulb fields but now also home to industry and a significant number of middle- and professional-class commuters. Sixty-six families participated in a larger study of parents' ethnotheories in Holland; all but 12 (with older children) are included here. The families were selected to yield 18 target children age 6 months and 12 at ages 18 months, 3 years, and 4.5 years. The sample is balanced by sex and birth order (firstborn vs. laterborn). Families were recruited through social networks centered on the neighborhood school attended by a child of the first two authors (C. M. S. and S. H.), with the restrictions that at least one parent be employed, that both parents be present, and that there be no major illness in the family. Occupations of the fathers, and of those mothers who worked (7% worked full-time, 53% part-time), varied over nearly the full range of income and status in this relatively egalitarian country, including cook and chemist, banker and baker, policeman and pilot, senior administrator in an international agency, worker in the bulb fields, businessman, teacher, sales clerk, and office worker. Both mothers and fathers tended to be in their early thirties (ranging from 23 to 61 years) and well educated (averaging 15 years of schooling for fathers and 13 for mothers, with a range from 6 to 25 years). About half the parents were from a Catholic background, a quarter Protestant, and a quarter said their parents had not followed any religions tradition.

Cambridge is one of several cities surrounding Boston, Massachusetts, the area our U.S. sample is from. Thirty-six families were recruited through a large health care provider based in Cambridge, but most of the families lived in surrounding towns. The same employment, health, and marital criteria were used for selection. Occupational levels of the fathers and the mothers who worked (nearly half worked full-time, and about one-quarter part-time) varied widely but do not represent the full range in this metropolitan area. Occupations included architect, lawyer, businessman, electronic technician, administrator, firefighter, service worker, teacher, and artist. Unlike the Bloemenheim study, samples here were in three cohorts (initial ages: newborn, 18 months, and 3 years) followed longitudinally and interviewed four times at 6-month intervals. The sample is balanced by sex and birth order (firstborn vs. laterborn) and as in Bloemenheim families with significant medical problems were excluded. The Cambridge parents were similar to those in Bloemenheim in age (averaging 33 years, ranging from 25 to 58). They were typically more educated, however, with both mothers and fathers averaging 16 years of school (the range was 12 to 21 years). The majority of parents came equally from Protestant and Catholic origins (about 40% each), with the remainder primarily from Jewish backgrounds. A separate U.S. sample, also from metropolitan Boston and generally similar by these measures, was used in an earlier study for the caretaker–child behavior observations reported here.

Beyond noting the general similarity of these two Western populations, and the application of similar recruitment and selection criteria, it is surprisingly difficult to derive comparable measures of demographic status for families in the two groups. Parental age is an exception, and statistical comparison indicates no reliable difference between the samples. The difference in maternal employment status is reliable and accurately reflects both daily life for the sample families and national differences in employment patterns. The differences in religious background are statistically significant, although one must also note that the history of religion in civil life, and therefore the current meaning of Catholic, Protestant, and none, is also different. The number of years of education is easily quantifiable but also does not reflect the same functions in the two nations. Postelementary schooling in the Netherlands is separated by academic and vocational level differently from that in the United States, for example, and some kinds of vocational training—for example, to manage a bakery—take place in formal educational settings that in the United States are more likely to take place on the job. On the other hand, university training in Holland is often shorter in years but more selective and more advanced than the comparable first postsecondary degree in the United States. More difficult still is measuring occupational status—the second traditional factor in social class—for the scales commonly used in the United States fit poorly the more egalitarian and homogeneous Dutch society. Nevertheless, if one calculates Hollingshead's two-factor index (Hollingshead & Redlich, 1958), two observations are relevant: First, the range in status is identical in the two samples (from the professional Class I through Class IV but not Class V, which includes uneducated laborers), and second, in both samples the dominant group is Class II. Beyond that, the Cambridge sample is weighted more heavily toward the upper end of the scale, as the small difference in education would suggest.

Two other aspects of the samples are central to the present concerns. First, each is a reasonably representative sample of an identifiable group that shares important features of lifestyle and cultural identification: a particular Dutch town, in one case, and U.S. families, in the other, who received a (then) distinctive kind of health care and parenting advice from a small group of pediatricians. Neither group is truly representative of their nation-state, or even of a region, but each does reflect the tendencies and variations of a specific community. Second, members of each group have shared for all their adult lives, and in virtually all cases in their origins, a common national culture with is historical meanings and current media. One purpose of the present research is to explore how this common cultural identity influences parental ethnotheories, despite of and in concord with intracultural variation.

## Data Collection Methods

Three methods of data collection were used. Parental interviews, carried out in the home, focused on parents' theories of infant care and development and on observations and explanations of their own infant's behavior. These semistructured interviews were conducted by the first two authors (C. M. S. and S. H.) in the parents' native language (the second and third authors [N. vT. and E. vdV.] assisted in the Dutch interviews). Parental statements in a variety of domains, including rest and arousal, were identified and coded for analysis. Weeklong diaries of infant experience were kept by the parents, who recorded on prepared forms the babies' activities as well as the location and other persons present. Entries were coded for analysis of time allocation. Behavior observations in the home were carried out on four occasions of 20 minutes each. Discrete caretaker and infant behaviors (such as vocalize, cry, give object), as well as the infant's state, were recorded in real time on a hand-held computer. Except for the advanced method of recording, this methodology is well established in the literature on parent–child interaction (Moss, 1967; Super et al., 1981). Reliability was established at .80 or greater, with the first author (C. M. S.) serving as the primary observer. The U.S. data for this one procedure come from an earlier study carried out by the first author (C. M. S.) on a comparable sample in the Cambridge area, but when the infants were either 4 or 10 months old (Super & Harkness, 1994).

## Results

### Themes of Rest and Arousal in the Parent Interviews

During the interviews parents in both samples expressed interest and concern about their child's patterns of rest and arousal; however, this topic was of much greater salience and specificity in Bloemenheim.

Several related themes illustrate the contrast, usually centered on questions of quality, duration, or regularity of sleeping, or on regularity of active and quiet periods during the day. First, when Cambridge parents discussed rest and arousal state, the most frequent themes of their comments was that some children are naturally or innately more or less regular in their sleeping or activities than are others. One Cambridge couple described the "natural cycle" of their 6-month-old this way:

MOTHER: She still has a good night cycle, which is great. Her fussiness is daytime, thank God. We could have it a lot worse.

FATHER: She's really very, very good about nighttime. She's on a pretty strict 11:00, 3:00 . . .

MOTHER: Not induced by us. She will generally take a feeding around 11:00, 11:30 and then you can set a clock by her. 3:00, bingo, she wakes up. 3:05, 3:06 is when I roll over and look at my clock and hear her crying, because it's taken her a few minutes to sort of wake up and realize that she is hungry. By 3:05 she's crying.

FATHER: She gets fed and changed and falls back to sleep again right away.

MOTHER: Bingo. And then she's out until about 6:30, 7:00. And then she's fussy all day long.

This theme of innateness arose in fully 30% of all Cambridge comments on rest and arousal, as illustrated in the left-hand bar in Figure 19.1 (for the data in this figure, $\chi^2 = 231.7$, $df = 5$, $p < .000$). In contrast, only 5% of the comments in Bloemenheim focused on innate characteristics (second bar from left).

The next three themes presented in Figure 19.1 form a particular cluster for the Cambridge parents. About 15% of the comments indicated that the parents found arousal and rest issues to be a real or potential problem (the third pair of bars). A somewhat larger percentage of the comments focused on specific strategies that would help the infant or child go to sleep and thus ameliorate the problem. Finally, a slightly smaller percentage focused on the attainment of regular sleep patterns as a major developmental achievement by the child.

Regularity as an individual accomplishment fits nicely with the larger U.S. themes of "independence" and of "stages" of development (Harkness, Super, & Keefer, 1992). The appearance of a predictable pattern marks the child's advancement toward the status of a self-regulating organism. This is an expectable, organic transformation that comes essentially from within according to a natural developmental

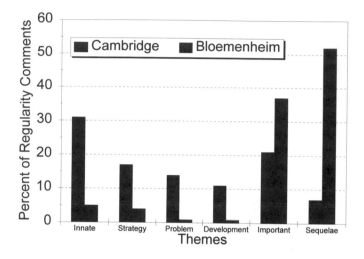

**FIGURE 19.1.** The frequency of selected regularity themes in parental interviews.

timetable (see Harkness, Super, Keefer, Raghavan, & Kipp, Chapter 12, this volume). It cannot be mechanically induced; it is simply to be noted and appreciated. "She is much more regular now in terms of her daytime sleeping," commented one mother of a 6-month-old. "She varies but I know what the patterns tend to be—she is starting to fall into a regular pattern."

If regular sleep patterns occur primarily with maturity, however, or as an innate characteristic of some children, at least some parents in Cambridge should be faced with the problem of an immature and irregular baby. This is the case, as the frequency of sleep problems indicates. But, according to these parents, there are still some specific strategies that can be employed to get the child to sleep, even though the basic disposition cannot be altered and maturation cannot be hurried. There are ample sources of advice on this topic, but finding just the right thing can take both time and luck. The following discussion captures one couple's sense of the problem with their 1-year-old, their identification of personal characteristics, and their success with little maneuvers while waiting for a developmental transformation.

MOTHER: He wakes up a couple times a night, [did it] right from the start. I kept waiting for him to start sleeping through the night.

Ever since he was born, he was up most of the night as a brand-new baby, and then he was up like four times a night, going to bed at 7:30 and he'd be up at 11:00 and he'd be up at 1:00, 3:00, 5:00. So the doctor said to let him cry. That was effective when we could stand it, but both of us—it drives us crazy. He could cry for 45 minutes. There were nights when he would not cry, but scream and shriek for 45 minutes.

FATHER: I know that you should just wait it out, but it's 3:00 in the morning and you know you've got to get up at 6:15.

MOTHER: And to know that he would go right back to sleep like that [snaps fingers] in our bed.

FATHER: It's a tough call.

MOTHER: Now usually he wakes up around 4:30 and he's hanging on to the headboard, jumping up and down. So finally at 5:00 I get up.

INTERVIEWER: What do you do with him?

FATHER: We both have different strategies. She'll put him in the walker down here and I generally put him in the playpen and try to keep him somewhat entertained, either by the TV or he loves the stereo. He loves music. If he's crying and he sees me going for the stereo, he'll stop crying and start to laugh in anticipation of the music. Even when he was a tiny baby, one night at 3:30 we discovered a particular song that would calm him down.

MOTHER: It was a psalm. We wondered if it was some divine intervention.

None of these themes—innate characteristics, developmental achievements, problems of irregularity, or short-term solutions—was frequent in the Bloemenheim interviews. The two dominant themes there (see right in Figure 19.1) were that parental maintenance or imposition of regularity, particularly regarding sleep, is very important, and that failure to impose these in the early months or years of life would have unfortunate sequelae later on. "To bed on time," explained one mother with reference to her 18-month-old, "because they really need rest to grow, and regularity is very important when they are so little. If she gets too little rest, she is very fussy."

It was in these discussions that the Bloemenheim parents explained to us "the Three R's" of childrearing: *Rust, Regelmaat,* and *Reinheid,* or rest, regularity, and cleanliness. These concepts were for many years a centerpiece of the official advice given to all new mothers by the national Consultation Offices (part of the national health service, which provides postnatal home visits, follow-up consultations, and comprehensive health care to all mothers and infants in the Netherlands). The official formulation is said to date from the 1920s, but it appears that it was drawn at that time in part from the folk culture. Although the Three R's have recently been removed from the formal curriculum for new mothers, the phrase is known to all the parents of Bloemenheim. A few make light of the idea as old-fashioned, and one parent suggested a new set of letters, the Three L's: "*Lucht, Licht, en Leifde*" (light, air, and love). Nevertheless, regularity and rest (as well as cleanliness) remain strongly valued traditions in organizing parental theories of early child care in Bloemenheim. One mother summarized it thus: "Regularity is important. The Three R's, you were brought up on that, and there has got to be a regular schedule."

## Diurnal Rest Patterns

The importance of parental ethnotheories stems in part, we have hypothesized, from their role in guiding customary parental behavior. The diary data kept by parents in this study illustrate this process and its consequences for diurnal patterns of rest and arousal.

Table 19.1 summarizes at each age several aspects of sleep behavior, as recorded in the daily diaries. The parents' notation of "sleep" may not accord exactly, of course, with demarcations that would have been derived from physiological data. Nevertheless, the present classification of sleep does indicate that the child is alone, quiet, and in bed, in a darkened room. Thus, the present data may overestimate true sleep, but they provide a reasonable estimate of rest and low arousal. As the methods of recording were identical in the two samples, the indices may be taken as valid comparisons of diurnal patterns of arousal.

It is evident, first, that infants and children in Bloemenheim get more rest in the opening years of life. The difference in total sleep is 2 hours per day at 6 months of age, diminishing to about 20 minutes in the fifth year. Second, the Dutch children are going to bed nearly an hour earlier than their U.S. counterparts. Finally, the timing of rest is less variable in the Bloemenheim group than in Cambridge in two senses. At the group level, there is less variance among individuals in Bloemenheim in when they are put to bed than there is in Cambridge (presented in the table as "*SD* bedtime w/in group")—this result speaks to the question of cultural homogeneity, discussed below. In addition, however, there is some evidence that bedtime is less variable for each Dutch child than is the case for U.S. children, at least at the oldest age (that is, the average standard deviation of recorded bedtimes is less, given in Table 19.1 as "*SD* bedtime w/in child").

### Caretaker–Infant Interaction

Observations of caretaker and infant behaviors suggest that parental ethnotheories concerning arousal and rest are instantiated not only at the level of daily routines but also in schemata, or scripts, for interaction on a moment-to-moment basis. The 80 minutes of observation were summarized in 10-second blocks; thus, the unit of reporting here is the percentage of 10-second units (out of 480) during which a particular behavior occurred. Figure 19.2 presents for each selected measure a triad of results: for the 6-month-old infants in Bloemenheim as the central bar, surrounded by bars for the 4- and 10-month Cambridge samples. There are, of course, substantial differences with increasing age during the first year of life, but because the age of observation in

**Table 19.1.** Rest and Regularity as Reflected in Daily Diaries

| Measure | Bloemenheim | Cambridge | $t/F$ | $df$ | $p$ |
|---|---|---|---|---|---|
| 6 months | | | | | |
| Total sleep/24 (hrs) | 14.9 | 12.9 | 2.9 | 26 | .006 |
| Mean bedtime | 6:56 P.M. | 8:32 P.M. | 4.0 | 15 | .001 |
| SD bedtime w/in group | 0.62 | 1.27 | 4.1 | 11,15 | .01 |
| SD bedtime w/in child | 0.91 | 0.81 | 0.5 | 26 | n.s. |
| 18 months | | | | | |
| Total sleep/24 (hrs) | 14.1 | 12.8 | 3.3 | 34 | .002 |
| Mean bedtime | 7:35 P.M. | 8:04 P.M. | 2.5 | 34 | .02 |
| SD bedtime w/in group | 0.45 | 0.94 | 4.5 | 23,11 | .01 |
| SD bedtime w/in child | 0.47 | 0.64 | 1.4 | 28.9 | .13 |
| 3 years | | | | | |
| Total sleep/24 (hrs) | 12.7 | 11.8 | 2.4 | 31 | .02 |
| Mean bedtime | 7:31 P.M. | 8:26 p.m. | 3.1 | 31 | .004 |
| SD bedtime w/in group | 0.61 | 0.85 | 2.0 | 21,10 | .004 |
| SD bedtime w/in child | 0.61 | 0.55 | 0.7 | 31 | n.s. |
| 4.5 years | | | | | |
| Total sleep/24 (hrs) | 11.6 | 11.3 | 1.0 | 22 | .31 |
| Mean bedtime | 7:26 P.M. | 8:17 P.M. | 4.6 | 22 | .0001 |
| SD bedtime w/in group | 0.40 | 0.51 | 1.6 | 11,11 | n.s. |
| SD bedtime w/in child | 0.32 | 0.65 | 3.3 | 22 | .003 |

Bloemenheim falls between the U.S. ages, it is easy to see that a hypothetical explanation of group differences based on monotonic age trends must be rejected. The primary result is contained in the first two triads of results, where it is shown that the infants in the Cambridge sample spent a majority of their observed time in a state of Active alertness (63% and 88%), whereas the infants in Bloemenheim are predominantly in a state of Quiet arousal (61%). (All group comparisons in Figure 19.2 are statistically reliable, $p < .05$.) In addition, infants in the Cambridge sample were observed to be in a Cry state about 1% of the time, but this extreme state of arousal was not observed in Bloemenheim. The definitions of state used here are standard behavioral ones, relying on motor, vocal, and visual activity (Brazelton, 1973). Results for one component index—gross motor movement in the arms and legs—is also presented in Figure 19.2. One reason for the higher state of arousal seen in the Cambridge infants may be a higher level of stimulation and interaction by their mothers. For example, as shown in

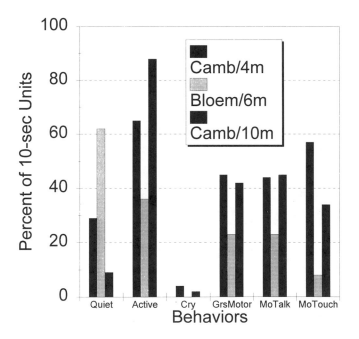

**FIGURE 19.2.** The frequency of infant and maternal behaviors during naturalistic observations.

Figure 19.2, the mothers in Cambridge talked more to their babies and touched them more.

There are probably several factors contributing to this difference in maternal behavior. One is a guiding ethnotheory in Bloemenheim that even young infants need to learn, and need help in learning, to organize their own behavior and "entertain" themselves; this is part of becoming "independent" or *zelfstandig*. The U.S. mothers, on the other hand, share a model of early development that postulates "stimulation" to be a critical ingredient for rapid social and cognitive growth (LeVine, 1980; Super & Harkness, 1994).

## Shared Concepts and Intracultural Variation

At the core of a cultural perspective lies the proposition that human environments are systematically organized such that individual or family variation within a culture is qualitatively different from the variability among cultures. Indeed, as Wallace (1961) set forth, one function of culture is the organization of internal diversity. In the realm of parental ethnotheories, this suggests that we should examine two further questions. First, to what degree does variation within each of the two present samples still revolve around shared ideas, even if some of the ideas are rejected or individually transformed by particular parents? Second, can differences between the two samples in parental beliefs or behavior be adequately accounted for by group differences in some *common* feature (e.g., social class) rather than require us to draw upon the concept of qualitatively distinct cultures?

With regard to internal variation around uniquely shared concepts, we must first note that the differences in spontaneous use of themes presented in Figure 19.1 are not an artifact of a few distinct and vocal parents in each group; rather, each of the themes we have indicated to be dominant in one group or another is in fact endorsed by a majority of families in that group. For example, in all the U.S. families at least one parent mentioned at least once the notion that differences in regularity are innate, whereas this is true in only one-third of the Dutch families. Conversely, all but one of the Bloemenheim families commented on the developmental sequelae of providing, or failing to provide, a regular routine of rest, whereas only slightly more than half the Cambridge families made this point.

There were also several instances in which a parent was explicit in rejecting the locally dominant concept, so that even though they did not endorse the cultural model being counted in the presentations here, they still used that model to some degree in organizing their thinking. Thus one father in Bloemenheim was definite in saying that rest and regularity were not so important, but no Cambridge parent did so. Likewise, no Dutch parent discussed particular strategies for getting an infant to sleep even though the underlying model used in Bloemenheim was one of environmental induction of rest. This particular version of environmental influence was relevant only in Cambridge, where strategies were seen as necessary to accomplish something that had not come about naturally, that is through disposition or maturity.

Authorities in the Bloemenheim school attended by the son of the first two authors provided a fine demonstration of how the parental ethnotheories of rest and regularity were in fact community-based models. Like elementary schools around the world, this school organized an evening of spring festivities to be presented by the children to the assembled families. The presentation was scheduled to take place after the dinner hour, at 7:00, so that fathers would be able to attend and the family meal would not be disrupted. This meant, however, that the children would be delayed in their bedtime until about 8:30, or an hour later than normal. Consequently, in order to ensure adequate rest for school the next day, school opening for the next morning was postponed by 1 hour. This was apparently a customary arrangement requiring no comment or discussion, except by the visiting Americans who were astonished and who subsequently realized that this custom was, like most, an instantiation of shared ethnotheories, now publicly at the community level.

## The Distinctness of Between-Culture Differences

Pooling data from the two samples allows a demonstration of the fact that differences between the two groups are not simply the consequence of sample differences in a common underlying variable such as social class. First, we calculated within each sample the correlations of belief (themes) and outcome (sleep) variables with father's education, the best single component of social class. There are a few correlations with this index in the Cambridge sample (couples with more educated fathers believe more in the innateness of regularity and have fewer problems with their children's sleep, and their children go to bed earlier and sleep more), but in Bloemenheim there are virtually none, despite the larger range in education. This result suggests the absence of a common underlying dimension of variation. The case is strengthened by combining data from the two samples, controlling for paternal education through regression, and then examining with analysis of variance the effect of group membership (Cambridge vs. Bloemenheim). The group differences would disappear if they were primarily an artifact of paternal education, but they do not. Rather, each of the variables listed in Table 19.1 remains reliably different between the two groups (except for the standard deviation in bedtime, within child, which does not give consistent results in Table 19.1). That is, when the data are adjusted to remove any effect of paternal education, the children in Bloemenheim are still seen to get more sleep, to go to bed earlier, and to be less variable as a group in their bedtime. Essentially the same results are obtained controlling for mother's education or for the Hollingshead social class score. This result reinforces the conclusion that the two groups comprise qualitatively distinct wholes and are not linear extensions along a single dimension of social class.

## Discussion

The present study demonstrates that parents in two communities with divergent cultural histories, but still within the Western tradition, hold different theories of sleep and arousal during the opening years of life, that these ethnotheories are reflected in the organization of daily life and momentary interactions, and that infants' patterns of arousal respond to these culturally organized differences. There are several implications of these results that warrant comment.

First, the operative ethnotheories in each group form an intricate thematic web. One strand in Cambridge unites the beliefs about innate regularity, the notion of maturational achievement, the identification of sleep problems, and the use of strategies to induce sleep. Although not all families focused on this full complex in their interviews, all four elements are widely shared in the community and are available for parents to draw upon if needed. Because parents draw differentially upon the shared cultural models to handle their specific child, the common corpus of ideas can contain elements that in the abstract might appear contradictory, such as the innateness and maturational ideas. The ultimate integration is done by individual parents to suit their particular needs, drawing on their personal background, network of peers, and access to "expert" advice (Harkness, Super & Keefer, 1992).

Second, the continuity of parental ethnotheories from one generation to the next takes place both at the individual level—a child is socialized—and through the sharing of cultural models among members of the community. In both Cambridge and Bloemenheim, for example, there were frequent references during the parent interviews to advice received from friends, family members, and expert sources. These two levels of intergenerational influence are mutually supportive. It is striking in this regard to compare the present results with Rebelsky's findings nearly 30 years ago (Rebelsky, 1967). Working as a

U.S. visitor in Utrecht, Rebelsky commented on the remarkable regularity of feeding and sleeping, compared to a U.S. sample from the Boston area, and also on a difference in attitudes and interactional behavior that parallels the present contrast. "American mothers looked at, held, fed, talked to, smiled at, patted and showed more affection to their babies more often than did Dutch mothers" (p. 3). "Even if a parent sees a child awake and wanting to play or look around, and Dutch parents do see this, he [sic] is not likely to respond to this wish or to the behavior which implies this wish, because of fear of 'spoiling' the baby or because of the belief that a baby in this age range should sleep and not play or stay awake" (p. 4). Rebelsky's concern in her study was to examine the critical role of "stimulation" in early development, and she found her results to be a challenge to contemporary U.S. thought. Theoretical developments since then have helped us appreciate the multiplicity of ways that parents and other environmental features can promote sound development, but the organization of environments remains a poorly understood aspect of the ecology of human growth.

Third, the present results contribute to our understanding of how environments work by illuminating the directive force of parental ethnotheories. In both Bloemenheim and Cambridge, parents' understanding of what their infants are capable of, and what they need, wields a powerful influence on the shape of arousal and rest throughout the day, and on the patterns of moment-to-moment stimulation and interactive processes. As has been observed in other reports (Super & Harkness, 1986a), it is the concordance and repetition of similar patterns through time, across domains, and over dimensional scales that gives systematic features of culture the power to influence human development so profoundly.

Finally, the present findings point to a new appreciation of environmentally induced patterns of arousal regulation. As reviewed at the beginning of this chapter, the research literature on infant arousal generally focuses on three areas: the maturation of arousal patterns; innate, constitutionally based differences in the regularity and level of arousal; and short-term effects of stimulation on arousal and short-term implications for response hierarchies. There is an interesting parallel between this view of the literature and the ethnotheories generated by the Cambridge parents. In each case there is the same set of concepts: maturation, temperament, and short-term management by the environment. The parallel is probably not coincidental and speaks to the question of the relationship between cultural models of development and scientific models of development (Harkness & Super, 1993; LeVine, 1980; Super & Harkness, 1995). More important, however, is the neglect in the literature of adaptation to culturally organized patterns of stimulation and rest during a sensitive period of early postnatal life. If the young organism is in effect setting parameters for the system of activation and arousal, the lifelong consequences cannot easily be accommodated by the three concepts outlined above. Rather, this concept incorporates features of the other three. Such early effects are a developmental phenomenon involving maturation; they result in constitutionally based differences and they coevolve in interaction with the environment. That is in fact what happens in the normal acquisition of sleep patterns by young children, although it has not always been evident in the absence of culturally variable examples. Such effects might also take place with the chronic elicitation of mood states, or the strong and highly elaborated socialization of arousal and affect. With regard to sleep, Weisbluth (1989) has argued that children's sleep patterns, particularly ones that involve moderate sleep deprivation, influence the chemical environment of the maturing brain and thus potentially alter cell reactivity. "Through their efforts to structure sleep," Weisbluth concludes, "parents have an opportunity to influence the neurochemical regulation of alertness, arousal, temperament, or emotionality" (p. 369). Kagan (1994), speaking of emotional disposition, has observed that contemporary theory does not make a distinction "between chronic emotional moods and temperamental biases" (p. 14), a failure that may limit our understanding of developmental phenomena. For both these domains the present study directs our attention to the power of culturally regulated experience, organized in large part by parental ethnotheories, to influence not only the patterns of arousal and affective expression but also, over the long run, the internal systems that are constructed for regulating these states.

# Acknowledgments

The work reported in this chapter was supported in part by research grants from the Spencer Foundation and the Center for the Study of Child and Adolescent Development at the Pennsylvania State University, and by a Senior Fulbright Fellowship Award to the first author (C. M. S.). The two senior authors (C. M. S. and S. H.), who held Visiting Professorships at Leiden University during the period of data collection, express their gratitude to the faculty, particularly to Professors G. Kohnstamm and T. van der Voort, for their gracious hospitality. Van Tijen, van der Vlugt, Fintelman, and Dijkstra received support from Leiden University and later were Visiting Scholars at the Pennsylvania State University. The authors are grateful to these institutions for their enabling support. All views expressed in this work, however, are the sole responsibility of the authors.

# References

Abbott, S. (1992). Holding on and pushing away: Comparative perspectives on an Eastern Kentucky child-rearing practice. *Ethos, 20,* 33–65.

Als, H., Tronick, E., Lester, B. M., & Brazelton, T. B. (1979). Specific neonatal measures: The Brazelton Neonatal Behavioral Assessment Scale. In J. D. Osofsky (Ed.), *Handbook of infant development* (pp. 185–215). New York: Wiley.

Berg, W. K., & Berg, K. M. (1979). Psychophysiological development in infancy: State, sensory function, and attention. In J. D. Osofsky (Ed.), *Handbook of infant development* (pp. 283–343). New York: Wiley.

Brazelton, T. B. (1973). *Neonatal Behavioral Assessment Scale.* Philadelphia: Lippincott.

Caudill, W., & Plath, D. W. (1966). Who sleeps by whom? Parent–child involvement in urban Japanese families. *Psychiatry, 29*(4), 344–366.

Cohen, J. F., & Tronick, E. Z. (1983). Three-month-old infants' reaction to simulated maternal depression. *Child Development, 54,* 185–193.

Elias, M. F., Nicolson, N. A., Bora, C., & Johnston, J. (1986). Sleep/wake patterns of breast-fed infants in the first 2 years of life. *Pediatrics, 77*(3), 322–329.

Gable, S., & Isabella, R. A. (1992). Maternal contributions to infant regulation of arousal. *Infant Behavior and Development, 15,* 95–107.

Harkness, S., Super, C. M., & Keefer, C. H. (1992). Learning to be an American parent: How cultural models gain directive force. In R. G. D'Andrade & C. Strauss (Eds.), *Human motives and cultural models* (pp. 163–178). Cambridge, UK: Cambridge University Press.

Harkness, S., & Super, C. M. (1985). Child–environment transactions in the socialization of affect. In M. Lewis, C. Saarni (Eds.), *The socialization of emotions* (pp. 21–36). New York: Plenum Press.

Harkness, S., & Super, C. M. (1992). Parental ethnotheories in action. In I. Sigel, A. V. McGillicuddy-DeLisi, & J. J. Goodnow (Eds.), *Parental belief systems: The psychological consequences for children* (2nd ed., pp. 373–392). Hillsdale, NJ: Erlbaum.

Harkness, S., & Super, C. M. (1993). The developmental niche: Implications for children's literacy development. In L. Eldering & P. Lesemen (Eds.), *Early intervention and culture: Preparation for literacy* (pp. 115–132). Paris: UNESCO.

Harkness, S., & Super, C. M. (1994). The "developmental niche:" A theoretical framework for analyzing the household production of health. *Social Science and Medicine, 38*(2), 217–226.

Hollingshead, A. B., & Redlich, F. C. (1958). *Social class and mental illness: A community study.* New York: Wiley.

Kagan, J. (1994). On the nature of emotion. In N. A. Fox (Ed.), *The development of emotion regulation: Biological and behavioral considerations* (*Monographs of the Society for Research in Child Development, 59*(2–3), Serial No. 240).

Korner, A. F. (1972). State as a variable, as obstacle, and as mediator of stimulation in infant research. *Merrill-Palmer Quarterly, 18,* 77–94.

LeVine, R. A. (1980). Anthropology and child development. In C. M. Super & S. Harkness (Eds.), *Anthropological perspectives on child development* (New Directions for Child Development No. 8). San Francisco: Jossey-Bass.

Morelli, G. A., Rogoff, B., Oppenheim, D., & Goldsmith, D. (1992). Cultural variation in infants' sleeping arrangements: Questions of independence. *Developmental Psychology, 28,* 604–613.

Moss, H. A. (1967). Sex, age, and state as determinants of mother-infant interaction. *Merrill-Palmer Quarterly of Behavior and Development, 13*(1), 19–36.

Parmalee, A. H., Wenner, A. H., & Schultz, H. R. (1964). Infant sleep patterns: From birth to 16 weeks of age. *Journal of Pediatrics, 65,* 576–582.

Pellegrini, A. D., & Stanic, G. M. (1993). Locating children's mathematical competence: Application of the developmental niche. *Journal of Applied Developmental Psychology, 14,* 501– 520.

Rebelsky, F. G. (1967). Infancy in two cultures. *Nederlands Tijdschrift voor de Psychologie en Haar Grensgebeiden, 22*(6), 379–385.

Sander, L. W. (1987). A 25-year follow-up: Some reflections on personality development over the long term. *Infant Mental Health Journal, 8*(3), 210–220.

Sroufe, A. (1979). Socioemotional development. In J. D. Osofsky (Ed.), *Handbook of infant development* (pp. 462–516). New York: Wiley.

Super, C. M. (1976). Environmental effects on motor development: The case of African infant precocity. *Developmental Medicine and Child Neurology, 18,* 561–567.

Super, C. M. (1987). The role of culture in developmental disorder. In C. M. Super (Ed.), *The role of culture in developmental disorder* (pp. 1–8). New York: Academic Press.

Super, C. M., Clement, J., Vuori, L., Christiansen, M., Mora, J. O., & Herrera, M. G. (1981). Infant and caretaker behavior as mediators of nutritional and social intervention in the barrios of Bogota. In T. Field, A. Sostek, P. Vietze & P. H. Leiderman (Eds.), *Culture and early interaction* (pp. 171–188). Hillsdale, NJ: Erlbaum.

Super, C. M., & Harkness, S. (1982). The infant's niche in rural Kenya and metropolitan America. In L. L. Adler (Ed.), *Cross-cultural research at issue* (pp. 47–56). New York: Academic Press.

Super, C. M., & Harkness, S. (1986a). The developmental niche: A conceptualization at the interface of child and culture. *International Journal of Behavioral Development, 9,* 545–569.

Super, C. M., & Harkness, S. (1986b). Temperament, culture, and development. In R. Plomin & J. Dunn (Eds.), *The study of temperament: Changes, continuities, and challenges* (pp. 131–150). Hillsdale, NJ: Erlbaum.

Super, C. M., & Harkness, S. (1993). Temperament and the developmental niche. In W. B. Carey & S. A. McDevitt (Eds.), *Prevention and early intervention: Individual differences as risk factors for the mental health of children—a Festschrift for Stella Chess and Alexander Thomas.* New York: Brunner/Mazel.

Super, C. M., & Harkness, S. (1994). The cultural regulation of temperament-environment interactions. *Researching Early Childhood, 2*(1), 59–84.

Super, C. M., & Harkness, S. (1995). *The metaphors of development.* Submitted for publication.

Symons, D. K., & Moran, G. (1987). The behavioral dynamics of mutual responsiveness in early fact-to-face mother-infant interactions. *Child Development, 58,* 1488–1495.

Wallace, A. F. (1961). *Culture and personality.* New York: Random House.

Weissbluth, W. (1989). Sleep-loss stress and temperamental difficultness: Psychobiological processes and practical considerations. In G. A. Kohnstamm, J. E. Bates, & M. K. Rothbart (Eds.), *Temperament in childhood* (pp. 358–375). Chichester, UK: Wiley.

CHAPTER 20

# *Imagining and Engaging One's Children:*
## *Lessons from Poor, Rural, New England Mothers*

Lynne A. Bond
Mary Field Belenky
Jacqueline S. Weinstock
Toni Cook

In this chapter, we will discuss a core hypothesis that has provided the basis for the Listening Partners Project, a large-scale preventive/promotive intervention program. The premise—ultimately supported by both quantitative and qualitative data—is that mothers' beliefs about child development and mothers' actual parenting strategies are strongly linked to their own broad epistemological perspectives (i.e., their conceptualization of the general nature of knowledge and of how they themselves come to know and understand themselves and their world). People's beliefs about the origins of knowledge, truth, and understanding provide frameworks for making meaning of the world and for conceptualizing the bases and trajectories of development. We imagined that women's assumptions about how people learn and their conceptions of *themselves* as knowers play a profound role in shaping their *parent* belief systems and the ways in which they approach and interpret their interactions with others, including their children.

Figure 20.1 (adapted from Bond, Belenky, Weinstock, & Monsey, 1992) provides a schematic diagram of the relations we have hypothesized. As the solid arrows illustrate, we imagine that women's own epistemological perspectives underlie their conceptions of child development, which, in turn, shape their conceptions of their roles as parents and their childrearing practices that ultimately contribute to their children's development. As the broken arrows illustrate, we expect that each of these components in the model (the women's epistemological perspectives, their conceptions of child development and parenting, their childrearing practices, and their child's development) contribute, in turn, to promoting personal and environmental contexts and characteristics that may shape opportunities for both mother and child to grow and understand themselves, their world, and their relationships

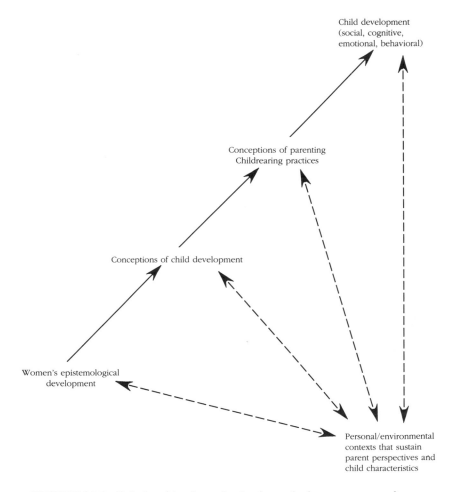

**FIGURE 20.1.** Relationships hypothesized to exist between women's epistemological frameworks, parenting, and child development.

in varied ways. For example, a given parenting strategy establishes a context that affects the child's development and understanding of himself as a thinker and at the same time, presents a setting that provides the mother with greater or fewer opportunities to engage in collaborative problem solving (one childrearing practice), observe her child's responsiveness to collaborative action (her understanding of child development), and reflect on her own reasoning skills, competence, and confidence with the tools of mind and voice (her own epistemological perspective). We provide illustrative examples later in this chapter.

We were especially interested in examining these notions within the context of a group of women who have been relatively unheard in U.S. society—isolated, rural, poor mothers of young children. Doubting one's intellectual capacity is all too common among the poor, among rural people, among women, and among mothers of young children—each a marginalized group within the United States. These overlapping populations—being widely seen as less capable and less worthy—are seldom supported to develop their intellectual potential. Doubts about one's capacities are often accompanied by social isolation and a sense of voicelessness that undercut one's potential for dialogue and connection with others. Mothers who are mired in self-doubt and uncertainty often discount what they, themselves, have to say, discouraging conversation with their own children (Bond et al., 1992). Because epistemological development is rooted in dialogue and relationships, the retreat into silence truncates their children's development as well as their own.

## Women's Epistemological Perspectives

### Ways of Knowing; Frameworks for Conceptualizing Their Children

How do women understand themselves as knowers? How do they conceptualize the origins of knowledge and truth? We use the term "epistemology" to refer to people's understanding of the basis of knowledge and the manner in which they think and come to understand their world. Unlike many traditional notions of "intelligence" that suggest a continuum of quantitative increments in degree of understanding and insight, epistemology is used to refer to qualitatively distinct frameworks or structures for organizing and making meaning of intellectual foundations and experience.

Intelligence and epistemology are interrelated but not identical. Intelligence tests are widely thought to measure, in part, innate intellectual ability, whereas epistemology indicates the way a person conceptualizes intellectual capacities and processes available to herself and to others. Genetic inheritance shapes one's intellectual potential, as does the way one conceptualizes that ability. Meanwhile, a person who has begun to articulate aspects of her intellectual powers is more likely to utilize and develop this potential than is someone who has not yet constructed such a theory of mind for herself.

Based on in-depth interviews with 135 women in the United States from highly diverse socioeconomic and educational backgrounds and ages, Belenky, Clinchy, Goldberger, and Tarule (1986) proposed a scheme of epistemological development—Women's Ways of Knowing. The scheme elaborates significantly on Perry's (1970) model of epistemological growth, which was based on an educationally and economically advantaged male sample of Harvard University undergraduates. The Ways of Knowing scheme identifies five perspectives that may well comprise a developmental course (for additional detail, see Weinstock, 1989).

1. *Silence.* Women think of themselves as "deaf and dumb" or as mindless and voiceless—unable to figure things out for themselves and unable to learn from others. Those who hold this view report an especially difficult time learning from words and lack confidence in their ability to speak their own thoughts, suggesting that their capacities for representational thought are not well developed. Indeed, words are thought of not so much as tools for conveying meaning between people but as weapons (e.g., "I deserved to be hit 'cause I was always mouthing off." "Why bother talking? What's it gonna get you but trouble?"). This perspective appears rooted in violence and social disintegration and is unlikely part of a typical sequence of development. Many Silent Knowers describe having been raised in social isolation with few mediated learning experiences. For them, the exclusion from the social community has likely hampered the development of representational thought and the skills necessary for participating in dialogue.

The lack of confidence in being able to pass meanings back and forth is profoundly isolating. As one woman explained, "When people talk and I don't understand, [long pause] I just say the heck with it, I'll just be by myself."

The use of raw power is more likely to proliferate when language fails to mediate meanings, desires, and differences. If people cannot represent their ideas in words they are more likely to rely on physical power-oriented means to express and achieve their goals. Moreover, not imagining that behavior can be guided by thought, people are more likely to act out of impulse rather than carefully reasoned longer-range plans.

2. *Received Knowledge.* Learning is equated with receiving, remembering, and returning the words of others. The ability to listen and to gain meaning from the words of others is of the utmost importance. It makes possible the entrance into the shared culture of one's community. Although Received Knowers possess these abilities and put great faith in language for transmitting knowledge their understanding of symbols and the interpretive powers of the mind are quite limited. They think of themselves as passive receptacles who learn automatically by hearing and memorizing material without mental modifications of any sort.

Truth is understood as absolute—eternal and singular. Any problem has only one right answer. Indeed, Received Knowers use many sets of dualistic concepts to characterize the world. Although contrasting illusive qualities in bold, clear terms may help in the initial stages of abstracting goals and values from one's experience in the world, such dichotomies ultimately obscure the complexities of reality (Perry, 1970).

The Received Knowing perspective may be relatively more functional in an intact agrarian society characterized by a slow rate of social and technological change. This way of knowing provides a sense of unity, continuity, and community that can be sorely missed in large segments of contemporary urban society. Dependence on elders and tradition for guidance, direction, and knowledge can be a severe handicap, however, when traditional agriculture is replaced by rapidly evolving scientific and industrial technologies (see, e.g., Hagen, 1962). Unquestioning conformity to the norms of one's community is particularly problematic for people presumed by others to be subordinate, submissive, and without the capacity for intelligence. Paulo Freire (1970) argued that this way of knowing justifies a "banking" notion of education that perpetuates the oppression of the poor. When teachers and authorities "deposit" their views of truth into the minds of passive recipients, the poor are kept from "naming" the reality of their experience and thus from transforming their relationship with the world.

The subsequent ways of knowing can be seen as steps involved in overcoming unquestioning conformity to the norms and dualisms of one's community—steps that allow women to see themselves as speakers as well as listeners, as capable of having thoughts as well as feelings, of leading as well as following.

3. *Subjective Knowledge.* Women come to appreciate that ideas can and do originate in the self and in understanding one's own experience. Seeing each person as having her or his own truth (lodged in the inner voice), there is no longer a belief in only one right answer. Believing in multiple realities, Subjective Knowers listen to others with a nonjudgmental view. Meanwhile, they hear and look to profit from others in

only limited ways because Subjective Knowers question the value of words to communicate personal truths and they understand truth to be nongeneralizable—knowledge is thought of as personal, private, and essentially incommunicable. Subjective Knowers conceptualize the source of knowledge as clearly lodged within the self; thus they value and focus on listening to their own inner voice rather than to the voices of others. Intuition and personal experience are now seen as *the* important sources of knowing; information that has been passed down from authorities is thought irrelevant.

4. *Procedural Knowledge.* The person understands knowledge and truth to emerge from systematic and communicable procedures. Two distinct types of procedures have been identified: the separate and connected approaches (see, e.g., Clinchy, 1989a, 1989b; Clinchy & Zimmerman, 1982, 1985).

In the *separate* procedural mode—highly characteristic of Western, scientific thought—the person works to remove the self from the knowing process, taking as impersonal a stance as possible by relying on impartial standards, rules, hypotheses, and so on, so that her or his own perspective will not bias the ability to perceive reality objectively. Unlike the constructed approach (described next), the importance of individuals' varied contexts for knowing may receive relatively little emphasis. The separate approach is often an adversarial one, focusing on critical analyses for proving and disproving arguments, as distinct from the constructed approach that more fully emphasizes the ongoing collaborative construction of new and improved procedures for seeing and understanding the issues at hand.

In the *connected* procedural mode, a mode many women seem to prefer, the goal is to understand and be understood rather than proving and disproving truths. The discourse is more contextual and narrative rather than logical and abstract. Connected Procedural Knowers emphasize collaboration rather than competition. Objectivity in the connected mode is sought by first drawing out others through interviewing and story telling so that they might be seen more fully. Then by drawing on this knowledge and her own empathetic capacities, the connected knower achieves objectivity by projecting the self *into* the other's perspective (rather than distancing herself) without superimposing her own perspective in the process. Connected Procedural Knowers' propensity for asking questions, drawing out and building up the ideas of others, has led us to think of them as "midwife teachers." Meanwhile, their personal views may get lost or set apart from the knowing process; thus new understanding may be "uncovered" but not fully "constructed" through a collaborative synthesis.

5. *Constructed Knowledge.* Individuals imagine that all knowledge is

continually constructed and evolving—that individuals of all ages and backgrounds are engaged in this construction process. Both separate and connected procedures are seen as invaluable tools to be used freely for deepening one's knowledge and understanding even when the goal of outdoing others through winning arguments has been firmly rejected. Constructivists have developed the ability to assert their own ideas while simultaneously absorbing those of others. It may well be that this capacity for listening while simultaneously marshalling one's own ideas makes it possible for the listener to take another's perspective without the loss of self often seen by both separate and connected Procedural Knowers. Because context is seen by Constructed Knowers as a vital force shaping what can be known, they feel responsible for examining, evaluating, and developing the frameworks they and others bring to the meaning-making process. The construction of knowledge and ways of knowing is perceived as a collaborative and dynamic process.

The Ways of Knowing scheme is not proposed as a fixed, universal sequence of epistemological development at this time. Currently, we know too little about the course of epistemological perspectives in diverse cultures; moreover, other ideal endpoints of epistemological development might be conceptualized besides the one specified here (see, e.g., Cirillo & Wapner, 1986). It is conceivable that these ways of knowing, their order of appearance, and their end points may vary under different cultural conditions (Shweder, 1991).

The Ways of Knowing scheme does, however, describe a series of outlooks in which each subsequent position seems more differentiated and more adequate for full participation in a society such as ours. As the world grows in complexity, as more and more people with markedly different world views interact, and as our knowledge base continues to change at an ever-accelerating rate, the importance of these epistemological achievements are impressed upon us with ever greater urgency.

Our ongoing examination of the developmental course of the epistemological perspectives among women in the United States does suggest that the Ways of Knowing framework may, in fact, present a relatively fixed sequence of epistemological outlooks in which each, in turn, is rejected and/or reorganized with movement to the subsequent perspective.

## Women's Epistemologies and Parenting

Building on the work of Loevinger (e.g., Ernhart & Loevinger, 1969; Loevinger, 1976), who attributed the rise and fall in mothers' authoritarian family attitudes to the mothers' ego development, we hypothesized a correspondence between mothers' ways of knowing and their conceptualizations of the child as a learner and thinker, and hence the parent–child relationship and the maternal role as teacher (see, e.g., Belenky, Bond, Weinstock, Burgmeier, & Monsey, 1990; Bond, Belenky, & Weinstock, 1991).

We imagine that the epistemologies described earlier provide powerful frameworks for the ways in which individuals conceptualize and experience the course of human development and interaction. Women who feel unable to use words to communicate and learn neither feel capable of nor value reflective dialogue. Because words come back to haunt, there is a fear of betrayal that encourages these women to be wary, distant, and silent. Relationships are guarded; it is safer to share activities rather than feelings and ideas. Interpersonal differences are scary because they are seen as neither potentially understandable nor resolvable; therefore, disagreements are to be avoided. In fact, differences or disagreements may be sufficient to define the relationship as critically flawed. In this environment of caution and restraint, it is difficult to discover or cultivate the powers of mind and voice—one's own or another's.

In contrast, a woman who sees herself as responsible for contributing to the creation of knowledge and full of ideas that can be articulated, evaluated, and revised is likely to search out the reflections of others, invite feedback, and look to others as important partners in the process of constructing, testing, and revising an understanding of the world. Articulation of differences and disagreements will be invited as providing rich opportunities for growth. Valuing others as a source of support and stimulation, these women will work to draw out the best of one another's thinking and, in so doing, promote their own and their partners' skills and confidence.

Related parenting patterns emerge. Women who rarely rely on words for problem solving and communication would be more likely to turn to power-oriented techniques for influencing their own children. Not feeling the power of their own minds and voices, these mothers would not imagine and draw out such capacities in their children. Not thinking and talking things through with their children, the mothers would be unlikely to explain what they themselves know or to ask their children questions that might help the children generate their own ideas, explanations, and choices. Mind and voice would be more likely to go unrecognized and unnurtured in both mother and child, and the child would be left with many of the thinking and parenting strategies of the parent, thus perpetuating these patterns and epistemologies through subsequent generations.

**Table 20.1.** Epistemological Perspectives of Self and Relations With Children

| Epistemological perspective | Mother's view of her mind and voice | Mother's view of child's mind and voice | Mother's view of childrearing |
|---|---|---|---|
| Silent knower | Feels stupid, mindless and voiceless; feels she can't teach others; words are weapons | Child as mindless and voiceless; child can't learn; child's feelings are dangerous, not understood | Use raw power to influence child; neither listen nor explain; much yelling; no dialogue; enforce absolute rules |
| Received knower | Goal is to receive, store, and transmit without modifying information; learns through memorization and recitation | Child learns by listening to elders; should be seen but not heard; child needs to be molded and filled with information | Inform child through lectures; teach right and wrong using rules, rewards, and punishments; emphasis on training and modeling |
| Subjective knower | Discover inner voice; truth comes from inner voice and experience, not authorities; values individuality | Child has own inner voice; each child is unique; delight in child's spontaneity | Let child think and speak for her/himself; laissez-faire; nonjudgmental |
| Procedural knower | Goal is to articulate and examine thoughts and feelings; uses procedures to evaluate and guide thinking | Child has thoughts and feelings to be developed; child can learn procedures for finding good answers | Ask for and provide reasoning and explanations; share processes behind each other's thinking |

In contrast, a mother who sees knowledge as the dynamic product of an active, constructive process—a transactional process that involves the self and others—is more likely to work to draw out her own and her children's thinking, to recognize and nurture their active involvement in discovering and, literally, constructing new truths. She is more likely to engage in the sorts of interactions that will both cultivate the thinking and expression of her child and exercise her *own* powers of mind and voice.

Table 20.1 (adapted from Bond et al., 1992) summarizes these hypothesized relations between women's epistemological perspectives of self and relations with children.

In summary, this project examined the premise that mothers' beliefs about child development and mothers' actual parenting strategies are strongly linked to their own broad epistemological perspectives—the women's conceptualization of the general nature of knowledge and how they themselves come to know and understand themselves and their world. We were especially interested in examining this premise among a group of isolated, poor, rural mothers—a group that has been marginalized and discouraged from recognizing the powers of their own minds and voices. By speaking with mothers about their epistemological perspectives and parenting beliefs and observing their interactions with their own children, we hoped to refine a framework that would guide us, ultimately, in supporting more constructive parent and child development.

# Method

## Study Participants

A total of 120 woman were recruited for the project from two contiguous and similar rural, impoverished, sparsely populated counties in northeastern Vermont. Participants were all 17–34 years of age with at least one child 6 years or younger, living below poverty in social/rural isolation with no involvement in support and self help groups, and identified by one or more referring agencies as having little family support and as being at risk for abuse or neglect of the children or under unusual stress. The women were recruited without regard for their marital status; pilot work revealed that mothers with partners as well as those without partners were raising children with limited social supports. Although mothers with partners sometimes have more adult supports within the home, they frequently have fewer formal supports offered to them from outside the home from, for example, local, state and federal agencies. Moreover, some single women have less access to informal supports, as well.

For the purposes of our investigation, a "study child" was also identified in each family, defined as the child living at home, under 7 years old, who was closest to 4.0 years old. This group included 51 girls and 69 boys who ranged in age from 0.2–6.8 years of age.

## Examining Maternal Epistemologies and Parenting Beliefs and Strategies

Using a variety of interview strategies, we explored the women's epistemologies and their beliefs about both their children and their responsibilities and goals in parenting their children. We also observed the women interacting with their children in semistructured and informal situations within their own homes.

### Maternal Self-Description/Background

We presented a brief series of interview questions in order to gather information about each woman's perceptions of herself and her children. This preliminary conversation also provided an introduction and focus for the remainder of the interview. Through these self-description questions, we attempted to elicit the "growing edge" of the respondent's ways of thinking about herself. For example, we asked: "How would you describe yourself to yourself?" "How do you see yourself differently now compared to the past?" "Who are the people you have really important relationships with right now?" "How would you describe X [that person] to me?" "How has your relationship with X changed over the years?"

### Ways of Knowing Interview

Belenky et al.'s 1986 interview was used to examine the women's epistemological perspectives—their thinking about truth, knowledge, authority, and themselves as thinkers. Using a semistructured interview format, the women were asked to talk about issues related to the ways in which they go about learning new things, how that has changed over time, people and experiences that have been important in shaping their approach to learning and understanding, and their understanding and handling of disagreements.

The coding procedures we used to infer a woman's epistemological perspective were based on the five general epistemological frameworks noted above and on the notion that structured wholes involve a "coming-into-being and a being" (Miller, 1989, p. 43). Specifically, we read and analyzed interview data for evidence of the major epistemological perspective as well as evidence of more minor epistemological assumptions. Individuals could thus be coded into one of 17 theoretically possible ordinal levels based on a major and minor epistemological code: Women who evidenced little transition from or toward a position besides the primary one (i.e., less than 20% of the epistemological assumptions expressed were reflective of an epistemological perspective other than the primary position) were coded with the major code only; women whose interviews suggested movement into or out of one of the general epistemological perspectives but predominant placement in another perspective (i.e., 60-70% of the epistemological assumptions expressed were reflective of that perspective) were coded with the predominant code as primary and the minor code as secondary; finally, women whose interviews suggested a fairly equal embeddedness in or transition between two primary epistemological perspectives were coded with both as primary.

The coding of each interview into one of the 17 theoretically possible ordinal levels was important to our goal of understanding the growing edge of a woman's thinking. For the purposes of certain statistical analyses, it was both useful and appropriate to collapse the first 10 levels (the only levels represented in our study population) into three epistemological groups: Any Silence, Full Received Knowing, and Any Subjective. Women who were coded with ordinal scores that reflected any Silent epistemological assumptions were categorized as "Any Silence"; "Full Received Knowing" included women whose epistemological scores reflected a clear embeddedness in Received Knowledge, with no strong evidence of any other epistemological assumptions. The Any Subjective group had scores that suggested at least some if not complete movement out of Received Knowledge and into Subjective Knowing. None of the study participants expressed predominantly Procedural or Constructed perspectives. In fact, in recruiting participants to this project, we had quite conscientiously worked to involve those community women who seemed to feel most silent and isolated.

## The Parent–Child Communication Strategy Interview

In the full version of this interview (McGillicuddy-De Lisi, Johnson, Sigel & Epstein, 1980), a series of 12 hypothetical situations are presented, each involving the interaction of a parent and 4-year-old child. Respondents are asked to indicate their preferred parent–child communication strategies, their rationales for their preferences, and their predictions as to which strategy they would actually use in each particular situation. Modifying this approach, we presented women with four of the scenarios. In the first, a child is playing with Lincoln Logs and begins to throw them around the living room when some of the pieces fail to fit; in the second, a child has refused to share her toys with the friend she has invited to her house to play; in the third, while the mother is bathing her child, the child wants to know whether the metal spoon he is playing with will float like his plastic bowl; and in the fourth, a child repeatedly asks her mother to play with her although mother has explained that she was very busy at that time.

For each scenario, we asked the mother to describe the strategy she would use to respond to that situation and her rationale for her selection; we also asked her to provide a follow-up strategy that she would use if her child did not respond and to present the rationale behind her follow-up approach. The women's responses regarding their preferred strategies and rationales were coded into nine categories, based on the work of McGillicuddy-De Lisi et al. (1980):

1. *Distancing*—interactional parent statements or question posing that places a mental demand on the child in order to elicit the child's active mental participation in a problem defined in the situation;
2. *Rational Authoritative*—communication strategies that provide the child with a statement of fact, rule, or information and that are accompanied by a supporting elaborative explanation that is an appeal to reason or to social norms;
3. *Direct Authoritative*—one-way communications that are directed toward shaping the child's behavior by providing a statement of fact or a rule without any further elaboration or explanation;
4. *Authoritarian*—communications that rely on physical manipulation of the child and/or her or his surroundings or the use of verbal threat or abuse;
5. *Diversion*—attempts to involve the child in some behavior or activity other than the one that is specified in the hypothetical situation, trying to alter the child's behavior by proposing a substitute activity that is not explicitly relevant to the problem at hand;
6. *Passivity*—refraining from intervening in any systematic way to modify the situation or the child's behavior;
7. *Parent Activity*—demonstrations and/or experimentation performed for or with the child in which the parent is an active participant and/or serves as a model (this category was originally part of a broader category termed "activity" by McGillicuddy-De Lisi, Johnson, Sigel & Epstein, 1980);
8. *Child Activity*—strategies that encourage experimentation by the child without significant input and without modeling by the parent (this category was not included in the work of McGillicuddy-De Lisi et al., 1980);

9. *Other*—strategies that did not fit with any of the previous categories.

As McGillicuddy-De Lisi et al.(1980) explained, these strategies vary along a continuum with regard to the degree to which they explicitly demand the child's active mental involvement. The Distancing strategies are conceptualized as encouraging the most active cognitive and verbal participation on the part of the child (i.e., they present the greatest mental operational demands on the child). The two authoritative strategies present decreasing cognitive demands on the child, first with Rational Authoritative including rationales and then Direct Authoritative presenting only statements without accompanying explanations. Finally, Diversion places no demand on the child to focus on the specific situation at hand. Our modified categories of Parent Activity and Child Activity fit into this continuum as well. Child Activity closely follows Distancing in the demands that it makes on the child while taking a more nonverbal approach; the message conveyed through the Child Activity strategy is that the child can and should work through the problem using active mental and physical experimentation on his or her own part. In contrast, Parent Activity is more closely in line with the authoritative strategies, with the parent assuming a central role in instructing the child (although at least in part nonverbally) as to how to proceed with the situation.

## Videotaped Mother–Child Interaction

Scenarios of mother–child interaction based, in part, on procedures developed by Sigel, McGillicuddy-De Lisi, and colleagues (e.g., McGillicuddy-De Lisi, 1982; McGillicuddy-De Lisi et al., 1980) were observed in each family. These sorts of episodes were selected because they represent, to varying degrees, interpersonal situations that require interpersonal communication, cooperation, negotiation and joint planning.

Each mother–child dyad was videotaped (with a small, hand-held portable recorder) in their home in 10 minutes of free play, two 5 minute teaching tasks, and up to 5 minutes of clean-up. During free play, the mother was asked to play with her child as she normally would with no particular restrictions put on the context of their interaction; for the first teaching task the mother was asked to help her child learn how to build a specified structure with Legos (plastic interlocking blocks); for the second teaching task she was asked to help her child learn how to assemble a particular (age-appropriate) puzzle; finally, during clean-up the mother was asked to engage the child in helping her to put the toys away. The complexity of these tasks varied so as to be age-appropriate but somewhat difficult for the child.

The videotaped interactions were coded using a scheme adapted from the Parent–Child Interaction Observation Schedule (PCI), originally developed by Flaugher and Sigel (1980), that categorized behavior into Child or Task Management; Low, Medium, or High Mental Operational Demands (see Bond et al., 1991, for additional details).

Child Management is defined as nonverbal and/or verbal parental efforts at stopping or modifying a child behavior, not necessarily related to the task, of which the parent does not approve (e.g., "Sit still now"). Task Management refers to specific verbal or nonverbal directions the parent gives the child that are directly related to accomplishing the task (e.g., "Put the big piece here"). Low Mental Operational Demands (MODS) are questions or statements that may or may not require a response from the child; they do not require the child to go beyond the concrete information before them. Medium MODs are questions or statements that require the child to retrieve information in order to give a response to the parent. High MODs are parent questions or statements that require the child not only to retrieve information but to organize and integrate it as well.

The middle 5 minutes of free play and of each teaching task were coded from videotapes by assistants unaware of the mother's epistemological perspective. Continuous, sequential coding of all relevant behaviors was conducted in teams of two and a minimum reliability of .80 was required between teams for each coding category. The number of responses in each behavior category was totaled for each participant on each task for further analysis. High MODs were infrequently and unreliably coded and thus were excluded from subsequent analyses.

# Results

We introduce our results by summarizing some quantitative analyses of our measures. Then we explore these findings further with the use of individual case examples.

## Quantitative Analyses of Women's Epistemologies and Parenting Strategies

### Hypothetical Parent–Child Communication Strategies

Important relations emerged between the hypothetical parent–child communication strategies and maternal epistemological perspectives. Tables 20.2 and 20.3 illustrate that with an increase in epistemological position, there was an increase in modal endorsement of Rational

Authoritative, Parent Activity, and Distancing parenting strategies and a decrease in the modal endorsement of Authoritarian strategies. Moreover, a firm footing in position 2 of epistemological reasoning (Received Knowing) appeared necessary, although not sufficient, for the modal endorsement of Distancing and Rational Authoritative strategies in the hypothetical scenarios.

Two different strategies were used to examine statistically the relationship between epistemology and modal communication response to the hypothetical scenarios. First, a rank number was assigned to each modal communication strategy based on the amount of parent control involved in the strategy as well as the amount of mental demand placed on the child. On a dimension from high parent control/low mental demand to low control/high mental demand, an Authoritarian modal response was ranked first, followed by Direct Authoritative, Parent Activity, Rational Authoritative, and finally, Distancing. (None of the women in this sample used Child Activity as their modal strategy.) A one-way Analysis of Variance (ANOVA) confirmed that women with Any Silent epistemological assumptions endorsed a more directive, less cognitively demanding communication strategy compared with women with more complex epistemologies, $F(2,73) = 4.29$, $p = .017$.

Given the large number of women in the study ($n = 41$) who endorsed Authoritarian strategies as their modal communication response in the hypothetical scenarios, we examined the degree to which women's epistemologies varied with their endorsement of Authoritar-

**Table 20.2.** Modal Parent–Child Communication Strategy as a Function of Primary Epistemological Position ($N = 81$)

| Primary epistemological Position | Parent–Child Communication Strategy | | | | |
|---|---|---|---|---|---|
| | Authoritarian | Direct Authoritative | Parent Activity | Rationale Authoritative | Distancing |
| 1 ($n = 11$) | 82% | 9% | 9% | — | — |
| $\frac{1}{2}$ ($n = 3$) | 100% | — | — | — | — |
| 2 ($n = 51$) | 49% | 4% | 29% | 10% | 4% |
| $\frac{2}{3}$ ($n = 5$) | 20% | — | 20% | 20% | 20% |
| 3 ($n = 11$) | 27% | 9% | 36% | 9% | — |

*Note.* Percents may not add up to 100 due to rounding error and the fact that not all possible communication strategies are included here. There were no women in the sample coded with epistemological scores greater than the primary position of 3 (Subjective Knowing).

ian ($n$ = 41) versus the non-Authoritarian ($n$ = 40) strategies. A one-way ANOVA revealed a lower mean epistemological score among women who endorsed an Authoritarian strategy as their modal response than among those who did not, $M$ = 4.66, $M$ = 6.00, respectively; $F(1,79)$ = 8.59, $p$ = .004. Specifically, among the former, the mean epistemological score fell between fully developed Received Knowing and a predominant Received Knowing epistemology but with a partial articulation of Silent epistemological assumptions as well. Meanwhile, women who did not endorse Authoritarian strategies as their modal response tended, on average, to articulate a fully developed Received Knowing perspective along with a partial articulation of Subjective Knowing assumptions.

One-way ANOVAs of women's *mean* use of the various communication strategies in the hypothetical scenarios revealed that women with more complex epistemological perspectives used more Distancing/Child Activity, $F(2,109)$ = 4.65, $p$ = .012; more Parent Activity, $F(2,109)$ = 3.47, $p$ = .035; and less Authoritarian communication, $F(2,109)$ = 4.07, $p$ = .020; see Tables 20.4 and 20.5. (Given the minimal use of both Distancing and Child Activity strategies and the similarities of these strategies with regard to the mental demands they place on the child, we chose to combine these strategies in examining their relation to epistemological position.)

**Table 20.3.** Modal Parent–Child Communication Strategy as a Function of Epistemological Group ($N$ = 81)

| Epistem-ological Group | Parent–Child Communication Strategy | | | | |
|---|---|---|---|---|---|
| | Authori-tarian | Direct Authori-tative | Parent Activity | Rationale Authori-tative | Distancing |
| Any Silence ($n$ = 19) | 79% | 5% | 5% | 5% | — |
| Full Received ($n$ = 30) | 47% | 7% | 33% | 10% | 3% |
| Any Subjective ($n$ = 32) | 38% | 3% | 31% | 9% | 6% |

*Note.* Percentages may not add up to 100 due to rounding error and the fact that not all possible communication strategies are included here. There were no women in the sample who were coded with epistemological scores greater than the primary position of 3 (Subjective Knowing).

Behavioral Mother–Child Communication Strategies
and Their Relation to Epistemological Perspectives

In addition to examining hypothetical scenarios, we examined mothers' actual behavioral strategies playing with and teaching their children as recorded in our videotapes. Mothers' use of Child Management strategies—a power-oriented behavioral communication strategy that focuses on nontask behavior—was negatively correlated with the mothers' epistemological perspectives ($p \leq .05$, Pearson product–moment correlation). A two-way Multivariate Analysis of Variance (MANOVA) (Epistemological Group x Task) revealed a similar finding, $F(2,37) = 4.21$, $p = .022$; women with Any Silence used more Child Management strategies than women with Received or Any Subjective knowing ($p \leq .05$). In addition, when teaching their children to work with Lego blocks, women with Any Silence tended to use fewer MODs overall with their children than did women in the other two epistemological groups, $p \leq .05$; $F(4,74) = 2.19$, $p = .078$ for the Group x Task interaction.

　　Thus, to summarize our quantitative analyses, mothers with more complex epistemological perspectives endorsed more cognitively demanding, nonauthoritarian, and nondirective parenting communication strategies—those that are more likely to draw children into active reciprocal collaboration and problem solving. Moreover, mothers with more complex epistemological perspectives used more cognitively engaging statements and questions while interacting with their children and focused less on controlling and/or restraining their children's non-task-related behaviors.

**Table 20.4.** Mean Parent–Child Communication Strategy Scores as a Function of Primary Epistemological Position ($N = 112$)

| Primary Epistemological Position | Parent–Child Communication Strategy | | | | | |
|---|---|---|---|---|---|---|
| | Authoritarian | Direct Authoritative | Parent Activity | Rationale Authoritative | Child Activity | Distancing |
| 1 ($n = 15$) | 3.0 | .8 | 1.5 | 1.3 | — | .1 |
| ½ ($n = 4$) | 3.6 | 1.6 | 1.1 | .9 | .5 | — |
| 2 ($n = 70$) | 2.5 | .6 | 1.9 | 1.1 | .5 | .1 |
| ⅔ ($n = 7$) | 2.2 | .2 | 2.0 | 1.4 | .5 | .7 |
| 3 ($n = 16$) | 1.8 | .7 | 2.0 | .8 | .7 | .3 |

Note. Scores can range from 0 to 8. Totals may not add up to 8 due to rounding error and the fact that not all possible communication strategies are included here. There were no women in the sample coded with epistemological scores greater than the primary position of 3 (Subjective Knowing).

## Case Examples

To understand further the relationships between women's epistemological perspectives and their concepts of parenting and children, let us listen to a few of the women themselves as they speak to us about themselves, their children, and their childrearing strategies.

### Susan

A woman we shall call Susan was among the many Silent Knowers who described having been raised in social isolation with few mediated learning experiences. Such exclusion from the social community likely hampers the development of representational thought and the skills necessary for participating in dialogue. Susan described her childhood:

> "I felt kind of dumb, very, very. 'Cause for when I went to school, I was picked on for, (*sigh*) I don't know how long.... "We don't want to play with you." You know, that kind of stuff.... All the kids always picked on me.... I felt dumb when I'd talk. You know, if I'd say something, it just didn't come out right. It just didn't sound right, and I felt like, oh, Susan, get out of here."

The lack of confidence in being able to pass meanings back and forth is profoundly isolating. The only kinds of learning projects that Susan

**Table 20.5.** Mean Parent–Child Communication Strategy Scores as a Function of Epistemological Group ($N = 112$)

| Epistemo-logical Group | Parent–Child Communication Strategy | | | | | |
|---|---|---|---|---|---|---|
| | Authori-tarian | Direct Authori-tative | Parent Activity | Rationale Authori-tative | Child Activity | Distancing |
| Any Silence (*n* = 25) | 3.1 | .9 | 1.4 | 1.3 | .2 | .1 |
| Full Received (*n* = 42) | 2.5 | .6 | 1.9 | 1.1 | .4 | .1 |
| Any Subjective (*n* = 45) | 2.2 | .5 | 2.1 | 1.0 | .5 | .3 |

*Note.* Scores can range from 0 to 8. Totals may not add up to 8 due to rounding error and the fact that not all possible communication strategies are included here. There were no women in the sample coded with epistemological scores greater than the primary position of 3 (Subjective Knowing).

feels really competent to undertake involve sensory–motor activities, not language. When asked how she would describe herself to herself as a learner or a thinker, Susan said:

"Well, I can cut hair but nobody's ever taught me. . . . I can knit, I can make slippers, and I don't even know how to do it. I couldn't even tell somebody how to do it because I don't even know how to do it myself. BUT YOU DO IT. [Words printed in uppercase letters within quotations indicate the comments of the interviewer.] Right. Well, um, I know how I do it but I couldn't tell you right now how to do it. You would have to watch me. YEAH, OKAY. Find out for yourself. Cutting hair. People ask me, 'How do you do it?' I say, 'You have to watch me.'"

Susan describes her own son as having difficulties learning from others as well:

"He's a very good kid but he has a problem on listening. He don't do nothing bad (UM HUM) but I'm saying, say if I told him to stay on the side [yard], like he'd adventure off a ways. I want to know where he is at all times. My older two, I know where they are; they have their boundaries too. They can't go out of the area. . . . He knows what's gonna happen [if he disobeys], that he will be put in bed or be sit down. Well, if that don't work, then I have to spank him."

It appears that Susan does not ask or expect her son to learn or understand the reasoning behind the rules she imposes; she does not imagine that her 5-year-old son can use relevant information to make appropriate judgments regarding reasonable behavior.

"I want to know where he is. There's a lot of things out here he could get hurt on that he's not aware of. UM HUM. A 5-year-old, to me they're not aware of it. And I want to know where he is all the time until I feel he might be even older until I feel he's capable of knowing right from wrong."

Asked about how she handles disagreements with her own son, Susan states, "Um, if he's right, then he's right but if he's wrong, then I have to take over, and I'll go, 'You did wrong.' 'You have to sit down,' or 'You have to give this back.'" Thus, notably absent from Susan's descriptions of her childrearing strategies are efforts to provide the child with explanations or rationales for the behaviors she expects, nor does she attempt to consider or explore the child's reasons for his behavior.

When we shared with Susan the story of a hypothetical 4-year-old named Billy who was playing with Lincoln Logs and began to throw them around the room when they wouldn't fit together (the Parent–Child Communication Strategy Interview of McGillicuddy-De Lisi et al., 1980), Susan stated that the mother should direct the child to "pick them up and try again . . . so that he'll realize he can't throw them around. . . . If he keeps throwing them, I just take them."

When Susan was videotaped "teaching" her 5-year-old son to assemble an animal with interlocking Lego blocks, there was a striking absence of both verbal and physical interaction between mother and son. In fact, rather than enter into any apparent teaching relation with her son, Susan focused quite intently and exclusively on her *own* construction with the blocks, seeming relatively unaware of her child and his attempts to manipulate the blocks. Throughout the entire period, Susan uttered literally only a few isolated, brief declarative statements (e.g., "Hang on to it [a block]," "Uh huh," "Let me try") as she took the blocks away from her son, disassembled those blocks he managed to clamp together, and resisted his attempts to manipulate the blocks with her, obstructing his view of her hands as she assembled the structure.

### Rachel

A second participant, whom we shall call Rachel, has a distinctly different perspective of herself. Unlike Susan, Rachel describes herself as able to acquire knowledge from the words spoken by others. When asked how she thought of herself as a thinker, Rachel said:

> "Well, I can understand things if somebody explains it to me. . . . I know I can do good in school, but I got in the wrong crowd and started goofing off. I knew I could do good if I would have just stuck to it. . . . The work and stuff I always understood. You know, I did good and stuff in my work and stuff.

But like other Received Knowers, Rachel sees herself acquiring knowledge from the words spoken by external authorities, not from the action of her own mind. In response to a question about the value of self-directed learning:

> "I don't think that's right. No. The teacher should be teaching you how to—what to learn and stuff. How can you learn on your own?

You have to have somebody teaching you. . . . The Teachers have, you know, been to school and stuff whereas they know how to teach it."

This view that you have to learn from others, combined with a confidence in her ability to learn from others, led Rachel to rely on explanations for educating children rather than punishment. Responding to the hypothetical scenario about the 4-year-old who throws the Lincoln Logs when they will not fit together, Rachel responds:

"I'd either explain to him that it wasn't right for him to throw it and not to get so mad over it, to ask for help if they need it you know, and ask somebody to help him to do it instead of getting made over it. I feel that you can teach a kid more by explaining to him why it's wrong than to hit him or something, than to holler at him."

Although Rachel describes how she explains things to her daughter, she does not present any images of drawing out her daughter's thoughts with good questions and mutual dialogue because she doesn't imagine her daughter—or anyone else—being capable of active thinking and problem solving. When asked at the initial interview to describe an important decision that she had made in her life, Rachel could think of none:

"CAN YOU THINK OF A TIME WHEN YOU HAD TO MAKE A DECISION, BUT YOU JUST WEREN'T SURE WHAT WAS RIGHT? I don't know. (*long pause*) A BIG DECISION? IT COULD BE RECENT, IT COULD BE ANYTIME IN THE PAST. Hum, I don't know. DID LEAVING SCHOOL SEEM LIKE A BIG DECISION? No, not really. IT JUST SORT OF HAPPENED? Yea. DID HAVING YOUR DAUGHTER SEEM LIKE A BIG DECISION? No. (*laughs*) Because it wasn't a decision, it just happened. WHAT ABOUT MOVING IN WITH YOUR BOYFRIEND? Uh huh. We've been together for over three years, it will be four years. WAS THAT A DECISION? No. (*laughs*) WELL, THAT'S INTERESTING!"

At that time in her life, Rachel's stance toward the future was equally passive. When asked, "What is your life going to be like in the future, say five years from now?" she responded:

"I don't know. HARD TO IMAGINE? I don't know for sure. I don't like to think about things and worry about what's it going to be like. If you worry about everything, then it's going to just bring you

down all the time, you know. IS YOUR LIFE LIKELY TO BE VERY
DIFFERENT? Probably not . . . I don't expect anything to change.
I only carry one day at a time."

Thus, while Rachel was confident in her ability to receive knowledge handed down by others, she did not imagine ideas springing up
out of her own mind. Her videotaped interaction with her 5-year-old
daughter fit within this Received Knowing framework. Unlike Susan,
who assumed physical control of the situation and the blocks themselves, Rachel maintained control over the activity through verbal
directions. Rachel drew her daughter into the building activity, but
under the guidance of Rachel's very specific verbal instructions regarding which block to put where. The assumption seemed to be that her
daughter could learn only from the transmission of specific, step-by-step
instructions from her mother, the expert. It is striking, however, that as
the learning session neared completion, Rachel loosened her verbal
grip upon her daughter and began to include open-ended questions to
guide the child's actions (e.g., "Where does this go?" "Does that open?"
"What goes in there?"). Perhaps Rachel felt her daughter had mastered
certain of the block-building skills through her mother's instruction and
was now ready to generalize these skills on her own.

### Pam

Procedural Knowers imagine themselves as constructing opinions—as
creators rather than conduits of ideas; moreover, they articulate some
of the methods they use in the process. A woman we shall call Pam was
one of the few women in the study who expressed some Procedural
perspective. For example, she explained:

> "I think better when I talk, if that makes any sense. YEAH, IT DOES
> . . . Um, just by talking about it. MMM. Just by talking about it, you
> know. It's the feedback I get that brings up ideas in my head. Or it
> brings up certain feelings that tell me what I'm thinking about it. . .
> . I can better come to a conclusion if I can talk to someone about it."

When asked to comment upon a statement made by another woman,
"The student is giving her opinion. It might not be the right one. The
teachers are always more or less right," Pam says:

> "No, I disagree with that. BECAUSE? Because the teacher—a lot of
> times—makes [up] an opinion, states an opinion to get the students
> thinking. MMMM. To get better feedback from the students."

Pam imagines the teacher manufacturing an argument to stimulate the student into active, independent thinking. She sees that conflict, disequilibrium, and good questions are powerful tools for drawing out embryonic thoughts.

Pam has begun developing some degree of both separate and connected Procedural approaches. When asked, "How do you go about understanding new things?" she replies, "I take on new ideas and things, with a very open mind. MMM. You know, I try to see the good in it before I begin picking it apart for all the bad." Pam tries to embrace an idea before beginning its dissection. She also sees that both approaches can provide useful tools for sponsoring the development of ideas and the intellectual growth of others. Although she recognizes the power of playing the devil's advocate for helping others clarify and develop their thoughts, she uses the connected approach when working with her almost 5-year-old daughter, Alice. By that we mean she draws out her daughter's thinking, listens, and confirms rather than argues. Asked about the ways she and Alice handle disagreements, Pam says:

> "We have to talk things out a little more than we used to. It used to be when we disagreed, Mommy was right and that was that. That was the way it was, you know. Now, I have to let her voice her opinion. I have to listen to how she feels about things because she's thinking more on my level than on a 4-year-old level, a lot of times. Not all the time, obviously, but a lot of times she sees it in a very logical way and, UM HUM. A lot of times she can be right. MMM. You know, lot of times. She understands more than I think the average 4-year-old kid understands. . . . Not all the time, obviously, but a lot of times she sees it in a very logical way."

There is a sense of equality and reciprocity between this mother and child. Pam gets down to her daughter's level, and she sees her daughter rising up to hers. She listens to her child and appreciates the logic that she hears. When Pam describes her daughter she sees the child's strengths, not the flaws:

> "Describe Alice? Alice is a beautiful little girl; very bright. She enjoys spending time with people and talking with people. She loves books. She's got a load of energy that just doesn't seem to quit. Um, she's a mother hen. Things have got to be just so and she knows the right way for them to be. And if they're not the right way, she gets concerned about it. (*laughs*) She's a responsible child. A very responsible child. I'm starting to look at her more as a little kid than baby. UH HUH. I realize that she's capable of doing things that, you know, that sometimes you don't become aware of and

suddenly there it is. You know, you realize that she's been doing it for 2 months. But you haven't just really noticed. RIGHT. UM, I'm letting her take on more little responsibilities and do the things that she wants to do."

Pam reaches for a kind of double vision. She tries to bring her daughter's "growing edge" into focus, seeing Alice as she is trying to become while also seeing her as she is at the moment.

The videotaped interactions of Pam and her daughter are extraordinary. In contrast to Susan and Rachel, Pam appears much less concerned with quickly and efficiently producing the animal we requested than she is with engaging Alice in mutual activity. For example, Pam begins by disassembling some of the Lego blocks that remained together from our previous session with another child, and she returns these blocks to the box so that Alice can take full control over selecting those she desires. Pam's conversation is rich with questions followed by full pauses, a pattern that encourages her child to participate as a full partner: "Can we try to make him?" "Is that this part here?" "Can you get it?" Pam provides Alice with guidance, yet does so through questions that draw her daughter into the activity: "Now on the bottom of that we need what?" "Is that the one we need?" "And now what do we need to do on the top of his head?"

In a step-by-step fashion, Pam orients her child through the task but slowly paces her guidance, allowing Alice to identify the next step and how to complete it. Daughter Alice performs all the manipulation of the blocks; even when she runs into difficulty, Pam refrains from taking over physically or verbally—although she offers her assistance. At several points, we observe Pam begin to interject words or actions and then "swallow" her words, or, in one instance, essentially sit on her hands to refrain from taking over. Despite temptation to the contrary, Pam seems to value her daughter working through the problems herself as much as she is able. Moreover, as the session proceeds, Pam's communication becomes increasingly less directive, shifting even greater responsibility and credit for progress to Alice. At the conclusion, Pam asks Alice to compare her construction with the picture we had presented—Alice herself is called on to analyze their similarities and differences and, ultimately, to claim success for her accomplishment.

## Summary

Our varied analyses describe an impressive relationship between, on the one hand, mothers' conceptions of child development and parent–

child relations in both hypothetical and real interactions and, on the other hand, women's epistemological perspectives. A woman's understanding of her children, her expectations for her relationships with them, and her images of the role of these relationships in her children's development appear closely tied to the mother's broader understanding of human development including her own life course and the role of relationships therein.

We have noted the likely bidirectional influences involved in the correspondence between epistemology and parents' "theories" of child development and their parent–child interactions (see Bond et al., 1992; and Figure 20.1 and Table 20.1). Epistemologies will frame a mother's understanding of both child development and her own role in supporting that development. These conceptions, in turn, influence the parent–child transactions. On the other hand, a mother's beliefs and parent–child transactions contribute to establishing contexts that reinforce and perpetuate the underlying assumptions and epistemologies. For example, not imagining the abilities of one's own mind and voice, a mother will be unlikely to draw on the minds and voices of others, including her children, further limiting opportunities for both her and her child to exercise, cultivate, and celebrate in the power of these personal and collective tools. Conversely, a woman who perceives herself as a capable collaborator in the construction of knowledge will be more likely to engage her children in the active and collaborative creation of ideas; this, in turn, will contribute to a situation of reciprocity and collaboration in which both mother and child can increasingly discover the powerful creations of which they are capable, and of which the *relationship* is capable.

This notion may explain some of the limitations of parent-training efforts that have focused on reshaping the mother's parenting behaviors and conceptions of her child's development without attending to her own developmental course. A woman's beliefs about child development and her parenting behavior do not exist in a vacuum. They rest within a broader developmental framework. We imagine that a significant elaboration and/or transformation of a parent's perspective on child development and childrearing requires a significant developmental transition on the part of the parent herself or himself.

Whence do people's epistemological perspectives emerge—these broad-scale frameworks that contribute so powerfully to mothers' notions of their children's development? We have talked extensively with isolated, impoverished women in the New England region of the United States about the people and experiences that have been important in shaping their understandings of themselves as thinkers and knowers. Although our analysis of this dialogue is not yet complete, it has become clear that certain types of experiences have been overwhelmingly important. With remarkable consistency, the women describe the roots of their epistemological perspectives by pointing to the degree to which they have felt truly heard and felt they have witnessed the power and/or impotence of their own minds and voices.

For example, for many of the women who grew up and continue to live in extraordinarily impoverished, rural, socially isolated settings, we found that experiences of feeling truly listened to and heard have been rare. As children, many remember a school system and a peer culture that demeaned the way they dressed, the way they lived, and the way they talked; many describe being treated as outcasts, condemned to the margins of the school and peer cultures because they did not have the economic resources or the social "know-how" to be accepted. Others describe the dramatic presence of this marginalization and voicelessness within their own families, perpetuated by parents and other adults in the household who appeared to feel threatened and voiceless themselves. Verbal and physical abuse were prevalent among these particular families. Intellectual dependency and personal isolation were working assumptions within many of these households; attempts to deviate from these norms were often treated as additional evidence of stupidity and insolence and met with greater rejection and isolation.

Clearly there are a host of social, political, historical, and economic forces on the global, national, community, and family levels that contribute to the greater marginalization and silencing of certain individuals as well as groups of peoples. These forces often propel and sustain belief and interactional systems that are, in many ways, self-perpetuating. If we hope to support parents' growth toward a rich understanding of their children's development, we might best focus on factors at the societal, community, family, and individual levels that support parents' own developmental course—promoting parents' opportunities to discover and cultivate their own social and intellectual powers, supporting a framework from which parents can imagine and engage their children in a fuller range of their potential. This strategy, which we have begun to develop in the Listening Partners Program (Belenky, Bond & Weinstock, 1995; Bond et al., 1991; Bond et al., 1992), has ripple effects that can be seen at a variety of levels of interaction within the family and community, with relationships and collaborative thinking assuming a central role in imagining and supporting the development of individuals, dyads, groups, and communities.

## Acknowledgments

This research is part of a larger project funded by a grant to Lynne A. Bond and Mary Field Belenky from the Bureau of Maternal and Child Health

(MCJ-500541) 10/86-6/91; and through support from the A.L. Mailman Family Foundation, and the Charles and Els Bendheim Foundation.

# References

Belenky, M. F., Bond, L. A., & Weinstock, J. S. *From silence to voice: Developing ways of knowing.* Manuscript submitted for publication.

Belenky, M. F., Bond, L. A., Weinstock, J. S., Burgmeier, P. T., & Monsey, T. V. C. (1990, April). *Mothers' ways of knowing and their conceptions of parenting.* Paper presented at the annual meetings of the American Educational Research Association, Boston.

Belenky, M. F., Clinchy, B. M., Goldberger, N. R., & Tarule, J. M. (1986). *Women's ways of knowing: The development of self, voice, and mind.* New York: Basic Books.

Bond, L. A., Belenky, M. F., & Weinstock, J. S. (1991). *Listening Partners: Psycho-social competence and prevention.* (Final Report of Grant MCJ-500541 [10/86-6/91] to the Maternal and Child Health Bureau). Rockville, MD: Department of Health and Human Services.

Bond, L. A., Belenky, M. F., Weinstock, J. S., & Monsey, T. V. C. (1992). Self-sustaining powers of mind and voice: Empowering rural women. In M. Kessler, S. E. Goldston & J. M. Joffe (Eds.), *The present and future of prevention: in honor of George W. Albee* (pp. 125–137). Newbury Park, CA: Sage.

Cirillo, L., & Wapner, S. (1986). *Value presuppositions in theories of human development.* Hillsdale, NJ: Erlbaum.

Clinchy, B. M. (1989a). The development of thoughtfulness in college women: Integrating reason and care. *American Behavioral Scientist, 32,* 647–657.

Clinchy, B. M. (1989b). On critical thinking and connected knowing. *Liberal Education, 75*(5), 14–19.

Clinchy, B., & Zimmerman, C. (1982). Epistemology and agency in the development of undergraduate women. In P. Perun (Ed.), *The undergraduate woman: Issues in educational equity* (pp. 161–181). Lexington, MA: D. C. Heath.

Clinchy, B., & Zimmerman, C. (1985, July). Connected and separate knowing. In *Gender differences in intellectual development: Women's ways of knowing.* Symposium conducted at the biennial meetings of the International Society for the Study of Behavioral Development, Tours, France.

Ernhart, C. B., & Loevinger, J. (1969). Authoritarian family ideology: A measure, its correlates, and its robustness. *Multivariate Behavioral Research Monographs, 69*(1).

Flaugher, J., & Sigel, I. (1980). *Parent–child interaction observation schedule.* Princeton, NJ: Educational Testing Service.

Freire, P. (1970). *Pedagogy of the oppressed.* New York: Seabury Press.

Hagen, E. E. (1962). *On the theory of social change: How economic growth begins.* Homewood, IL: Dorsey Press.

Loevinger, J. (1976). *Ego development: Conceptions and theories.* San Francisco: Jossey-Bass.

McGillicuddy-DeLisi, A. V. (1982). The relationship between parents' beliefs about development and family constellation, socioeconomic status, and parents' teaching strategies. In L. M. Laosa & I. E. Sigel (Eds.), *Families as learning environments for children* (pp. 261–299). New York: Plenum Press.

McGillicuddy-DeLisi, A. V., Johnson, J. E., Sigel, I. E., & Epstein, R. (1980). *Communication strategy administration and coding manual.* Princeton, NJ: Educational Testing Service.

Miller, P. H. (1989). *Theories of developmental psychology* (2nd ed.). New York: W. H. Freeman.

Perry, W. G., Jr. (1970). *Forms of intellectual and ethical development during the college years: A scheme.* New York: Holt, Rinehart & Winston.

Shweder, R. A. (1991). *Thinking through cultures.* Cambridge, MA: Harvard University Press.

Weinstock, J. S. (1989). Ways of knowing coding manual. In *Epistemological expressions among college women in two contexts: Conflicts with friends and authorities* (pp. 109–183). Unpublished master's thesis, University of Vermont, Burlington.

# CHAPTER 21

# American Cultural Models of Early Influence and Parent Recognition of Developmental Delays

## Is Earlier Always Better Than Later?

Thomas S. Weisner
Catherine C. Matheson
Lucinda P. Bernheimer

There comes a time for some parents which they never forget. It is when they first come to have a serious concern about their child's health and normal developmental status. Parents may recall this time as a series of events, or as a particular moment when they talked with a relative, friend, physician, teacher, or psychologist and had prior suspicions confirmed or doubts mirrored. It is the time when parents recognize that their child may have a serious developmental problem. Such concerns about one's child combine profound emotional dread and fears, uncertainty, and informational ambiguity and confusion. Parents begin to recognize that the child may not be able to learn skills necessary to be able to earn a living or marry. They have concerns that the child will not have sufficient social and cultural knowledge and communicative skills to enable it to act in the world as a competent, morally appropriate person. These concerns strike at every parents' hopes for their child's very survival, and at parents' goals for their child's competence and the continuity of family. Such goals are what parents everywhere want for their children, and are a part of every society's cultural models of normal development. These concerns are at the core of what LeVine (1977, 1988) has identified as universal goals parents everywhere have for their children—survival and health, subsistence competence, and social and moral appropriacy.

Initial concerns and recognition of delay are like "flashbulb memories" (Neisser, 1982) of unique and emotionally powerful events, never forgotten. Although there might be a particular period that parents remember as the time when they had their first real concerns, or had concerns confirmed by professionals, such concerns usually develop gradually and depend on their child's age, their access to information, the nature of the child's developmental delays, and many other circumstances. There may be stages in the development and evolution of such concerns and the responses to them in the United States. Miller (1993), for example, suggests that there are four: surviving, searching, settling in, and separating. Although in this broader sense there is no defined beginning or end of "recognition" and its continuous negotiation, our families do recognize a delimited period of time when their concerns began. Here are some family situations and parents' comments about that initial recognition.

Jimmy was born full-term, by Caesarean section due to fetal distress. He experienced anoxia and had seizures while in the hospital. The parents were told, "Well, he is maybe going to live and maybe going to die." After he had stabilized, according to father, "They painted a picture for us that he was going to be in a really bad mental condition, possibly [go] straight into a mental institution." Jimmy came home from the hospital with a diagnosis of severe cerebral palsy and severe mental retardation.

In the case of Annie G, there was nothing remarkable about mother's pregnancy, labor, or delivery. The parents thought she was a normal baby. They first became concerned between 6 and 8 months, when they noticed that Annie was much less active than her cousin, who was only 6 weeks older. She "wasn't moving and getting around." This is when their initial concern began. Their physician, a general practitioner, told them not to worry: "She's going to get up with the other kids, she's going to be fine." But their recognition that their child might be delayed gradually grew from that time. By the time Annie was 15 months they were "real worried," and were being urged by friends and family members to have her seen by someone else. They switched to a pediatrician who "knew right away something wasn't right" and referred them to a pediatric neurologist. The neurologist diagnosed Annie as hypotonic and referred her to physical therapy. The parents described their reaction as "'Oh my God—now what do we do?' We just didn't know what to think."

"Sharon was born fine. She came out healthy. She was about 14 months before she really started walking. She was slow, but, you know, so was my son. When she was about 2 years old, we started noticing that she was talking like my son when we first noticed his problem. And we found out that there were speech problems in the family that we weren't even aware of. We were hoping Sharon didn't have it. And sure enough about 2 years old we noticed the problem. And we started early with therapy."

Brett's family did not begin to worry until he was 3. Brett was the second of three children with disabilities (his older and younger sisters both had significant hearing losses). In part because of the attention focused on the older sister, the parents were not concerned about Brett in his first 2 years; in fact, they felt very fortunate that he did not have a hearing loss. Mother had some concerns regarding difficult behavior from about 18 months on, but it was a surprise and a shock to her when the older sister's teacher suggested Brett might be "aphasic" when he was 3. An evaluation at the university clinic confirmed the teacher's hunch, and Brett started in a special education preschool. His mother expressed concerns about the future: "I look at Ellen [older sister] now and I say, 'She's a normal kid except her ears don't work.' She's normal in every way . . . but with Brett it's a little harder, because I'm not sure that he will be normal. . . . I'm going to give myself time to see how it goes."

By age of recognition we mean the age of the child when the parents' concerns emerged and were mirrored or negotiated with professionals. In Jimmy's case, parents were aware right at birth that their child might have developmental problems of some kind. Such children typically require biomedical interventions very early. Annie's, Sharon's, and Brett's parents were unaware of any developmental problems until they became concerned later on or a teacher or doctor or relative noticed something and asked the parents about the child. The age of recognition ranged in these four families from birth, about 8 months, about 2 years, and age 3. Such a range is not uncommon in studies of the emergence of these kinds of developmental concerns.

Does earlier or later age of recognition make a difference in how families adapt to their child with delays or in children's developmental status? Recognition at earlier rather than later ages seems almost self-evidently desirable because earlier recognition fits with both professional models of intervention and folk cultural models of development. These models can be summarized as follows: The earlier the age of recognition the better because the early months and years of life are uniquely important stages for human development, and so the sooner we recognize delay, the better for interventions and parental adaptive responses, because parents and family members would respond even more urgently and deeply to their child's problems. However, another hypothesis, derived from ecocultural theory, is that a child growing up in the midst of a family practicing its implicit, normative cultural model of family life and development *is* protected. A young child's everyday participation in that family's daily routine is protective even when, later on, the child will be identified as delayed in some way. Excluding families with clear family pathology or abuse or those children with early biomedical concerns, and with certain other cautions, our prospective longitudinal study of families with children with delays tends to support the latter hypothesis.

This chapter first considers the professional and folk cultural model, that early recognition and response are better. Then we review ecocultural theory, which provides a rationale for why earlier is not always or necessarily better. We then describe our sample of 102 families with children with delays that were recognized at different ages and present evidence that the children's developmental status, and the family's adaptation to their child, is not uniquely influenced by the age of recognition (leaving aside that group of children with biomedical problems recognized at birth or soon thereafter). We conclude with implications for parents and for policy.

## Cultural Models and Early Recognition of Delays

D'Andrade (1987) defines a cultural model as "a cognitive schema that is intersubjectively shared by a social group" (p. 112) and which is hierarchically organized. Cultural models motivate actions because they include cultural and personal goals that organize action (D'Andrade, 1992, p.28). "Buying something," for example, is a cultural activity that is schematically organized, involves shared knowledge, and includes such concepts as money, seller, price, and so on, organized in a hierarchy of such schemata. Similarly, "early stimulation and attention to a child" is a cultural activity that includes (in Euro-American middle-class culture and also in other groups) verbal stimulation, mirroring, contingent responsiveness, treating the child as imagined coequal interlocutor, intentional changes by caretakers in the child's physical environment and visual field for the purpose of enrichment, and so forth. These activities are part of the cultural model of appropriate parenting, and the model includes the goal of enhancing social and intellectual competence later in life. "Stimulation" of infants and young children very *early* in life is an inherent part of this model because the early stages of life are thought to be uniquely important and the effects of inattention may be irreversible later on.

One reason cultural models (e.g., the notion that the very earliest periods of life are the most important) are so powerful is that they are implicit or procedural rather than explicit, formalized, and declarative (D'Andrade,1987). Implicit cultural models include deep cultural rules and beliefs underlying actions, which cannot necessarily be fully articulated even when researchers try to elicit them. They are "transparent" most of the time; they are taken to be reality (D'Andrade, 1992, p. 38). Implicit cultural models are in many ways even more forceful in directing behavior than models consciously held and explicitly analyzed and articulated. As D'Andrade (1992) states, "The very transparency of some schemas helps give them motivational force because, although the person sees the world a particular way, it is experienced as an undeniable reality" (p. 38).

Another reason for the power of cultural models is that they are tools for the mind—they assist in personal and familial adaptation to life. Cultural models matter for family adaptation. These models evolved in part in response to human problems, and they serve as tools to solve human problems. As tools for family adaptation, then, cultural models have a dual implication for families recognizing delays in their children at different ages. On the one hand, existing cultural models and family adaptations have a protective value for parents and children and might well have this same result for a child with delays. On the other hand, when concerns about possible developmental delay for the child appear, these implicit, understood cultural models, used as tools for assisting families in parenting, at the least will be questioned and probably will be changed in some ways by parents. Professionals and others may encourage changes in parents' beliefs and practices. New cultural models (of delay, handicap, special needs, etc.) will then emerge and interact with existing models. These new models do not replace more general ones but rather are applied specifically to the child with delays. Earlier recognition of delay may or may not be more adaptive for families and children generally, depending on whether the changes, absence of changes, or use of new, specific cultural models assists in family adaptation to the child with delays.

When parents recognize delays, implicit cultural models shift to explicit and are forced to change. Such shifts can be difficult and dangerous and produce suffering and dis-ease in their own right. But parents' cultural models change continually in any case. Establishing and sustaining any cultural model involves continual social construction. Harkness, Super, and Keefer (1992) studied U.S. parents with infants and toddlers, for instance, and note that "learning cultural knowledge is an active, constructive process that continues throughout the life-span . . . [and] the system from which cultural knowledge is drawn is itself dynamic and constantly changing" (p. 176). The emergence of enduring concerns about one's child's development (as painful as this is), and the resultant changing understandings based on that recognition, seem to be based on these more general processes of establishing and maintaining a cultural model of parenting and family life, rather than being dramatically different from them.

The cultural model of parenting and early child development emphasizing early stimulation and recognition of delays or developmental problems is associated with a number of ecological and sociohistorical circumstances. These include declining mortality threats and total fertility; changing work and work scheduling requirements for men, women, and children alike; increasing years and universality of schooling for children; and increasing biomedicalization and professionalization of birthing and child development practices, among other reasons (e.g., Ehrenreich & English, 1978; Mintz & Kellogg, 1988; Shorter, 1975). Of course, this contemporary model of infancy and childhood developmental periods and of the family have changed historically and vary dramatically cross-culturally (e.g. Scheper-Hughes, 1990). Although threats to infant mortality have dramatically declined for Euro-Americans, birth and infancy are still seen as potentially dangerous periods of life for mortality and health, as well as a time of unique and irreplaceable learning and stimulation opportunities for children.

The importance of early recognition and response, including the unique dangers and importance of very early periods in development, seems to be a widely shared cultural model in North America–important in scientific research and among professional clinicians, as well as among parents and laypersons. Professional or scientific models of early intervention influence folk models and vice versa; they share the same sociohistorical context and so have many concerns in common. But, of course, they differ in many other ways—evidentiary bases, methods, breadth of knowledge, and the way information is stored and presented, for example. We are not conflating professional/scientific with folk/cultural models by pointing to the similar emphasis on early recognition and responsiveness common to both but rather observing how these different but related bodies of knowledge have mutually influenced one another and share the same sociohistorical context.

Scientific and folk models share the implication, for instance, that earlier recognition of delays might be more conducive to family adaptation, cognitive precocity, a more secure sense of self, and physical health, compared to later ages of recognition. The folk/cultural model that earlier recognition is always better certainly fits with some research findings. The infant and toddler appear in contemporary research as precocious learners, actively exploring their environment (e.g., Kaye, 1982). Verbally responsive interactions and the developmentally sensitive mirroring of the child's explorations by caregivers are widely shared contemporary cultural models for optimal infant and young child care among professionals and parents alike (e.g. White, Kaban, & Attanucci, 1979). A virtually unchallenged scientific point of view in the field of developmental delay assumes that awareness and recognition at an earlier age leads to earlier action and intervention, which in turn leads to benefits (Cunningham, Morgan, & McGucken, 1984). For instance, Bristol and Schopler (1985) and Seligman and Darling (1989) suggest that the earlier parents become aware of a developmental problem, the better, since the process of redefining as disabled a child previously defined as normal is very difficult. This position assumes that awareness of delay is accompanied by a diagnosis, and that a convincing diagnosis, no matter how bleak, may reassure parents who have begun to question their competence as caregivers due to the developmental delays of their child (Featherstone, 1980). The earlier a family receives a diagnosis in this view, the earlier intervention can begin, and the less likely it is that the diagnosis will have a deleterious effect on parent–child interaction.

There is no question that a number of benefits of early intervention have been documented. For instance, children in early intervention spend fewer years in special education (Garland, Stone, Swanson, & Woodruff, 1981), and the special education services they require are less intense than those required by children who never get it. There are other associations between early intervention and somewhat better developmental and educational outlooks for children (Moxley-Haegert & Serbin, 1983; Shonkoff & Hauser-Cram, 1987; Shonkoff, Hauser-Cram, Krauss, & Upshur, 1988; Weiss, 1981). Thus, there are certainly reasons to encourage early recognition of delays, in cases in which such interventions would substantially increase the child's and family's ability to survive, function, and adapt.

Other studies in the early intervention and special education fields, however, suggest that for some children with developmental delays, earlier recognition does not lead to normal cognitive scores later on (Bernheimer & Keogh, 1988). The great majority of such children end up in special education in any event (88% in our sample, for instance)

(Bernheimer, Keogh, & Coots, 1993). Hence, although early recognition and intervention clearly have considerable value for many children and families, they are not likely to lead to a normal developmental status later on for most children. Further, for some kinds of delays, it may not matter whether the benefits of intervention begin at, say, age 3 months or 18 months for the same ultimate benefits to accrue later on for the child and family. These data are congruent with another view of development in infancy and early childhood: that normative cultural models and family adaptations that go with these models are themselves protective of children, even if it is later recognized that the child has a delay.

If our evolved normative cultural models can have this protective use for parents, then early recognition, particularly when associated with early labeling of the child as delayed, may lead to less than optimal actions and attitudes on the parents' part. Early recognition can alter what would have been parents' normal family routines of everyday life with their child and change their otherwise implicit cultural models, schemata, and scripts for parenting. Without early recognition, the child would be nested within the larger family system, and the family's resources and energy would be spread across all members and perhaps other kin as well, thereby benefiting the wider family system within which the young child is embedded. Parents' everyday routines, absent any recognition of delays, presumably would not involve more than the normal, expectable stress and struggle involved in establishing and sustaining the family routine of life. Nor would there be any of the possible stigma that might attach to the child or family. The costs of early interventions for families might be greater than the benefits *if* there is no evidence that interventions would substantively increase the child's and family's abilities to function and adapt in their communities, and if there is an absence of compelling medical/physical reasons to intervene early. Early recognition could in such situations produce more problems for families and children than solutions, as long as recognition eventually occurred at a later time appropriate for that child and family.

## Ecocultural Theory, Family Adaptation, and Age of Recognition

Our interest in the importance of cultural models, the ecocultural circumstances of families, and their effects on family adaptation to children with delays is based on more than 8 years of longitudinal studies of 102 Euro-American families and children in the Los Angeles, California area participating in Project Child (Weisner, 1984; Gallimore, Weisner, Kaufman, & Bernheimer, 1989; Gallimore, Weisner, Guthrie, Bernheimer, & Nihira, 1993; Nihira, Weisner, & Bernheimer, 1994). Project child focuses on families with a young child who exhibits developmental delays of unknown or uncertain cause (Bernheimer & Keogh, 1982, 1988). Delays can occur in speech, motor, cognitive, behavioral, or socioemotional behavioral domains. Studies of family adaptation processes in these families in fact have found that even after concerns appear and delays are recognized, families select and implement changes and new practices drawn from the same cultural repertoire of family practices that is found generally in Euro-American culture (Gallimore, Weisner, Kaufman, & Bernheimer, 1989). This repertoire seems to be similarly available to parents regardless of the age of recognition of the delay. Of course, substantial changes in family adaptation also occur due to having a child with delays, although these changes seldom involve an entirely new repertoire (Gallimore et al., 1989; Gallimore et al., 1993; Weisner, 1993). It seems that most families with children with delays alter neither their basic cultural model of parenting and development nor their repertoire of cultural practices. Rather, changes are usually specific to the situations of their child and family. The proactive change efforts families make to alter their everyday routines we call family accommodation.

This adaptive task of accommodation occurs in a local cultural ecology (Weisner, 1984, 1993; Gallimore et al., 1989; Keogh & Weisner, 1993). Ecocultural theory proposes that the adaptive problem faced by families with children with delays is the same as that faced by all families: *constructing and sustaining a daily routine of life that has meaning for culture members, and that fits with the competencies of available members of the family and community.* Cultural models provide families with powerful, socially and historically inherited tools to assist in this adaptive task in a local ecocultural niche. The construction and maintenance of a meaningful daily routine is an adaptive problem that challenges all families, whether or not they have a child with developmental delays. "Sustaining" a daily routine means adapting it to a local ecology and the family resource base. That is, it refers to survival, work, and wealth. To sustain a routine means dealing with the resources and constraints available and perceived in the world. It requires an assessment of class, gender, and power and the physical and geographic ecology surrounding the family and community. A "meaningful" routine is one that has moral and cultural significance and value for family members. It is also a routine of life that is interpretable within some shared cultural model in a community. The "competencies" of family members are defined by such maturational and cultural indicators as age, gender, temperament, kinship status, cultural beliefs about competencies and status, the developmental status of children, and many others. Competencies include those that emerge as a part of a child's culturally defined developmental career, as well as those individually inherited capacities afforded by genetic inheritance. Competencies within a developmental period such as infancy and early childhood can be defined either as a maturational, biological period in the life course or as a "stage" defined within a particular cultural tradition (Harkness et al., 1992, p. 177). In either case, however, these require responses by the family.

Ecocultural theory draws on anthropological and cross-cultural human development research (Whiting, 1976, 1980; Whiting & Edwards, 1988; Munroe, Munroe, & Whiting, 1981; LeVine, 1977; Nerlove & Snipper, 1981; Super & Harkness, 1980, 1986; Weisner & Gallimore, 1985; Weisner, Gallimore, & Jordan, 1988; Whiting & Whiting, 1975). The focus on cultural context, parental goals and family adaptation, the daily routine, and behavior settings—and their power to shape interaction and cognition—comes from this research tradition. The ecocultural model also draws on sociocultural and activity theory and research (e.g., Ochs, 1988; Vygotsky, 1978; Cole, 1985; Rogoff, 1982, 1990; Tharp & Gallimore, 1988; Wertsch, 1985). This work emphasizes the socially constructed nature of cognition and mind, as well as the role of activities and practices as the constitutive elements of the daily routine producing developmentally sensitive interactions.

Ecocultural theory treats families as proactive agents, not hapless victims of implacable social and economic forces. Families do not merely "have" an ecology and a daily routine around them; they also actively create their family ecology and routine (Weisner, 1986). The notion of "constructing" a routine reminds us that families shape, as well as are shaped by, the social world around them as they create their routines. It also emphasizes, of course, the power of cultural models, because these models are tools parents use to construct their routines. Ecocultural theory proposes that cultural models are powerful tools for adaptation, but only insofar as they can be found instantiated somewhere in the child's and family's everyday routine. From the perspective of ecocultural theory, a child's participation in his or her routine, everyday family activities is the preeminent experience shaping the child's development. The construction of the daily routine by families provides these activities for children.

The cultural place and daily routine are certainly not the only important influences on child development and family adaptation, however. Ecocultural theory requires a multidetermined approach to the course of developmental delay. Cultural models and the age of recognition have their effects within a multivariate set of causes. With regard to the *relative* importance of cultural models particularly, the following remark is *apropos*:

> As most anthropologists in moments of intellectual sobriety recognize, action, the self, emotion, etc., are influenced by many things besides culture—the way the human body is constructed, the way the brain works, social factors of many kinds, economic considerations, individual interests, etc. To trace out the process by which culture influences action requires a theoretical multi-causal vocabulary which can encompass variation and similarity. . . . (D'Andrade, 1992, p. 41)

## Parents' Cultural Models and Adaptive Responses to Children with Delays: A Prospective Naturalistic Longitudinal Study of the Effects of Differing Ages of Recognition

Our studies in Project Child show that parents' cultural models are absolutely critical to family adaptation. Parents do implement a common cultural repertoire of practices and beliefs in adapting to their child with delays. For instance, we studied the influence of religious commitment—belief, formal affiliation, prayer, attendance at a church or temple—on family accommodation to children with delays (Weisner, Beizer, & Stolze, 1991). The more religious parents had a clearer sense of the meaning of why they had a delayed child and reported a greater peace of mind about what they were trying to do with regard to accommodations, professional involvements, supports, and so forth. But these families did not in fact have more support as measured by independent questionnaire and interview data. Their children were not easier to handle according to other fieldwork data, nor did their children have higher developmental assessments according to a completely independent testing assessment. Nor did these families have more professional involvements or more income. It was their construction of the meaning of their child's condition that gave them a greater sense that they did have many of these things in their life.

We also examined the parents' beliefs regarding the roles of siblings (Weisner, 1993). Here again, parents' cultural models of sibling's roles clearly influenced their practices. When the child with delays was age 3, parents were concerned about "equal treatment" of siblings and giving "attention" to siblings; siblings were also used as a normative developmental reference standard. By age 6, parents were more concerned about providing meaningful activities for their family as a unit and handling behavior management problems. Family adaptation and goals relating to interdependence increased, whereas concerns over equal treatment and normative development declined.

Cultural models of "careerism" also influenced parents' adaptations. Mothers' goals of having a career, rather than "just having a job" or being a homemaker, led to extensive accommodation activities by families when children were age 3—an effect stronger than that of socioeconomic status itself (Gallimore et al., 1993).

Finally, we also have found that it is the parent's perceptions of the child's impact on the family daily routine—the child's "hassle" and social and physical disruptiveness—that matters most in terms of patterns of family adaptation. "Hassle" is a term we borrowed after hearing it used by a number of our parents. It describes the parents' and other family members' experience of managing the daily routine with a sometimes difficult and disruptive child. This is relevant to our more general argument regarding the importance of cultural models for family adaptation because parents' beliefs about hassle are more strongly associated with family adaptation than standardized developmental test scores for the children.

Because differences in parents' cultural models clearly do matter for family adaptation to delay, would the age at which parents recognized the possibility of delay influence family adaptation and cultural models as well? Would children with later-recognized delays have similar developmental outcomes, and would their patterns of family adaptation, ecocultural circumstances, beliefs about development, and patterns of interaction with their child be similar to those of children recognized earlier? To explore these questions, we required a prospective, naturalistic, longitudinal design such as Project Child's, in order to compare families in which parents' initial age of recognition differed.

An ideal design, however, would randomly assign children with similar delays recognized at different ages to different families, perhaps first controlling for gender, socioeconomic status, or other features. Such a design, of course, is ethically and practically impossible. Hence, of necessity, the kind of delay the child has is confounded with the age of recognition and the family's response. For instance, children born prematurely, with medical problems at birth or in the early months, immediately were of concern to parents and physicians and others, and so had ages of recognition beginning at birth or very soon thereafter. Children not born prematurely, or with more subtle cognitive, speech or motoric delays, had later ages of recognition. These children varied in age of recognition across a three-year age range. This group of children not recognized right around birth provides a rough (albeit not the ideal) kind of natural experiment. These children grew up for varying lengths of time in families in which their parents had a normative cultural model of parenting and development for their child. Given this variation in age of recognition, did subsequent patterns of family adaptation, or child status, differ due to the age at which parents developed their recognition of delay?

## Sample[1]

Each family in Project Child has a child with delay. "Developmental delay" is a term of relatively recent vintage and lacks definitional specificity (Bernheimer & Keogh, 1986). The term is essentially a nonspecific "clinical" one with less ominous overtones for the future than "retarded." There is much less information about the developmental course of these children as compared to children with other developmental disabilities (e.g., Down Syndrome and cerebral palsy). Children with developmental delays of uncertain etiology comprise the majority of school-age children with "mental retardation." The longitudinal data from Project Child indicate that whereas some children with early delays "catch up," the majority continue to lag behind age norms on standardized tests of development and cognition, and the majority are placed in special education classes once they enter school (Bernheimer, Keogh, & Coots, 1993).

Each family in our cohort has a child who had been judged to be "developmentally delayed" by a professional or an agency by the age of 3 or earlier. Children were excluded from the sample if they were known to have chromosomal abnormalities and/or genetic conditions associated with mental retardation, or if the delay was associated with known prenatal drug or alcohol usage or postnatal neglect or abuse. Hence, this group of children does not necessarily have a single clear "diagnosis" and known etiology; their delays can be quite ambiguous and uncertain. Unlike parents of children with Down syndrome, cerebral palsy, or autism, parents of children with developmental delay have no books or parent groups to turn to for specific information and support. Thus there is no preexisting specific set of beliefs and practices already set down, socially modeled, and available to these parents from which to directly model their own changing beliefs and practices. Given our interest in understanding a wide range of family adaptations, this seemed an appropriate population from which to draw a sample.

One hundred and three children in 102 families were recruited into our cohort. Seventy-three different agencies in the greater Los Angeles metropolitan area assisted in the assembly of the cohort. Public schools and private intervention programs constituted two-thirds of the cooperating agencies. Only 5% of an original pool of 313 children was not included due to self-selection (the parents declined to participate, or the agency "decided" the parents would not be interested). All the remaining cases initially mentioned or referred that did not eventually participate in the study did not participate because they did not meet our screening criteria. This suggests that selection bias is present in the final cohort, but at an acceptable level of 5%.

At entry, the mean child chronological age was 41.8 months ($SD$ = 6.2; range = 32 to 55). The mean Gesell developmental quotient (DQ) was 72.32 ($SD$ = 15.97; range = 38 to 117). All but 18 of the children had DQs below 90, and all 103 had significant delays in one or more areas (motor, speech, behavior, or cognition) in spite of some relatively high DQs; 58.3% of the children were boys. At age 6–7, the mean Stanford–Binet IQ was 71.40 ($SD$=18.26; range = 24 to 114). The cognitive–developmental scores were remarkably stable (Bernheimer et al., 1993) with a correlation from entry to the second data collection period 3 years later of .69, although, of course, individual children had moved up or down.

The 102 families in our study cohort consisted predominantly of married couples in their thirties in middle-class circumstances; however, there is a wide range of variation and heterogeneity surrounding this central tendency. For example, 12% were mothers living independently (due to divorce, separation, widowhood, or never having married) or in a variety of other residential and marital circumstances (e.g., living with parents). Altogether, 19.4% of the children were in a single-parent household (mother, father, grandmother, or other relative). About 25% of the mothers were employed full-time when the children were age 3–4. The mean family socioeconomic level, assessed with the Hollingshead, was 44.7 ("middle-middle-class"), with a range from below poverty level in a number of families to a family with income over $150,000 a year. About 25% described practices and beliefs that indicated strong religious commitment to Protestant, Catholic, and Jewish traditions, and about 25% indicated little or no such commitment, with those families in between reporting moderate levels of religious beliefs and practice.

# Methods

## Interviews

All families were visited by a trained interviewer when the developmentally delayed child was ages 3–4 and 6–7. The interviewer conducted semistructured interviews with the parents; each interview was tape recorded and lasted 2 to 3 hours. Interviewers were provided both open-ended and specific questions and topics to be covered regarding ecocultural constraints and opportunities, accommodation to the delayed child, child behavioral problems and hassles encountered in raising the child, and family functioning and adaptation. Interviewers were trained to use systematic probes to ensure clarity and comparability of data obtained from all families and to ensure that there would not be missing information on any specific topic at the conclusion of the interview and family visit. The interview materials were then scored for content, including parents' reports regarding their developmental beliefs and the extent of their active efforts to change their family practices and daily routine due to the delayed child. Most parents spontaneously brought up the process by which they became concerned about their child's development. We also probed systematically for diagnoses, length of time the process took, and professional contacts.

## Reliability of Interview Scoring

Coders reviewed all the tape-recorded interview and written field note materials, and scored each family using a coding manual. Reliability was established by independent, "blind" rating of 12.5% of the cases ($N = 13$). Each case was coded by at least two blind raters, trained by one of the authors (T.S.W.). The raters were blind to the research questions and had no knowledge of the specific purposes of their task. No items used in research studies had reliability under 70% agreement; overall reliability averaged 82%.

## *Family and Child Assessment Data*

Information obtained from formal measures, standardized scales, and independently rated tasks was used in statistical analyses of the influence of the age of recognition. This information included several measures.

## Interactional Measures

We used measures developed by Levine, Schneider, Haney, and Hall (1987), who examined mother–child interaction by coding behaviors during a book-sharing task when the child was between 3 and 4 years of age (Hecht, Levine, & Mastergeorge, 1993). Variables included number of mothers' directives, number of mothers' requests for responses from the child, number of child responses, and total numbers of mother and child utterances. These measures were used in order to investigate potential differences in mother–child interaction style relating to age of first concern. The interactional measures were done by independent raters using videotape analyses. These researchers were entirely unaware of the other measures being used to explore the effects of age of recognition.

### Children's Assessments

To obtain a standardized measure of child status, each child was tested by a trained psychologist using the Gesell (age 3–4) or Stanford–Binet (age 6–7) and Vineland. These developmental assessments were obtained by independent testers. These testers were entirely unaware of the other measures being used in the study and did not know the parents' age of recognition.

### Family Assessments

Three formal measures of family and child functioning were used. These measures included the Family Environment Scale (FES; Moos, Insel, & Humphrey, 1974), the Family Adaptability and Cohesion Evaluation Scale (FACES; Olson, Parnter, & Lavee, 1985), and the Home Observation for Measurement of the Environment (HOME; Caldwell & Bradley, 1983). The FES and FACES were administered to parents in a mailout questionnaire when children were age 3–4 and again at age 6–7.[2] The HOME was completed by fieldworkers at both age points.

## Dimensions of Family Adaptation and Parental Beliefs

Dimensions used in our analyses cover a wide range of information regarding families' circumstances, beliefs, and actions which may be influenced by age of recognition. The dimensions included the following measures.

### Family Accommodation

Our measures of family accommodation to the child with delays have been presented in Gallimore et al. (1993). We used a set of 12 domains likely to be important in family accommodation (described in Gallimore et al., 1989) and scored each family for the amount of accommodation activity in that domain on a 9-point scale. Two domains were ultimately dropped, one due to low variance and one due to low item reliability.

A higher accommodation score in a given domain indicates a greater amount of activity in that domain related to the delayed child.[3]

## Ecocultural Factors

Details of the construction of the 12 ecocultural factors have been reported in Nihira et al. (1994). Briefly, 127 items from our interview and questionnaires were subjected to factor analyses using the theoretical model derived from ecocultural theory. The maximum likelihood factor extraction and varimax rotation yielded a total of 12 statistically significant and interpretable factors, which we used in our analysis of the effects of age of recognition regarding delay on family adaptation.[4]

## Parents' Developmental Beliefs

We discussed seven beliefs about general child development with parents. The beliefs we asked parents to discuss included the importance of early experiences, the salience of parental versus societal responsibility for the child's development, whether or not the family should adjust to the child's needs, the significance of environmental versus genetic influences; the importance of integration into the non-handicapped world, whether the child should or should not be independent as an adult, feelings about the opportunity versus burden of childrearing, and whether or not religion is a positive force in coping with a handicapped child. We also asked about what parents thought their child's future developmental course would be and whether the child would be in regular educational classes or whether the child would be in some kind of special educational program. General ratings of parents' expectations of their child's educational future were collapsed into three categories at age 3 (Parents are uncertain, Child will be mainstreamed/integrated but may still have some problems, and Child will outgrow problems) and four categories at age 6 (Parents are uncertain, Child will be mainstreamed/integrated but may still have some problems, Child will outgrow problems, and Parents consider that their child is developing normally).

## Child Status Groups

The children were grouped into one of four categories, depending on the type of problems and the degree of impact on the family's daily routine: high medical problems/high impact on the daily routine; high behavioral problems/high impact; low(mild) developmental delay/low impact; and high (significant) developmental delay/low impact (Bernheimer, Gallimore, & Kaufman, 1993). These groups were unrelated to both children's test scores and to family socioeconomic status.

## How Does Recognition of Delay Develop in Parents' Experience?: Five Age Periods of Recognition

We defined an *initial* concern as that point at which the concerns appeared to parents as persistent rather than transient and they were unable to quickly dismiss their initial worries. Concern may have been expressed first by parents or professionals. However, if professionals expressed concerns first, parents had to express agreement with concerns (either explicitly or indirectly by following professional recommendations). For example, after a pediatrician tells a parent that the child is developmentally delayed, parents indicate that "that's when we recognized that she was behind in certain areas."

If first concerns were biomedical, the problems appeared to parents as life-threatening or serious and ongoing in nature and involving major surgery, extended hospital stays, long-term medication, and/or home treatment (e.g., apnea monitors, oxygen, shunt implantation, heart or kidney surgery, and seizure activity). Medical problems that resolved or were seen as transient or normal (e.g., a "cold") were not included. Biomedical problems trigger recognition of a delay right at birth or before (although later speech or behavioral concerns may not develop), motor problems during the first year and communication and behavioral concerns in the second and third years. However, many children show several kinds of delays, and parents' adaptations, in most cases, are subsequently based on multiple problems.

If first concerns were nonbiomedical, parents said that their child did not appear to be developing as expected in some or all areas (motor skills, language skills, social skills). Less specific comments by parents, for instance, "we knew something was wrong," also seemed to be evidence of initial concern at that age.

Recognition and subsequent labels, diagnosis, and validation by others occurred slowly, in stages, and through negotiation by all parties. Being social constructions, concern, recognition, diagnosis, and validation shift and change in the minds of parents. Hence, only a few families identified a single point at which the parents came to recognize that their child was delayed. Further, parents' recognition of delays involved their prior cultural model regarding normative development, as well as their own expectations regarding goals for their child. Recognition as a process often involved matching this prior cultural model and particular developmental beliefs to their child's development, as some of our quotes from parents illustrate. Consequently, we did not usually find a single, exact age of recognition measured in months or days.

Instead, families were grouped into five age ranges as follows: Recognition at birth; Recognition at or by year 1; Recognition at or by year 2; Recognition at or by year 3; and finally a group with No parental recognition, even though there were professional concerns and diagnoses.

In the Recognition at birth group ($N = 29$), many of the children were born prematurely or were born with medical complications. Although most families became concerned because of something they were told by professionals (usually physicians), some families suspected on their own that "something was wrong." The group included children who were given a poor prognosis for survival ("the doctors told us he might not make it"), children with extremely negative developmental prognoses (a doctor saying "the child will be a vegetable"), and children born with hydrocephaly or heart problems requiring surgery. Other children in this group included those whose parents had general concerns about their prematurity and those whose parents had an immediate feeling that "something is wrong" ("she seemed funny looking").

In the group with Recognition at or by year 1 ($N = 40$) most infants had delayed or atypical motor development ("he did funny creeping"). Several of these parents reported comparing their child's development unfavorably with that of an older child, usually a sibling or a relative or friend's child ("the other baby was active, kicking the arms, moving the head, and facial movements and stuff and Mark just lay there, not trying to pull his arms up, but just lay there"). In other cases, concerns were recognized after a discrete event (e.g., the child was given a routine DPT shot, followed by seizures). There were also general developmental concerns represented in this group ("the tracking [visual] thing was one of the things we noticed she wasn't doing"). Although some of these parents became concerned within a couple of months of birth (and so were quite similar to the Recognition at birth group), others raised their child as a normal infant right up to the end of the first year.

In the group with Recognition at or by year 2 ($N = 20$) concerns were focused primarily on atypical or delayed communication, with a smaller subset concerned about behavioral characteristics ("we thought he was deaf because he didn't acknowledge anything . . . he was just like in his own little world"). Again, many parents began to recognize delays because of comparisons with other children ("I knew I had several friends who had children within a month of Danny and they were just going in leaps and bounds in language and . . . he wasn't"). All the parents in this group raised their infants without any recognition regarding delays well into the second year of life, and many only developed recognition of delays later in the toddler stage.

Whereas the majority of parents recognized concerns by 24 months, there were two remaining groups. The Recognition at or by year 3 (N = 4) group included families who were not concerned until a professional suggested there might be a problem. As with the year 2 group, concerns tended to be communicative or behavioral ("[the doctor] . . . was starting to compare my son with other average kids . . . he said he [should] be able to phrase stuff"). The final group, No recognition of delay (N = 5) includes a group of our parents who expressed no developmental concerns regarding their children, although in all these cases, the possibility of developmental problems had been raised by others. In some cases these professional concerns resulted from a premature birth; in other cases professionals noticed and commented on developmental delays or differences. The parents, however, were confident that their child would catch up, or they did not agree with the professional assessments.

## Does Age of First Recognition Influence Subsequent Child Developmental Status and Family Adaptation?

Using these five age-of-recognition groups we looked for possible variance due to the different ages of recognition, in mother–child interactions, family home environment, family accommodations and ecocultural resources and constraints, parental beliefs about development, and the child's developmental status.

### Mother–Child Interactions

Analysis of variance revealed no significant differences among the five recognition groups on the ways mothers interacted with their children on the reading task for any of the five interactional measures scored from the videotapes.[5] These results are particularly important, because they represent completely independent data on the children and families. The raters of videotapes were unaware of the age of recognition categories we subsequently developed and were not involved in the interviews with families.

However, there were significant associations between age of recognition and developmental test scores at child age 3–4 and 6–7 years (Table 21.1). Children with concerns at birth or within the first year had lower Gesell or Stanford–Binet scores, with the order of magnitude of the difference being from a half to a full standard deviation, due

**Table 21.1.** Developmental Test Scores at Ages 3–4 and 6–7 by Age of First Concern

|  | Concern at birth | Concern 1–12 mos. | Concern 13–24 mos. | Concern 24 mos./none | F |
|---|---|---|---|---|---|
| Gessell DQ Age 3–4 | 68.26a (14.5) | 69.37a (16.2) | 82.58b (15.0) | 76.78 (16.2) | 4.12[*] |
| Stanford–Binet IQ Age 6–7 | 68.51 (14.3) | 68.09 (17.5) | 81.29 (17.6) | 86.83 (23.1) | 4.09[*] |

*Note.* Means with different subscripts are significantly different.
[*]$p < .01$.

primarily to their biomedical problems and prematurity complications. However, most pair-wise comparisons between means within each child age were not statistically significant. Furthermore, DQ scores were not related to other measures of child functioning: the DQ scores at age 3–4 were unrelated to the child's "hassle" level ($r = -.05$), for example. By age 6–7, hassle was statistically associated with IQ ($r = -.33$), however, because school entry decisions evidently made such scores more salient for parents.

## Home Environment

We compared the recognition groups by scores on several of our standard measures of the quality of the family home environment. We also looked at our own judgments of the families' adaptation over time, which were constructed by fieldworkers from qualitative information regarding family strengths and vulnerabilities. Analyses of variance again indicated that none of these measures were directly related to age of first recognition of delays. No particular group of families showed significant differences in the ways they arranged their home environments or in the specific adaptive strengths they possessed as families, due to the age of recognition.

## Family Accommodation and Ecocultural Resources and Constraints

Next, we looked for associations between age of recognition and family resources/constraints and their use and the activities families instituted in their daily routines to accommodate to the delayed child. Specifically, we wanted to know whether parents who were concerned at earlier ages made more, fewer, or different changes in their daily routines (our

Accommodation Scales) or made differential use of resources (our Ecocultural Scale dimensions) compared to parents whose concerns originated later in their children's lives.

Results of analyses of variance indicated no statistically significant differences among the five recognition groups on any accommodation domains when children were ages 6–7 or 3–4 (Figure 21.1 illustrates the age 6–7 data). Parents whose recognition that they had a delayed child began very early in the child's life did *not* adjust the daily routines of their families significantly more or less, or in a different pattern, than parents whose recognition did not arise until the child's second or third year. However, Figure 21.1 shows clearly that there is a trend for accommodation activities by parents (i.e., adaptive efforts made due to their child with delays) to become proportionally less the later the age of recognition. Moderate accommodation activity by parents steadily declines as age of recognition increases. High activity, however, declines less consistently.

Two significant effects were noted for our ecocultural measures of resources and constraints, however. For Socioeconomic Status and Use and Availability of Services families who expressed concern by the age of 12 months (i.e., earlier in the child's life) received higher scores than did families who did not express concern ($F[4,86] = 2.5$, $p < .05$; $F[4,95] = 4.43$, $p < .01$, respectively) until later. Families who showed concern at earlier ages tended to be from higher socioeconomic levels, and made greater use of services for their delayed children than did families who did not express concern about their delayed children as early. It is of interest to note that the 10 other domains of ecocultural resources and constraints were *not* associated with age of recognition.

## Parental Beliefs about Development

Next we looked for possible associations between parents' beliefs, attitudes, and expectations about their delayed children on one hand and the age of first recognition on the other. We assessed (1) cultural models reflected in parent's general beliefs about child development (the seven beliefs described in the methods section) and (2) specific parental beliefs and attitudes regarding their own child's delayed status, as well as a general rating of how optimistic parents were about their child's future at child ages 3–4 and 6–7 years, specific beliefs about whether children would "outgrow" their handicaps, and whether their child would remain in special education throughout their school careers (rated at child age 6–7 years only).

Analyses of variance indicated no significant relations between beliefs about child development in general, and age of recognition. We

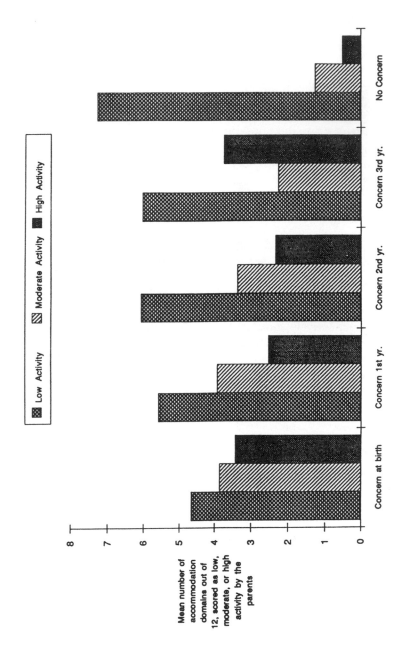

**FIGURE 21.1.** Amount of accomodation activity at child age 6–7 by age of first concern.

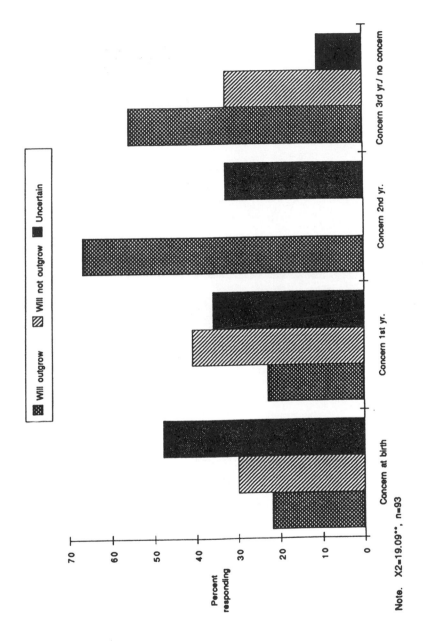

Note.   X2=19.09**, n=93

FIGURE 21.2.   Parents' beliefs about child's future development by age of first concern about the child.

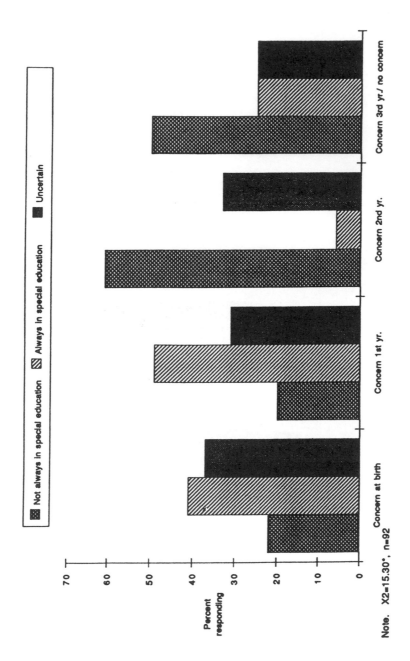

FIGURE 21.3. Parents' beliefs about use of special education by age of first concern about the child.

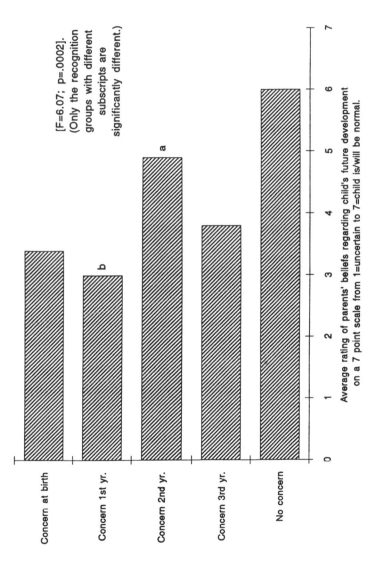

[F=6.07; p=.0002].
(Only the recognition groups with different subscripts are significantly different.)

Average rating of parents' beliefs regarding child's future development on a 7 point scale from 1=uncertain to 7=child is/will be normal.

521

**FIGURE 21.4.** Average parent rating of child's future development at child age 6–7 by age of first concern.

believe this to be an important result: It suggests that these parents' cultural models regarding normal development have not significantly shifted due to having a child with delays, regardless of the age of recognition for that child and regardless of the nature and severity of the delay.

However, a number of significant results were noted for beliefs *related specifically to their child with delays.* Chi-square analyses indicated significant differences in parent beliefs about outgrowing handicaps and staying in special education which were related to the age of recognition. Parents whose concerns did not originate until the child's second year of life or later were significantly more likely to believe that their child *would* outgrow his or her problem or handicap ($\chi^2 = 19.1$, $p < .01$) and be placed in regular education ($\chi^2 = 15.3$, $p < .05$) than were parents whose recognition of the child's delays originated at birth or in the first year of life (Figures 21.2 and 21.3).

Analyses of variance also showed significant differences between the recognition groups for parents' ratings of their child's future development, both at child age 3–4 years and at 6–7 years (Figure 21.4). Parents who did not become concerned until their child's second year gave more positive, optimistic ratings regarding their child's future at later child ages than did parents who became concerned during their child's first year (at child age 3: $F = 4.43$, $p < .01$; at child age 6: $F = 6.07$, $p < .001$).

## Developmental Status

Parental beliefs and age of recognition are of course also influenced by the nature of the child's delay: The child's medical status, after all, is confounded with age of recognition, particularly for any child with birth complications or more severe and visible delays. To compare children's developmental status and parents' beliefs, we grouped families according to the severity of the child's developmental and/or medical disabilities. There was indeed a pattern of associations between the impact of the child's problem and the parent's rating of the child's future. Parents with a child whose delays were biomedically based and had a high impact on the family tended to rate their children *less* optimistically. However, close to half (46%) of even these highly impacted parents felt at child age 3 that their children *would* be mainstreamed, integrated in school, or outgrow their problems. This number decreased at child age 6, to 33%, probably reflecting some degree of reaction to experience with professionals and schools. Similarly for the *low*-impact groups, one-quarter of the parents still felt *uncertain* about their child's future development, both at age 3 and at age 6.

Furthermore, parents' developmental expectations clearly seemed influenced by much more than DQ or IQ alone. Recall from Table 21.1 that there were only scattered associations between DQ or IQ scores and the age of recognition. Although the *F*'s are significant at both ages, small differences in these test scores were unlikely to be noticeable in everyday interactions. Furthermore, some parents were not even aware of these scores, and there were children with test scores even a half standard deviation below or above what would be expected who none-theless felt their children would or would not outgrow problems. For instance, there were some parents with children with DQ or IQ scores substantially lower (or higher) than would be expected based on the mean scores for their age of recognition group who nonetheless felt their children would outgrow their delays (or, conversely, thought their child would always be in special education) even though their child's test score was lower (or higher) than expected.

Finally, a recent study conducted by Keogh and Bernheimer (1994) supports the relatively weak associations between age of recognition, family adaptations, and standardized DQ or IQ tests (except for those children recognized at birth). They compared cognitive and behavioral characteristics of two etiology groups in the Project Child sample at ages 3–4 and 6–7. The first group consisted of 28 children with clear evidence of perinatal or neonatal stress. The second sample was composed of 41 children with no histories of early biological stress—the children in our study with truly "unknown" etiology. *There were no significant differences between the two etiology groups on DQ or IQ measures of cognitive development.* Of course, by definition there was substantial overlap between the 28 children in the perinatal or neonatal etiology group and our Recognition at birth group. However, the 41 children with no etiological histories of early biological stress were spread across all four of our later recognition groups (i.e., all the groups other than our Recognition at birth group). These findings suggest that DQ or IQ measures, although certainly not entirely irrelevant to age of recogni-tion, are unlikely to represent a major confounding influence on our findings regarding relationships between age of recognition, parental beliefs, and family adaptation.

Although the nature of the child's medical conditions influenced both the age of recognition and parents' beliefs about their child's developmental future, much more was involved. Parents varied widely in their developmental beliefs within each age-of-recognition category, for instance. Age of recognition influenced beliefs net of biomedical severity, as confirmed by our qualitative data and case materials. Parents' age of recognition, family resources and constraints, and cultural models of development and parenting appear to play complementary roles and interact in shaping parents beliefs and new cultural models of development of their child with delays.

## Conclusion: Family Adaptation, Cultural Models, and Age of Recognition of Delays

This pattern of findings supports the view that a young child's everyday participation in his or her family's daily routine can be protective even when, later on, the child will be identified as delayed in some way. Our study found, for instance, that ecocultural circumstances, parents' beliefs about their child's delay, and the nature of the child's delay were stronger influences on family adaptation than was age of recognition. A recognition, or "labeled" identification, of a child as potentially or actually delayed is a deeply powerful message for parents. But the age at which this occurs during the first 3 years of life, excluding biomedical concerns and conditions of family pathology or abuse, does not seem to matter as much as the family's overall adaptation in their daily routines. The lack of association between age of recognition on the one hand and a variety of other measures of children's development and families' adaptations is a very consistent finding. For example, a summary list of our findings on which measures of children and families were *not* associated with the five age-of-recognition groups includes: mother–child interaction in a structured book-reading situation, the family and home environment assessed using standard scales, family use of supports, resources and constraints, family accommodations in response to their child's delay, and parents' *general* beliefs about child development.

Nor had the parents in our study *replaced* a prior, standard cultural model of development with a different model once they recognized they had a child with delays. This standard model presumably operated before the parents developed a concern about their child and still is present after the recognition of delays, regardless of the age when concerns emerged. Families also used culturally available adaptive strategies, rather than culturally unusual ones. This suggests that the changes in parents' more specific developmental beliefs regarding their delayed child that did occur were focused primarily on their delayed child's particular developmental course, not on beliefs about development generally.

There were some relationships between age of recognition and certain parental beliefs or concerns, however. Particularly for those parents with recognition at birth or soon thereafter, age of recognition and the nature of the delay are confounded (these children have more immediate and severe biomedical and related developmental problems, for instance), and such circumstances did influence subsequent beliefs and adaptations although they were certainly not determinative. Our findings also suggest that parents with later ages of recognition were more likely to believe that their child will outgrow some problems and be in regular classes. In general, however, these associations between specific developmental beliefs about one's child on the one hand and age of recognition on the other were the exceptions.

All the children in our study *had* been recognized as delayed or possibly delayed by ages 3 to 4, and most were receiving some sort of professional assistance. Hence, when we talk about correlates of earlier or later age of recognition, this should be understood within the context of our sample—a group of children who all had eventually been identified by age 3 to 4. We are not suggesting, obviously, that if these children had never been recognized, this nonrecognition would have made no difference to the child's development and to the family's cultural beliefs and adaptive responses. To the contrary, we feel certain that for the great majority of these children and families, recognition of delays was important for parents and children alike.

Whenever the age of recognition, recognition always led parents to seek some sorts of assistance, unless of course, as sometimes occurred, professionals had already initiated the first concerns. The impact of that assistance depends on its quality and availability. Our study is in the context of the *existing* levels of social investment in families and children in Los Angeles County. One might imagine a far deeper, better-funded network of comprehensive and continuous interventions, services, schools, and parental supports. If such a network existed, it might make earlier interventions more effective and, hence, earlier ages of recognition more relevant for some children. In such a situation, an earlier age of recognition might have made a difference for the children or families, but we have no way of knowing this.

More funds and personnel do not necessarily lead directly to better family adaptations and child status, however. Even if more money and people were to be available, the question would remain: What kinds of interventions would work best for these children and families? For this question as well, we believe that cultural models and ecocultural theory have much to offer. Any intervention has to diffuse into the existing everyday routines and parental cultural models present in a community. No matter how desirable interventions might be, they will not assist in family adaptation if they do not diffuse in families and communities and motivate parental action. Interventions and services have to fit into the slots in families' daily routines and fit into the goals and schemata and cultural models that motivate parents (Gallimore, Goldenberg, & Weisner, 1993).

In this respect, as in others, ecocultural research with families with children with delays has implications similar to those for all families. Cultural models assist in a challenge facing all families, whether or not they have children with delays: the families' adaptive task of organizing their everyday routine, gaining new information, and reallocating their ecocultural resources and constraints. It is this human adaptive task that cultural models assist in achieving. The role of general cultural models as well as more specific parental beliefs in this adaptive process would be a fruitful topic for new research to assist in improving the quality of life of *all* families and children.

Parents of children with delays sometimes worry that they should have recognized the possible delays in their child earlier than they in fact did. These concerns originate from the very cultural model among so many parents (and scientific model among researchers and professionals)—"the earlier and more the stimulation, the better." Our data suggest that parents and professionals did remain appropriately vigilant regarding these children's development—after all, the children in our study *were* identified by age 3. For the later-age-of-recognition groups, our data suggest that parents who developed concerns somewhat later should not worry that they became concerned "too late." For that particular subgroup of children (those without biomedical or other conditions requiring very early intervention), the age of recognition does not appear related directly to subsequent child developmental status or family adaptation. Parents of children with delays certainly have many very real concerns and difficult adaptations to make, but it appears from our prospective longitudinal data that differences in age of initial recognition for children without biomedical or related conditions necessitating specific interventions need not be one of those worries. To a measurable degree, these parents already offer protection to their children by undertaking their common cultural project of shaping a sustainable, meaningful daily routine for their families.

# Acknowledgments

The authors appreciate the many contributions of the participating families. This research was supported by Grant Nos. HD19124 and HD11944 from the National Institute of Child Health and Human Development. The Sociobehavioral Research Group of UCLA's Mental Retardation Research Center (MRRC) and the Division of Social Psychiatry, Department of Psychiatry and Biobehavioral Sciences also provided support. The assistance of the Statistical Resources

Group (D. Guthrie, Coordinator & G. Gordon, Senior Statistician) was provided with the support of a Mental Retardation Center Grant (No. HD04612) to the MRRC at UCLA. Fieldworkers included Bernheimer, Monique DeCicco, Sandra Z. Kaufman, Laura Beizer Seidner, Lori Stolze, and Matheson. Dr. Jennifer Coots provided important statistical assistance. Barbara Keogh and Ron Gallimore gave valuable comments on earlier drafts.

# Notes

1. Sample description adapted from Weisner, (1993).

2. Scores were obtained for all 18 subscales. The HOME consists of eight subscales which we used in our analyses: Learning Stimulation, Language Stimulation, Physical Environment, Warmth and Affection, Academic Stimulation, Modeling and Encouraging of Social Maturity, Variety in Experience, and Acceptance.

The FES consists of 10 dimensions of "social climate in the home":

Cohesion, Expressiveness, Conflict, Independence, Achievement Orientation, Intellectual–Cultural Orientation, Active–Recreational Orientation, Moral–Religious Emphasis, Organization, and Control

3. The 10 accommodation domains scores used in our analyses were: Family subsistence base, Services, Home/neighborhood, Domestic workload, Child-care tasks, Child peer groups, Marital roles, Instrumental/emotional support, Father/spouse role, Parent information.

4. The 12 ecocultural factors were: Socioeconomic Status, Career Orientation of Couple, Use/Availability of Services, Attempts to Structure Home Environment for Delayed Child, Family Workload Related to Delayed Child, Use and Availability of Help for Family, Use and Availability of Help within Family, Connectedness of Family, Amount and Variety of Formal/Instrumental Support for Family, Involvement of Child into Non-Handicapped Networks, Involvement of Child into Handicapped Networks, Information-Seeking from Professionals Regarding Delayed Child.

5. $F$-tests ranged from 0.41 for children's responsiveness, to 2.60 for mother's requests for verbal responses from the child; all $p$ levels were greater than .05.

# References

Bernheimer, L. P., Gallimore, R. G., & Kaufman, S. Z. (1993). Clinical child assessment in a family context: A four group typology of family experiences with young children with developmental delays. *Journal of Early Intervention, 17*(3), 253–269.

Bernheimer, L. P., & Keogh, B. K. (1982). *Research on early abilities of children with handicaps* (Final report, longitudinal sample). Los Angeles: University of California Press.

Bernheimer, L. P., & Keogh, B. K. (1986). Developmental disabilities in preschool children. In B. K. Keogh (Ed.), *Advances in special education* (Vol. 5) (pp. 61–93). Greenwich, CT: JAI Press.

Bernheimer, L. P., & Keogh, B. K. (1988). The stability of cognitive performance of developmentally delayed children. *American Journal of Mental Retardation, 92,* 539–542.

Bernheimer, L. P., Keogh, B. K, & Coots, J. J. (1993). From research to practice: Support for developmental delay as a preschool category of exceptionality. *Journal of Early Intervention, 17*(2), 97–106.

Bristol, M. M., & Schopler, E. (1985). Developmental perspective on stress and coping. In J. Blacher (Ed.), *Severely handicapped young children and their families* (pp. 91–142). New York: Academic Press.

Caldwell, B. M., & Bradley, R. H. (1983). *Home Observation for Measurement of the Environment* (rev. ed.). Little Rock: University of Arkansas Press.

Cole, M. (1985). The zone of proximal development: where culture and cognition create each other. In J. Wertsch (Ed.), *Culture, communication, and cognition* (pp. 146–161). New York: Cambridge University Press.

Cunningham, C. C., Morgan, P. A., & McGucken, R. B. (1984). Down's syndrome: Is dissatisfaction with disclosure of diagnosis inevitable. *Developmental Medicine and Child Neurology, 26,* 33–39.

D'Andrade, R. (1987). A folk model of the mind. In D. Holland & N. Quinn, (Eds.), *Cultural models in language and thought* (pp. 112–148). New York: Cambridge University Press.

D'Andrade, R. (1992). Schemas and motivation. In R. D'Andrade & C. Strauss (Eds.), *Human motives and cultural models* (pp. 23–44). New York: Cambridge University Press.

Ehrenreich, B., & English, D. (1978). *For her own good. 150 years of the expert's advice to women.* Garden City, NY: Anchor Press/Doubleday.

Featherstone, H. (1980). *A difference in the family.* New York: Basic Books.

Gallimore, R., Goldenberg, C., & Weisner, T. (1993). The social construction and subjective reality of activity settings: Implications for community psychology. *American Journal of Community Psychology, 21*(4), 537–559.

Gallimore, R., Weisner, T. S., Kaufman, S. Z., & Bernheimer, L. P. (1989). The social construction of ecocultural niches: Family accommodation of developmentally delayed children. *American Journal of Mental Retardation, 94*(3), 216–230.

Gallimore, R., Weisner, T. S., Guthrie, G., Bernheimer, L., & Nihira, K. (1993). Family response to young children with developmental delays: accommodation activity in ecological and cultural context. *American Journal of Mental Retardation, 98*(2), 185–206.

Garland, C., Stone, N. W., Swanson, J., & Woodruff, G. (Eds.). (1981). *Early intervention for children with special needs and their families: Findings and recommendations* (WESTAR Series No. 11). Seattle: University of Washington Press.

Harkness, S., Super, C. M., & Keefer, C. H. (1992). Learning to be an American parent. In R.G. D'Andrade & C. Srauss, (Eds.), *Human motives and cultural models* (pp. 163–178). New York: Cambridge University Press.

Hecht, B. F., Levine, H. G., & Mastergeorge, A. B. (1993). Conversational roles of children with developmental delays and their mothers in natural and semi-structured situations. *American Journal of Mental Retardation, 97*(4), 419–430.

Kaye, K. (1982). *The mental and social life of babies. How parents create persons.* Chicago: University of Chicago Press.

Keogh, B. K., & Bernheimer, L. P. (1994). Etiological conditions as predictors of children's problems and competencies in elementary school. *Journal of Child Neurology, 10* (Supplement 1), S100–S105.

Keogh, B., & Weisner, T. (1993). Ecocultural perspectives on risk and protection. *Learning Disabilities Research and Practice, 8*(1), 3–10.

LeVine, R. (1977). Child rearing as cultural adaptation. In P. Leiderman, S. Tulkin, & A. Rosenfeld (Eds.), *Culture and infancy* (pp. 15–27). New York: Academic Press.

LeVine, R. (1988). Human parental care: Universal goals, cultural strategies, individual behavior. In R. A. LeVine, P. M. Miller, & M. M. West, (Eds.), *Parental behavior in diverse societies* (pp. 3–12) (New Directions in Child Development No, 40). San Francisco: Jossey-Bass.

Levine, H. G., Schneider, P., Haney, M., & Hall, E. A. (1987). *Maternal scaffolding, child ability, and performance of developmentally delayed children on an everyday task analogue.* Paper presented at the biennial meeting of the Society for Research on Child Development, Baltimore.

Miller, N. B. (1993). *Nobody's perfect. Living and growing with children who have special needs.* Baltimore: Paul Brookes.

Mintz, S., & Kellogg, S. (1988). *Domestic revolutions: A social history of American family life.* New York: Free Press.

Moos, R. H., Insel, P. M., & Humphrey, B. (1974). *Family Environment Scale.* Palo Alto, CA: Consulting Psychologist Press.

Moxley-Haegert, L., & Serbin, L. (1983). Developmental education for parents of delayed infants: Effects on parental motivation and children's development. *Child Development, 54,* 1324–1331.

Munroe, R., Munroe, R., & Whiting, B. (Eds.). (1981). *Handbook of cross cultural human development.* New York: Garland STPM Press.

Neisser, U. (1982). *Memory observed. Remembering in natural contexts.* San Francisco: W. H. Freeman.

Nerlove, S., & Snipper, A. (1981). Cognitive consequences of cultural opportunity. In R. H. Munroe, R. L. Munroe, & B. B. Whiting, (Eds.), *Handbook of cross-cultural human development* (pp. 423–474). New York: Garland STPM Press.

Nihira, K., Weisner, T., & Bernheimer, L. (1994). Ecocultural assessment in families of children with developmental delays: construct and concurrent validities. *American Journal of Mental Retardation, 98*(5), 551–566.

Ochs, E. (1988). *Culture and language development. Language acquisition and language socialization in a Samoan village*. New York: Cambridge University Press.

Olson, D. H., Partner, J., & Lavee, Y. (1985). *Family Adaptability and Cohesion Evaluation Scales*. St. Paul: University of Minnesota, Family Social Science.

Rogoff, B. (1982). Integrating context and cognitive development. In M. E. Lamb & A. L. Brown (Eds.), *Advances in developmental psychology* (Vol. 2, pp. 125–170). Hillsdale, NJ: Erlbaum.

Rogoff, B. (1990). *Apprenticeship in thinking: Cognitive development in social context*. Oxford, UK: Oxford University Press.

Scheper-Hughes, N. (1990). Mother love and child death in northeast Brazil. In Stigler, J., Shweder, R., & Herdt, G., (Eds.), *Cultural psychology. Essays on comparative human development* (pp. 542–565). New York: Cambridge University Press.

Seligman, M., & Darling, R. B. (1989). *Ordinary families, special children: A systems approach to childhood disability*. New York: Guilford Press.

Shonkoff, J. P., & Hauser-Cram, P. (1987). Early intervention for disabled infants and their families: A quantitative analysis. *Pediatrics, 80*, 650–658.

Shonkoff, J. P., Hauser-Cram, P., Krauss, M. W., & Upshur, C. C. (1988). Early intervention efficacy research: What have we learned and where do we go from here? *Topics in Early Childhood Special Education, 8*, 81–93.

Shorter, E. (1975). *The making of the modern family*. New York: Basic Books.

Super, C., & Harkness, S. (Eds.). (1980). Anthropological perspectives on child development (*New Directions for Child Development No. 8*). San Francisco: Jossey-Bass.

Super, C. M., & Harkness, S. (1986). The developmental niche: A conceptualization at the interface of child and culture. *International Journal of Behavior Development, 9*, 1–25.

Tharp, R. G., & Gallimore, R. (1988). *Rousing minds to life: Teaching, learning, and schooling in social context*. Cambridge, MA: Cambridge University Press.

Vygotsky, L. (1978). *Mind in society: The development of higher psychological processes* (M. Cole, V. John-Steiner, S. Scribner, & E. Souberman, Eds.). Cambridge, MA: Harvard University Press.

Weisner, T. S. (1984). Ecocultural niches of middle childhood: A cross-cultural perspective. In W. A. Collins (Ed.), *Development during middle childhood. The years from six to twelve*. Washington, DC: National Academy Press.

Weisner, T. S. (1986). Implementing new relationship styles in conventional and nonconventional American families. In W. Hartup & Z. Rubin (Eds.), *Relationships and development* (pp. 185–206). Hillsdale, NJ: Lea Press.

Weisner, T. S. (1993). Siblings in cultural place: ethnographic and ecocultural perspectives on siblings of developmentally delayed children. In Z. Stoneman & P. Berman (Eds.), *Siblings of individuals with mental retardation, physical disabilities, and chronic illness* (pp. 51–83). Baltimore: Brooks.

Weisner, T. S., Beizer, L., & Stolze, L. (1991). Religion and the families of developmentally delayed children. *American Journal of Mental Retardation, 95*(6), 647–662.

Weisner, T. S., & Gallimore, R. (1985, December). Ecocultural and neo-Vygotskian models of cultural acquisition. Washington, DC: American Anthropological Association.

Weisner, T. S., Gallimore, R., & Jordan, C. (1988). Unpackaging cultural effects on classroom learning: Hawaiian peer assistance and child-generated activity. *Anthropology and Education Quarterly, 19,* 327–353.

Weiss, R. S. (1981). INREAL intervention for language handicapped and bilingual children. *Journal of the Division for Early Childhood, 4,* 40–51.

Wertsch, J. V. (1985). *Vygotsky and the social formation of mind.* Cambridge, MA: Harvard University Press.

White, B., Kaban, B., & Attanucci, J. (1979). *The origins of human competence.* Lexington, MA: Lexington Books.

Whiting, B., & Edwards, C. (1988). *Children of different worlds. The formation of social behavior.* Cambridge, MA: Harvard University Press.

Whiting, B., & Whiting, J. W. M. (1975). *Children of six cultures. A psycho-cultural analysis.* Cambridge, MA: Harvard University Press.

Whiting, B. (1976). The problem of the packaged variable. In K. Riegel & Meacham (Eds.), *The developing individual in a changing world: Historical and cultural issues,* (Vol. 1) (pp. 303–309). Netherlands: Mouton.

Whiting, B. (1980). Culture and social behavior: A model for the development of social behavior. *Ethos, 8,* 95–116.

# Author Index

Abbott, S., 366, 448
Abelson, R., 323
Abelson, R.P., 336
Acker, J., 209
Adewale, S.A., 419
Agiobu-Kemmer, I., 409, 412
Ahmed, M., 429, 442
Ahmet, N., 429, 442, 446
Aina, T.A., 409, 412, 425
Akinware, M., 408, 424
Alessandri, S.M., 221, 240
Allen, K., 49
Allport, G.W., 57
Als, H., 448
Alwin, D.F., 65
Anderson, R.E., 177
Angleitner, A., 41
Aoki, M., 174, 182
Aronson, D.R., 410–411
Aronsson, K., 291
Attanucci, J., 502
Azuma, H., 217, 272, 275, 279, 280

## B

Babatunde, E.D., 407, 409, 415–416, 417, 425
Backett, K.C., 328, 339
Bakeman, R., 230

Baldwin, A., 4
Ban, P., 387
Barry, H. III, 365
Bascom, W.A., 411, 422–423
Batchelder, W.H., 246
Bates, J.E., 42, 173, 188
Bateson, G., 141
Baumrind, D., 387
Bausano, M., 5
Bayles, K., 173
Bayley, N., 409
Becker, W.C., 111
Beiser, M., 429, 442
Beizer, L., 362, 506
Belenky, M.F., 467–495
Bell, R.Q., 3, 111, 378
Belsky, J., 318, 360
Bengtson, V.L., 241
Benigni, L., 77, 392
Bentley, M.E., 442, 443
Berg, K.M., 448
Berg, W.K., 448
Bernhardt, E., 195, 202
Bernheimer, L.P., 5, 496–531
Bernstein, M., 243
Berry, J.W., 31
Besevegis, E., 45
Best, D.L., 29
Bijur, P.E., 370
Black, W.C., 177

# Subject Index

Abortion, 86, 195
Accumulation belief, 93
Activity belief, 93
Activity level, 185
Adolescents, 241
 gender differences, 236–237
 ideas of, 227–230
 modern, 229
 traditional, 229
 uncommitted, 229–230
Advice, expert. *See* Experts; Pediatricians
Africa
 Kenyan Gusii parents, 149
 Nigeria. *See* Yoruba culture, Nigeria
 Tanzania. *See* Tanzanian mothers' beliefs
African-American families
 cosleeping in, 365–366, 378–379
 matriarchal structure, 378–379
 sleep practice study, 381
  alternative factors in, 374, 375
  parental approach to sleep practices, 371–375
  procedure for, 370–371
  qualitative analysis, 375–376
  samples for, 367–370
Agreeableness, 37

Allowances, for household work, 332–336, 338
ALSCAL procedure, 279, 280
American mothers' beliefs. *See also* United States
 on child cognitive development
  content of questions, 152–154
  research setting for, 150–152
 children's school behavior ratings and, 161–163
 on intellectual development, 157–159
 on knowledge acquisition, 217
 *vs.* Tanzanian mothers' beliefs, 159–161, 163–165
Anglo-American mothers, 219–220
 *vs.* Lebanese-Australian mothers, household work and, 318–320
Anglo-Australian parents, 339–340
Attitudes toward school, 39
Authoritarian communication, 479
Authoritarianism, 219
Autonomy, 20, 41

## B

Bangladeshi cultures, 418
Bayley Scales of Infant Development, 409

- 543 -